Oral Medicine

Disclaimer

The authors and publishers have taken all precautions to ensure that drug selection and dosage given in the text are according to the current recommendations and practice at the time of publication. However, due to continuous research, change in government regulations and flow of information regarding drug therapy and drug reactions, the readers must read the package insert for each drug regarding changes in the indications, dosage, warnings and precautions, etc. before its use.

Authors

Oral Medicine

Satish Chandra
Director and Professor
Sardar Patel Postgraduate Institute of Dental and Medical Sciences, Lucknow

Ex-Professor and Head of the Postgraduate Department and Dean
Dental Faculty (Formerly KG Medical College and KG Medical University, UP KG Dental University)
CSM Medical University, Lucknow

Ex-Professor, Dean, Head and Principal
DJ Postgraduate College of Dental Sciences and Research, Modinagar, UP
Ex-Professor, Dean, Head and Principal, Institute of Dental Sciences, Bareilly

Paper setter and Examiner for BDS, MDS and PGME Examinations in many Universities
Ex-Member, Dental Council of India
Best Teacher Awardee

Shaleen Chandra
Professor and Head of the Department
Saraswati Postgraduate Dental College and Hospital, Lucknow
Ex-Professor and Head of the Department
Sardar Patel Postgraduate Institute of Dental and Medical Sciences, Lucknow
Ex-Assistant Professor, Rama Postgraduate Dental College and Hospital and Research Centre, Kanpur
Ex-Lecturer, Dental Faculty (formerly KG Medical College, UP KG Dental University and KG Medical University)
CSM Medical University, Lucknow
Ex-Lecturer, Budha Postgraduate Institute of Dental Sciences, Patna
Paper setter and Examiner of BDS, MDS and PGME Examinations in many Universities

Girish Chandra
Rajendra Nagar Dental Clinic, Lucknow

Kamala R
Professor and Head of the Department of Oral Medicine and Radiology
Sardar Patel Postgraduate Institute of Dental and Medical Sciences, Lucknow
Paper setter and Examiner of BDS and MDS Examinations in many Universities

JAYPEE BROTHERS MEDICAL PUBLISHERS (P) LTD
New Delhi • Ahmedabad • Bengaluru • Chennai • Hyderabad • Kochi • Kolkata • Mumbai • Nagpur

Published by
Jitendar P Vij
Jaypee Brothers Medical Publishers (P) Ltd
B-3 EMCA House, 23/23B Ansari Road, Daryaganj, **New Delhi** 110 002, India
Phones: +91-11-23272143, +91-11-23272703, +91-11-23282021
+91-11-23245672, Rel: +91-11-32558559   Fax: +91-11-23276490
+91-11-23245683, e-mail: jaypee@jaypeebrothers.com
Visit our website: www.jaypeebrothers.com

Branches

- 2/B, Akruti Society, Jodhpur Gam Road Satellite
  Ahmedabad 380 015   Phones: +91-79-26926233, Rel: +91-79-32988717
  Fax: +91-79-26927094   e-mail: ahmedabad@jaypeebrothers.com
- 202 Batavia Chambers, 8 Kumara Krupa Road, Kumara Park East
  Bengaluru 560 001   Phones: +91-80-22285971, +91-80-22382956, 080-22372664
  Rel: +91-80-32714073   Fax: +91-80-22281761
  e-mail: bangalore@jaypeebrothers.com
- 282 IIIrd Floor, Khaleel Shirazi Estate, Fountain Plaza, Pantheon Road
  Chennai 600 008, Phones: +91-44-28193265, +91-44-28194897
  Rel: +91-44-32972089   Fax: +91-44-28193231, e-mail:chennai@jaypeebrothers.com
- 4-2-1067/1-3, 1st Floor, Balaji Building, Ramkote, Cross Road,
  Hyderabad 500 095   Phones: +91-40-66610020, +91-40-24758498,
  Rel: +91-40-32940929   Fax:+91-40-24758499,
  e-mail: hyderabad@jaypeebrothers.com
- Kuruvi Building, 1st Floor, Plot/Door No. 41/3098, B & B1, St. Vincent Road
  Kochi 682 018 Kerala   Phones: +91-484-4036109, +91-484-2395739
  +91-484-2395740   e-mail: kochi@jaypeebrothers.com
- 1-A Indian Mirror Street, Wellington Square
  Kolkata 700 013   Phones: +91-33-22651926, +91-33-22276404, +91-33-22276415
  Rel: +91-33-32901926   Fax: +91-33-22656075
  e-mail: kolkata@jaypeebrothers.com
- 106 Amit Industrial Estate, 61 Dr SS Rao Road, Near MGM Hospital, Parel
  Mumbai 400 012   Phones: +91-22-24124863, +91-22-24104532
  Rel: +91-22-32926896   Fax: +91-22-24160828, e-mail: mumbai@jaypeebrothers.com
- "KAMALPUSHPA" 38, Reshimbag, Opp. Mohota Science College, Umred Road
  Nagpur 440 009   Phone: Rel: +91-712-3245220, Fax: +91-712-2704275
  e-mail: nagpur@jaypeebrothers.com

Oral Medicine

© 2007, Jaypee Brothers Medical Publishers

All rights reserved. No part of this publication should be reproduced, stored in a retrieval system, or transmitted in any form or by any means: electronic, mechanical, photocopying, recording, or otherwise, without the prior written permission of the authors and the publisher.

This book has been published in good faith that the material provided by authors is original. Every effort is made to ensure accuracy of material, but the publisher, printer and authors will not be held responsible for any inadvertent error(s). In case of any dispute, all legal matters are to be settled under Delhi jurisdiction only.

First Edition: **2007**
ISBN 81-8448-145-4
Typeset at   JPBMP typesetting unit
Printed at   Replika Press Pvt. Ltd.

Contributors

Arun V Subramaniam
Professor and Head
Department of Medicine and Radiology
Padmashree Dr DY Patil Dental College and Hospital
Pimpri, Mahesh Nagar
Pune 411 018
(Maharashtra)

Ashok L
Professor and Head
Department of Oral Medicine and Radiology
Bapuji Dental College and Hospital
Devangere 577 004
(Karnataka)

Karjodkar FR
Associate Professor
Head of the Department of Oral Medicine and Radiology
Nair Hospital Dental College
Mumbai 400 008

Karthikeya Patil
Professor and Head
Department of Oral Medicine and Radiology
JSS Dental College and Hospital
Sri Shivarathruaswara Nagar
Mysore 570 015
(Karnataka)

Shashi Kanth MC
Professor and Head
Department of Oral Medicine and Radiology
College of Dental Sciences
Devangere 577 004
(Karnataka)

S Jayachandran
Professor and Head
Department of Oral Medicine and Radiology
Tamil Nadu Govt Dental College, Opp Fort Railway Station
Chennai 600 003
(Tamil Nadu)

Subrata Kr Talukder
Professor and Head
Department of Oral Medicine and Radiology
Subharati Dental College, Subharati Puram
Delhi-Haridwar Bypass Road
Meerut 250 003
(Uttar Pradesh)

Sumanth KN
Professor
Department of Oral Medicine and Radiology
College of Dental Surgery, Light House, Hill Road
Mangalore 575 001
(Karnataka)

K Vinay Kumar Reddy
Professor
Department of Oral Medicine and Radiology
Mamata Dental College, 4-2-161, Police Housing Colony
Giriprasad Nagar, Opp Rotary Nagar
Khamam 507 002
(Andhra Pradesh)

Vidya
Professor
Department of Oral Medicine and Radiology
SRM Dental College, Bharathi Salai, Ramapuram
Chennai 600 089
(Tamil Nadu)

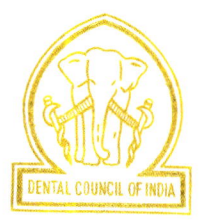

भारतीय दन्त परिषद

DENTAL COUNCIL OF INDIA
(CONSTITUTED UNDER THE DENTISTS ACT 1948)
Aiwan-E-Ghalib Marg, Kotla Road, New Delhi-110 002

DR. ANIL KOHLI
MDS (Lko), DNBE (USA)
President
Awardee :
- **Padmashri**
- **Padmabhushan**
- **Dr. B.C. Roy National Award**

Telephone : 23220204 Direct
23238542, 23236740
Fax : 0091 - 11 - 23231252
0091 - 11 - 23220204
E-mail : dciindia@hotmail.com
Website : http://www.dciindia.org

No. DE-118-2007/A-4340

Dated the 25th July 2007

Foreword

I feel pleasure in writing foreword for the *Oral Medicine* by Prof Satish Chandra and others. In the last three decades the fundamentals, theories and practice of oral medicine have undergone drastic changes due to advancements in the diagnostic and management techniques.

The knowledge about the impact of medical conditions and the diseases on the dental health care has dramatically increased in the last three decades. The average life expectancy has very much increased in recent years, which has also increased the importance of oral medicine due to the increased demand of dental treatments in medically compromised patients, especially the aged.

This book has completely covered all the topics of the subject with the basic fundamentals, theories and recent advances. The language is very simple, clear and lucid. Different stages of all the lesions have been illustrated with colored photographs. For pin-point identification the lesions have been pointed by the arrows and the arrow heads. The well illustrated presentations have made the reading very informative and interesting for the undergraduate and postgraduate students, teachers and practitioners. The very special feature of the book is the multiple choice questions, which are very useful especially to the students preparing for various competitive examinations.

The book has completely covered the syllabus of Dental Council of India. Overall this is an excellent book. I strongly recommend this book to all BDS and MDS students, teachers, researchers and the practitioners.

Anil Kohli

Professor AP Tikku
Faculty of Dental Sciences
CSM Medical University
Ex-Dean, Student Welfare
UPKG University of Dental Sciences, Lucknow
Executive Committee Member
Dental Council of India, New Delhi
President—Federation of Operative Dentistry, India
Vice President–Indian Endodontic Society

Residence
A-1, River Bank Colony
Lucknow - 226 018

Foreword

I am very much pleased to write the foreword for the *Oral Medicine* by Prof Satish Chandra and others. Since last three decades the subject of Oral Medicine has undergone revolutionary changes. There have been remarkable developments in the diagnostic techniques and the managements of the oral diseases. Many new diagnostic techniques which give informations in the objective forms, i.e. in numericals have been developed.

This book has comprehensively covered all the topics of the subject with basic fundamentals and recent advances. The language in this book is very simple and crystal clear. The well illustrated and labelled presentations with basic fundamentals and recent advances have made the reading very informative and interesting for the undergraduate and postgraduate students and teachers and practitioners. For self-evaluation multiple choice questions have been given in the end. This is a very special feature of the book. The MCQs are very useful especially to the students preparing for various competitive examinations.

The book provide up-to-date information and a rational approach to the chair-side and bed-side diagnosis and comprehensive management of the patient of oral medicine. The book has completely covered the syllabus prescribed by the Dental Council of India. There are many colored photographs presenting the rare advanced stages of the lesions.

I strongly recommend this student-friendly book to all for BDS and MDS students and the practitioners.

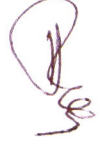

AP Tikku

Preface

It is essential for dental surgeons to have thorough knowledge of Oral Medicine to understand the etiology, predisposing factors, prevention, diagnosis and management of oral diseases and recognition of underlying systemic diseases and also the management of dental and oral diseases of the patients with complicating medical diseases.

It has been a great pleasure to write the book on Oral Medicine with MCQs. Our goal has been to prepare a standard textbook and to simplify and update all the aspects of the subject. The purpose of this book is to teach the principles and practice of oral medicine to undergraduate and postgraduate students, teachers, research workers and practitioners. The text is the combination of basic fundamentals with latest research and its clinical applications. Latest diseases have been described in detail.

The book contains chapters on latest topics. This book is very useful for having thorough knowledge of all the aspects of oral diseases and their management. Simple and lucid language and plenty of colored clinical photographs have been used to make the subject matter crystal clear and interesting. In the end MCQs have been given which are very useful for self-evaluation and for various competitive examinations.

We are thankful to all the persons involved in this book without whose help this book would not have been possible. We are grateful to Shri JP Vij, Chairman and Managing Director and Mr Tarun Duneja, General Manager (Publishing) and the devoted staff of M/s Jaypee Brothers Medical Publishers (P) Ltd, New Delhi for publishing the text in the excellent book form.

Authors

Contents

1. Introduction, Scope and Role of Oral Medicine in Dental Practice 1
2. Evaluation of Patient and Psychology 4
3. Oral Physiology, Anatomy and Histology Related to Oral Medicine 6
4. Nutrition and Oral Diseases 10
5. Pathology Related to Oral Medicine 14
6. Oral Examination and Diagnosis 18
7. Developmental Disorders Affecting Oral and Para Oral Structures 21
8. Diseases of Teeth and Supporting Tissues 30
9. Diseases of the Pulp and Periapical Tissues 38
10. Ulcerative and Vesiculobullous Lesions of the Oral Cavity 44
11. Red and White Lesions of the Oral Mucosa 57
12. Pigmented Lesions of the Oral Tissues 76
13. Benign Oral Tumors 84
14. Malignant Oral Tumors 95
15. Diseases of the Tongue 112
16. Diseases of Salivary Gland 119
17. Temporomandibular Joint Disorders 134
18. Orofacial Pain and Abnormalities of Taste 143
19. Cardiovascular Diseases Related to Oral Medicine 153
20. Diseases of Respiratory System Related to Oral Medicine 159
21. Gastrointestinal Diseases Related to Oral Medicine 166
22. Renal Diseases and Oral Medicine 170
23. Relation of Immunologic Diseases with Oral Medicine 174
24. Neuromuscular Diseases Affecting the Orofacial Region 182
25. Diabetes Mellitus and Its Oral Manifestations 188
26. Hematological Disorders 193
27. Disorders of Hemostasis and Oral Medicine 203
28. Infectious Diseases Related to Oral Medicine 209
29. Endocrine Diseases and Orodental Health 215
30. Orodental Medicine in Geriatrics 217
31. Orodental Considerations in Organ Transplantation 222

   Multiple Choice Questions 226
   Appendices 245
   Index 251

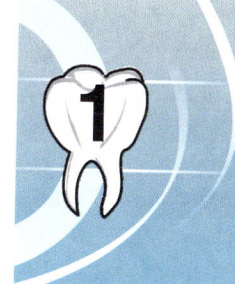

Introduction, Scope and Role of Oral Medicine in Dental Practice

DEFINITION

Mosby's Dental dictionary has defined oral medicine as "The discipline of dentistry that deals with significance and relationship of oral and systemic diseases. According to Taber's Medical dictionary "Oral medicine is the branch of medicine concerned with the preservation and treatment of the teeth and other orofacial tissues". The American Academy of Oral Medicine has defined the specialty as 'Oral Medicine is the speciality of dentistry that is concerned with the oral health care of the medically compromised patients and with the diagnosis and nonsurgical management of medically related disorders or conditions affecting the oral and maxillofacial region. However, oral medicine is the branch of dentistry that deals with the diagnosis and medical treatment of the diseases of oral cavity and surrounding structures and their relationship with systemic diseases.

The specialists of oral medicine deals with nonsurgical medical aspects of dentistry. They are concerned with the diagnosis and medical treatment of oral diseases which normally are not treated by routine dental or maxillofacial surgical procedures. Oral medicine also includes the diagnosis and treatment of oral manifestations of systemic diseases. In oral medicine special attention is paid to the dental treatment of medically compromised patients.

INTRODUCTION

Only in the middle of twentieth century dental surgeons recognized oral medicine as a specialized branch. All the diseases are correlated to each other. The dentists are concerned only with the conditions in the mouth and the general clinicians ignore this part of the body as outside their area of jurisdiction.

Sir Jonathan Hutchinson (1828-1900)—Surgeon in London Hospital, is regarded as the father of oral medicine. He was first to describe number of conditions such as oral manifestation of syphilis and intraoral pigmentation. FW Brondrick (1928) published a book "Dental Medicine" and introduced the biochemical basis for understanding the dental diseases.

Hubert H Stones (1935) described the oral manifestation of systemic diseases and his book "Oral and Dental diseases" emphasized on medical aspects of oral diseases. Lester W Burket (1907-91) devoted his life to oral medicine and published first book on Oral medicine in 1964. The majority of these teachers were medically and dentally qualified. All of them emphasized on the fact that all the basic sciences which are necessary for the practice of medicine are also necessary for the practice of dentistry. Thus, oral medicine got a foundation as a specialized branch.

SCOPE

The physical body of man is composed of various parts, but functions as a whole unit. Its parts are interrelated to each other and with the body as a whole. Likewise dentistry cannot be considered separately from other health sciences and services, as far as diagnosis, treatment planning and treatment of the patients are concerned. Although dental surgeon is a specialist of the oral cavity, but it must be clearly understood that the patient is one single biologic unit. All the organs and systems of a body play a role in the development of a clinical lesion in the mouth. Further, local lesions of the oral cavity have a direct effect on systemic health.

Oral cavity is considered as a mirror of the body because many systemic diseases manifest first in oral cavity. Some manifest in oral cavity along with their manifestation in the body. Hence dental surgeon has an opportunity and also a professional responsibility to identify such systemic diseases observed in patient and refer to appropriate place for the treatment. This responsibility becomes more important if an oral health care provider is the only health care provider in contact with the community for a considerable period. His field should not be restricted to oral diseases, if he has the training, knowledge and practical ability to recognize common medical disorders requiring urgent attention like cholera, diarrhea and dysentery. The oral health practitioner must care for the oral and maxillofacial complex for the purpose of maintaining good health, motor sensory and psychosocial functions. The oral and maxillofacial complex includes the teeth, gums, oral cavity, jaws, salivary glands and contiguous craniofacial structures. The clinical responsibilities of oral health care practitioner include an understanding of the causes, risk factors, prevention and diagnosis of oral diseases and disorders. He should be regarded as a person who cares for the health and welfare of the community. He must have good abilities and knowledge for oral health maintenance and general living conditions such as habits, diet and sanitation.

Oral medicine concerning the common medical disorders and their diagnosis and treatment enables the dental students to understand the patient in a better way and they can provide better dental treatment. Their duty is not restricted to oral diseases but they have to deal with other medical disorders and their oral manifestations. So, the knowledge of oral medicine enables dental surgeons to understand the etiology, risk factors, prevention and diagnosis of oral and systemic diseases and their manifestations.

ORAL MEDICINE IN HOSPITAL PRACTICE

The most complex cases of oral medicine are frequently seen in the hospital practice. Hospitalized patients may have oral and dental complications which are the manifestations of diseases like HIV infection, diabetes, bleeding disorders and heart diseases. So, every hospital must have a dental department which can provide dental treatment for patients with severe systemic diseases. The oral medicine procedures can be best performed in the hospital because there is availability of both diagnostic and life saving equipment and expert clinicians of all areas of health care for consultation, if need arises. The commonly seen dental problems in hospitalized patients are oral ulcers, oral bleeding and oral infections secondary to chemotherapy or blood dyscrasias. The commonly provided services are dental care to prevent osteoradionecrosis prior to radiotherapy and dental care to prevent infection in open heart surgery and organ transplant patients.

MANAGEMENT OF DENTAL PATIENTS HAVING SEVERE MEDICAL PROBLEMS

The dental patient with severe medical problems, which may need emergency resuscitation, care of consultants of other medical fields before and after the dental procedure, and laboratory facilities before and after the dental procedures, should be hospitalized by a dental surgeon. Further private dental practitioners have to decide whether the dental procedure should be carried out in a hospital or in his own clinic. This depends upon the condition of the patient.

The patient with the following disorders for dental treatment may be admitted in the hospital:
a. Severe cardiovascular diseases
b. Need of general anesthesia or heavy sedation
c. Bleeding disorders
d. Prone to infection due to immunodeficiency
e. Susceptibility to shock
f. Neuromuscular or other physical disability.

Dental patients who are admitted to the hospital should have a complete medical history and head and neck examination. The hospital dental surgeon is responsible for the total well-being of the hospitalized patient, though the dental surgeon may not be able to treat all the problems that arise, he should know whom to consult in the particular situation. The dental surgeons must have a knowledge of physical diagnosis, laboratory diagnosis and advanced oral medicine which could help them to manage dental patients with severe medical problems. The dental surgeons must be able to understand the language, abbreviations etc. used by the cardiologists and the physicians. The dental surgeon should write, the necessary instructions to the nursing staff and to the patient. He should also write frequency of vital signs, medications, radiological and laboratory investigations, diet and bed rest follow-up treatment and home care by the patient.

Proper precautions, home care, follow-up instructions, details of procedure performed results of the investigations and medications etc. should be written on the discharge card. During internship and residency programs in oral medicine department, dental students and surgeons must be trained in all the above hospital procedures. These programs must train interns and residents to provide oral health and dental care for patients with complex medical disorders as well as solve the difficult diagnostic problems of the mouth and jaws. On the proper training of interns and residents in hospital procedures, depends the future of oral medicine and hospital dentistry. Therefore the routine hospital procedures should be the integral part of dental internship and residency programs.

BIBLIOGRAPHY

1. Bader JD, Ismail Al. (Univ of North Carolina, Chapel Hill). A primer on Outcomes in Dentistry. J Public Heath Dent 1999;59:131-5.
2. Carr AB, McGivney GP. (Ohio State Univ, Columbus; State Univ of New York, Buffalo). Measurement in Dentistry. J prosthet Dent 2000;83: 266-71.
3. Cooke BE. History of Oral Medicine. Bri Dent J 1981;131:11-13.
4. Jacob RF, Carr AB. (MD Andersom Cancer Ctr, Houston; Ohio State Univ, Columbus). J Prosthet Dent 2000;83:137-52.
5. Soberman A. Dedication-Lester W Burket. J Oral Med 1978;33.

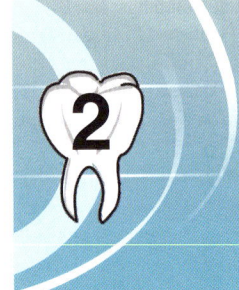

Evaluation of Patient and Psychology

With the increasing health awareness, availability of medical facilities and better living conditions the mean age of individuals is increasing almost all over the world. The oral health status of the population in the advanced countries is also undergoing changes. Due to awareness and increased use of dental services more people are going to retain their dentition. The adult and elderly patients will have a continuous need to improve masticatory function along with the demand of superior esthetics. It has been proved that there is intimate relationship between dental, oral and systemic health. Therefore in the years to come the number of dental patients having chronic medical problems like blood pressure, diabetes and multiple medications but still demanding good oral and dental health will increase.

The oral cavity and face in the human being are of great psychic importance. These are used to express a number of emotions from fear, anger and determination to tenderness, joy and happiness. Many emotional disorders may reveal their manifestations in oral cavity, without the patient's being aware of the cause, thus other parts of the body do not have so much psychologic importance.

There is a correlation between oral complaints and emotional stress.

DOCTOR-PATIENT RELATIONSHIP

In the diagnosis and treatment of oral diseases, the dental surgeons work on the basis of scientific methods and principles but they must learn and master the art of psychology in dental practice. The practitioner's primary and traditional objectives should be of utility, which includes the prevention and cure of lesions, diseases and suffering of the body and of mind.

The dental surgeon can treat easily the well-behaved sensible patient having classical symptoms and lesions, but it becomes difficult to treat psychologically disturbed person who is tense, nervous with typical symptoms and lesions; they require special consideration and attention. Almost all the patients have emotional problems, which are expressed, in the form of diseases. When they appear before a dental surgeon they are fearful and suspicious and want more comfort, consoling words and relief rather than cure.

The clinician should solve the problems of patient as a person as well as according to his pathologic condition. The patient must recognize that his problems are meaningful so that the doctor should be able to understand them. The practitioner must be well trained in all dental sciences and knowledge of oral diseases. He must have capacity to understand the problems of patient as a human being and patient should be comfortable with him. In treating the sufferings of the patients he must have technical and scientific knowledge, experience as well as human understanding.

PSYCHOSOMATIC ORAL DISEASES

The term psychosomatic implies a physical disorder that is caused by or influenced by emotional state of the patient. These psychosomatic disorders are the result of those emotional controversies, which are not resolved. Emotions that fail to be expressed may be converted into somatic symptoms so as to relieve tension.

Usually the human being cannot freely express his emotional problems in the society because of social restrictions necessary to live in harmony. This results in increased tension leading to frustration. In an effort to live within his environment, the individual develops psychosomatic disorders. Since the oral cavity has high psychologic potency, it unconsciously becomes the recipient of somatic symptoms and diseases.

Some of the common psychosomatic diseases of the oral cavity are burning mouth, burning tongue, dry mouth, bruxism, trismus, aphthous ulcers, stomatitis and temporomandibular joint pain. These suppressed emotions can also be converted into oral psychoneurosis which is an emotional disorder in which feeling of anxiety, compulsive acts and physical complaints without any evidence of disease, dominate the personality. For example, in such condition patient can complain of gagging in perfectly constructed denture or there may be complaint of inability to chew food even though patient have a well functioning and efficient natural dentition.

Oral habits such as cheek biting, tongue thrusting and lip biting are also the result of unresolved emotional conflicts. These symptoms and complaints are caused by emotional problems and form the essential cause of psychosomatic oral diseases.

ORAL AND DENTAL MANIFESTATIONS OF ANXIETY

Anxiety can have oral and dental manifestations which can be divided into following categories.

Faulty Oral Behavioral Patterns

Anxiety may lead to abnormal behavior regarding the care of teeth, eating habits, or attitude towards the dentist, that have an effect on oral health. For example, some patients will brush their teeth vigorously that will cause wearing of enamel and dentin, and another group of patients do not brush their teeth at all, that leads to accumulation of plaque and debris, causing dental decay and gingival diseases. Faulty dietary habits like excessive eating of sweets and failure to eat nutritious food, contributes to caries. Vigorous chewing of food is necessary for maintenance of periodontal tissues, otherwise it may lead to low-grade inflammation of gingiva with resulting periodontal diseases.

Effect on Autonomic Nervous System

There can be dysfunction of autonomic nervous system as a result of anxiety that may lead to pathologic changes in oral cavity. Autonomic over activity may lead to changes in vascularity of gingiva or changes in the chemical content and volume of salivary flow. Xerostomia or an excessively dry mouth is a characteristic symptom of depressed patients. Anxiety and tension reduce salivary flow. The autonomic nervous system also have interaction with the gingiva. People working under the conditions of continuous fatigue, strain and tension frequently have acute necrotizing ulcerative gingivitis.

Relationship of Pain and Anxiety

Anxiety can greatly change the patient's response to pain. The patient may feel the pain without presence of any stimulus. Anxiety can lead to pain that results from spasm or dilation of blood vessels, with consequent hyperemia or ischemia of tissue cells. Tension, fatigue and stressful life situations may lead to habits like bruxism and jaw clinching which produce muscle spasm and consequent pain of temporomandibular joint.

PSYCHOLOGICAL CONSIDERATIONS IN DENTAL TREATMENT

A successful dental treatment requires a wide approach to the patient as a whole, along with establishing the dentition in a state of health and rapid relief of symptoms. The dental surgeon should not show overenthusiasm, in making a diagnosis or in treatment. This may increase tension or muscle spasm and lead to more difficulties. If the patient is having emotional problems, only necessary procedures should be carried out. The dental surgeon can give best results if he handles the patients conservatively and moderately and gives them reassurance and useful information about the psychology and physiology of their condition. The dental surgeon should attentively listen to anxiety—ridden patient and should avoid over treating and over straining them. He should give them simple but reasonable explanations of their symptoms. The patient will surely respond to such a warm and intellectual dental surgeon. Patient-doctor relationship and patient's condition are improved when the dentist is understanding, confident and competent.

BIBLIOGRAPHY

1. Behar-Horenstein LS, Dolan TA, Courts FJ, et al. (Univ of Florida, Gainesville): Cultivating Critical Thinking in the Clinical Learning Environment. J Dent Educ 2000; 64:610-5.
2. Facts and comparison. St. Louis (MO). A Wolters Kluwer Co. 2000.
3. PDR for nonprescription drugs and dietary supplements. Montvale (NJ): Medical Economics Co. 2000.
4. Physician's desk reference. Montvale (NJ): Medical Economics Co. 54th edn., 2000.
5. Wynn RL, Meiller TF, Crossley HL. Drug information handbook for dentistry. Cleveland: Lexi-Comp, 6th edn., 2000.

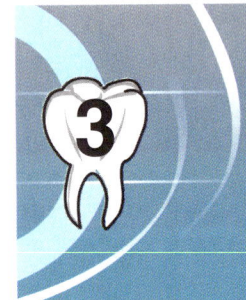

Oral Physiology, Anatomy and Histology Related to Oral Medicine

Oral physiology, anatomy and histology provide a basis for understanding the structure and functions of the oral cavity and surrounding structure on the macroscopic and microscopic level. The dental surgeon should have the knowledge of the anatomic terms of structure and functions of tissues and organs in health and in disease. Without this knowledge, he would be unable to communicate, think and reason in a right way when faced with a clinical problem. The understanding of nonclinical and paraclinical sciences like anatomy, histology, biochemistry, physiology, pathology, microbiology and pharmacology enables the dental surgeon to deal successfully with the etiology, pathology, diagnosis, treatment and prognosis of oral diseases.

SALIVA

Saliva maintains the aqueous environment of the oral cavity. It is clear, slightly acidic secretion formed in parotid, submaxillary, sublingual and accessory salivary glands.

The daily secretion of saliva varies from 1 to 1.5 liters. Its pH varies between 6.8 and 7.

Composition of Saliva

Water accounts for 99% of the saliva. The remaining 1% consists of inorganic ions, secretory proteins and glycoproteins. Major inorganic ions of saliva are Na^+, K^+, Cl^- and HCO_3^-.

Secretory proteins present in saliva include enzymes, mucins, and antibacterial substances. Albumin, blood clotting factors and immunoglobulin are also found in saliva.

Role of Saliva in Oral Health

a. Salivary secretions are protective in nature as they contain antibacterial factors such as lysozyme, lactoferrin and myeloperoxidase and antibodies like immunoglobulin G (IgG) and M (IgM), which help in controlling the bacterial colonization, breakdown of bacterial cell wall and oxidation of susceptible bacteria.
b. The cleansing action of saliva has a major influence on plaque by mechanically cleaning the tooth surfaces and helping to remove debris and dead cells.
c. Saliva also contains coagulation factors VIII, IX and X that fasten coagulation and protect wound from bacterial invasion.
d. Minerals and glycoproteins present in saliva maintain the integrity of tooth by mechanism of remineralization and mechanical protection.
e. Saliva moistens and lubricates the food and mucous membrane and thus helps in deglutition and speech.

ORAL MUCOUS MEMBRANE

The oral mucous membrane lines the oral cavity. Based on functional adaptation oral mucosa is divided into (a) masticatory mucosa (gingiva and hard palate), (b) lining mucosa (cheek, floor of mouth and soft palate) and (c) specialized mucosa (dorsum of tongue and taste buds).

Histology of Mucous Membrane

Oral mucous membrane consists of two layers epithelium and connective tissue. The connective tissue is termed as lamina propria. It is attached to periosteum of alveolar bone, or it may cover the submucosa which is present in soft palate and floor of mouth. The submucosa attaches the mucous membrane to the underlying structure. Glands, blood vessels, nerves and adipose tissue are present in this layer.

The epithelium of the oral mucous membrane is of stratified squamous type. It may be keratinized, parakeratinized or nonkeratinized. The epithelium of gingiva and hard palate is keratinized, whereas cheek, faucial and sublingual tissues are nonkeratinized.

The mucous membrane of the hard palate is tightly bound to the periosteum and is immovable. It is pink in color. The mucous membrane on the floor of mouth and vestibule is loosely attached to the underlying structures and does not limit the movement of lips, cheek and tongue. The mucous membrane of the soft palate is highly vascularized and reddish in color.

There should be thorough knowledge of structures and functions of oral mucosa in order to understand the characteristic changes that are caused by systemic diseases.

GINGIVA

The gingiva is that part of oral mucosa which covers the alveolar processes and encircles the teeth. It is divided into marginal, attached and interdental gingiva. The marginal gingiva is unattached coronal end of gingiva. Attached gingiva extends from gingival groove to mucogingival junction and is firm, dense, stippled and tightly bound to underlying periosteum, tooth and bone. The interdental gingiva occupies the interproximal space between two contacting teeth. In healthy conditions the color of gingiva is coral pink, consistency is firm and resilient and surface texture is stippled.

Histology of Gingiva

Histologically, gingiva consists of connective tissue covered by stratified squamous epithelium.

Epithelium

The principal cell of gingival epithelium is keratinocyte along with Langerhans cells, Merkel cells and melanocytes. The outer epithelium that covers the surface of marginal gingiva and attached gingiva is generally parakeratinized. The sulcular epithelium that lines the gingival sulcus is thin and nonkeratinized. The functional epithelium that is attached to the tooth surface and to the gingival connective tissue consists of stratified squamous nonkeratinizing epithelium.

Connective Tissue

The connective tissue of gingiva is known as the lamina propria. It mainly contains collagen fiber bundles called gingival fibers. The principal cells present in gingival connective tissue are fibroblasts, mast cells, macrophages and histiocytes.

PERIODONTIUM

Periodontium is the connective tissue that attaches the roots of the teeth to the bone. The connective tissue present in periodontium are classified as follows:

Fibrous Tissues

a. Periodontal ligament
b. Lamina propria of gingiva.

Mineralized Tissues

a. Cementum
b. Alveolar bone.

Periodontal Ligament

Periodontal ligament is a fibrous connective tissue that occupies the periodontal space between cementum and alveolar bone. Principal fibers are the important elements of periodontal ligaments which are collagenous and arranged in bundles.

Fibers: The principal fibers of periodontal ligament are arranged in six particular groups that include transseptal, alveolar crest, horizontal, oblique, apical and interradicular.

Cells: The principal cells present in healthy periodontal ligaments are as follows—

a. Connective tissue cells
    i. Fibroblast
    ii. Cementoblast
    iii. Osteoblast
b. Resorptive cells
    i. Osteoclast
    ii. Fibroblast
    iii. Cementoclast
c. Epithelial rest cells
d. Defense cells
    i. Macrophages
    ii. Mast cells

Functions: The periodontal ligament has a number of functions, which are as follows—
- Periodontal ligament attaches the teeth to the bone.
- Periodontal ligament transmits occlusal forces to the bone and acts as a shock absorber.
- Cells of periodontal ligament help in synthesis and resorption of cementum and bone which occur in physiologic tooth movement.
- The periodontal ligament supplies nutrients to cementum, alveolar bone and gingiva through blood vessels.

PULP

The dental pulp occupies the central portion of the tooth contained within the dentinal walls. It consists of blood vessels, nerves and connective tissue. The dental pulp is composed of (a) coronal pulp located centrally in the crowns of teeth and (b) radicular pulp that extends from cervical region of crown to root apex.

Structure of the Pulp

The pulp is divided into (A) Odontoblastic zone, (B) Cell-free zone, (C) Cell-rich zone and (D) Central zone.

Odontoblastic Zone

Odontoblastic zone surrounds the periphery of the pulp. It consists of odontoblast, the second most prominent cell in the pulp. The primary function of the odontoblast is the production and deposition of dentin throughout the life of pulp.

Cell-free zone

The cell-free zone contains some fibroblasts, mesenchymal cells and macrophages. The main constituent of this zone is the plexus of capillaries, nerve plexus of Raschkow and ground substance. Fibroblasts help in production of the reticular fibres. Mesenchymal cells differentiate into new odontoblasts when the old ones are destroyed by any injury. The nerve plexus of Raschkow is concerned with the neural sensation of the pulp. The ground substance is involved in exchange of metabolites and restricts the spread of infection.

Cell-rich zone

The cell-rich zone is located between cell-free zone and central zone. It is composed of ground substance, fibroblasts, undifferentiated mesenchymal cells and defense cells. Ground substance supports the cells of the pulp and serves as transport medium for nutrients, metabolites and waste products.

Fibroblasts are the principal cells in the pulp. Their main function is the production of collagen fibers. Undifferentiated mesenchymal cells are the totipotent cells and are derived from dental papilla. They help in repair and regeneration of odontoblasts, fibroblasts and macrophages. The defense cells such as macrophages, histiocytes, mast cells and neutrophils are also present in cell-rich zone. They act as a phagocyte and remove necrotic debris and foreign material.

Central Zone

The central zone contains blood vessels and nerves. The blood vessels transport nutrients, fluids and oxygen to the tissues and remove metabolic waste from the tissues. The majority of nerves that enter the pulp are nonmyelinated. These nerves transmit the sensation of pain in response to stimuli such as heat, cold, pressure and chemical agents.

MICROBIAL FLORA OF ORAL CAVITY

Oral cavity is colonized by a large and different types of microorganisms. Microbial flora present in oral cavity can be divided into indigenous flora and transient flora.

Indigenous Flora

The organisms which are almost always present in the oral cavity are referred as indigenous flora. The common indigenous organisms found in oral cavity are *streptococcus*, *lactobacillus*, *neisseria* and *actinomyces*.

Transient Flora

These organisms reach the oral cavity through extraoral substances and last only for a short time, as the oral environment may not be suitable for their survival.

Factors which Influence Growth of Microorganisms

The factors which influence growth of microorganisms are as follows:

Temperature: The oral temperature of 37°C is optimally favourable for the growth and multiplication of organisms.
Hydrogen-ion concentration: The hydrogen ion concentration (pH) of the oral cavity is about 7, which is most suitable for most of the bacteria for their growth.
Nutrient sources: The diet, saliva, gingival crevicular fluid, microbial products and host products are the nutrient sources for microorganisms.

Microorganisms Present in Oral Cavity

Usually the following microorganisms besides others are present in the oral cavity.

Bacteria

i. Gram-positive bacteria
   – *Streptococcus mutans*
   – *Streptococcus sanguis*
   – *Streptococcus salivarius*
   – *Staphylococcus albus*
   – *Staphylococcus aureus*
   – *Lactobacillus*
   – *Actinomyces*
   – *Eubacterium*

ii. Gram-negative bacteria
   - *Bacteroids*
   - *Neisseria*
   - *Entero-bacteria*
   - *Actinobacillus*
   - *Treponema*
   - *Pseudomonas*
   - *Mycoplasma*

Fungi

i. *Candida albicans*
ii. *Candida tropicalis*

Protozoa

i. *Entamoeba gingivalis*
ii. *Trichomonas tenax*

DEPOSITS ON TEETH

Deposits on teeth are normally formed around the teeth in majority of population. These deposits are materia alba, dental plaque and calculus. Most of the dental diseases are originated from these deposits and they are the most frequent cause of pain and loss of teeth in the oral cavity.

Materia Alba

Materia alba is a yellow or grayish white, soft deposit found on tooth surface. It consists of microorganisms, epithelial cells and a mixture of salivary proteins and lipids. It generally accumulates on the gingival third of the teeth and on malposed teeth. It is easily removed with spray of water. The irritating effect of the materia alba on the gingiva is due to bacteria and their products. (Fig. 3.1)

Dental Plaque

Dental plaque is defined as the soft deposits adherent to the tooth surface. It is classified as supragingival, marginal and subgingival, according to its position on the tooth surface. The plaque found at or above the gingival margin is supragingival plaque whereas the plaque found below the gingival margin is subgingival plaque. The plaque that is in direct contact with gingival margin is referred as marginal plaque. Dental plaque consists mainly of microorganisms within an intercellular matrix along with epithelial cells, macrophages and leucocytes.

Plaque appears on those teeth that are least accessible to oral hygiene measures and when removed, develops on teeth again after 1 to 2 days. The location and rate of plaque formation depends upon oral hygiene measures as well as factors like diet, salivary composition and salivary flow rate.

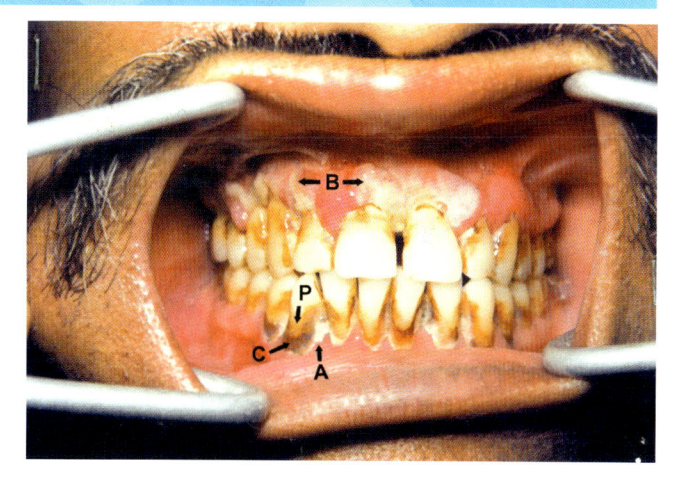

Fig. 3.1: Materia alba (shown by A), dental plaque (shown by P) and supragingival calculus (shown by C). Maxillary gingiva is also showing burns due to chemicals (shown by B)

The plaque present at different regions is responsible for different diseases of teeth and periodontium. For example supragingival and tooth associated plaque are related to calculus formation and root caries, whereas subgingival and tissue-associated plaque is responsible for development of gingivitis and periodontitis. (Fig. 3.1)

Calculus

Calculus is a calcified mass that adheres to the tooth surface. Calculus results from mineralization of bacterial plaque. It is classified according to its position on tooth surface. The calculus located coronal to gingival margin is supragingival calculus. It is white and yellowish-white in color and of hard clay-like consistency. Subgingival calculus is located below the marginal gingiva hence it is not visible. It is dark-brown or greenish black in color and denser than supragingival calculus.

Supragingival and subgingival calculus have the same composition but differs in source of minerals. The saliva is the main source of minerals for formation of supragingival calculus, whereas the gingival fluid or sulcular fluid supplies minerals for subgingival calculus. (Fig. 3.1)

BIBLIOGRAPHY

1. Bosch FX, Ouyahoun JP, Bader BL, et al. Extensive changes in cytokeratin expression patterns in pathologically affected human gingiva. Arch VB Cell Pathol 1989;58:59.
2. Chavier C. Elastic fibers of healthy human gingiva. J Periodontal 1990;9:29.
3. Sawada T, Yamamoto T, Yanagisawa T, et al. Electron immunochemistry of laminin and type IV collagen in the junctional epithelium of rat molar gingiva. J Periodontal Res 1990;25:372.

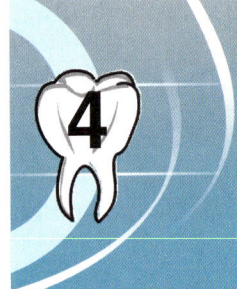

Nutrition and Oral Diseases

Nutrition is referred to as assimilation and use of essential food elements from the diet required for physiologic growth and metabolism. A balanced diet is necessary for structural and functional efficiency of every cell of the body. The human body transforms the nutrients of food into energy which is of prime importance in life. Nutrients necessary for maintenance of status of body cells can be categorized as follows.
   i. Energy—yielding nutrients which are carbohydrates, fats and proteins.
  ii. Water, electrolytes and minerals.
 iii. Vitamins.

CARBOHYDRATES

Carbohydrates are the principal source of energy in the diet. They provide 50% of energy and heat required by the body. The carbohydrates that are essential for proper nutrition are of the following three types.

Monosaccharides

These are simplest carbohydrates that cannot be hydrolysed, e.g. glucose, fructose and galactose.

Disaccharides

Disaccharides are water soluble, crystalline sugars consisting of two molecules of monosaccharides, e.g. sucrose, maltose and lactose.

Polysaccharides

These are complex carbohydrates consisting of more than two monosaccharide molecules linked to each other. Starch is nutritionally the most important polysaccharide which is a major source of energy. Other polysaccharides are glycogen, dextran and cellulose.

Functions of Carbohydrates

   i. Carbohydrates provide energy to the body cells in the form of glucose.
  ii. Carbohydrates are necessary for the oxidation of fats.
 iii. Glycogen, a polysaccharide provides a food storage system. It is found in higher concentration in liver and also in muscles.
  iv. Carbohydrates provide fibers for normal peristalsis.
   v. They provide energy for normal bacterial flora of oral cavity.

Role of Carbohydrates in Dental Caries

Dental caries is the microbial disease in which demineralization of the inorganic portion and destruction of the organic substance of the tooth takes place. The dental and oral environmental factors like amount of salivary flow, types of dental plaque, bacteria, nature of carbohydrates eaten and frequency of food intake are causative agents related to initiation and extension of dental caries.

Carbohydrates plays a role in the production of dental caries in following ways:
   i. The bacteria present in the dental plaque breakdown the fermentable carbohydrates by their enzymes into acids like lactic acid, pyruvic acid and formic acid, which initiate demineralization of enamel or cementum.
  ii. Sucrose is the most cariogenic carbohydrates as it has capability to penetrate the dental plaque and produce acids by fermentation. It also stimulates plaque formation and its attachment.
 iii. Retention of food in the mouth is the major factor in production of dental caries. The sticky and sugar-rich foods that remain on and around the teeth for long period of time ultimately breakdown into organic acids and contribute in demineralization phase of dental caries.

iv. The caries producing bacteria like *Streptococcus mutans* and *Streptococcus sanguis* have the ability to synthesize and store polysaccharides for their future use. These polysaccharides help bacteria to adhere together as a tenacious material on the tooth surface.

v. Normally the carious process is intermittent, but when the frequency of sugar intake increases in between the meals it becomes a continuous process and thus incidence of dental caries increases.

ROLE OF FATS IN ORODENTAL HEALTH

A pure fat is composed of a molecule of glycerol to which fatty acids are linked. Fats are the excellent source of energy; they maintain body temperature by insulating against cold. Fats also helps in prevention of caries by the following mechanism.

a. It coats the surface of the tooth with oily substance due to which food particles are not easily retained.
b. A thin layer of fat over the plaque prevents the fermentable sugar to penetrate into the plaque and to be degraded into acids.
c. High concentration of fatty acids may delay the growth of cariogenic bacteria.
d. The presence of a thin layer of fat on the fermentable sugar particle prevents its fermentation and production of acid.

Fats also have some effect on periodontium. The diet consisting of more than 30% of fat may show degenerative changes in the gingiva, irregular bone resorption and replacement of bone and cementum by proliferative tissue. A diet consisting of less than 2% of fat may give rise to inflammatory changes in periodontal ligament.

RELATIONSHIP OF PROTEINS WITH ORAL HEALTH AND DISEASE

Proteins consist of number of amino acids joined together by peptide bonds. Proteins are the essential constituent of the cytoplasm and nuclei of cells and act as a building block of the cell membrane and tissue structures. They are the essential components of enzymes and hormones and the precursors of antibodies.

Proteins play a significant role in health and diseases of teeth and periodontium which is as follows:

a. Proteins are essential during active growth period.
b. Deficiency of proteins in children may cause inadequate development of the jawbones which leads to crowding and rotation of the teeth.
c. Due to protein deficiency in mother's diet, the child's teeth may be smaller in size and will be more prone to caries.
d. Protein deficiency affects the activity of fibroblasts, osteoblasts and cementoblasts.
e. Protein deprivation may cause degeneration of connective tissue of gingiva and periodontal ligament, osteoporosis of alveolar bone and retardation in deposition of cementum.

VITAMINS AND THEIR ORAL MANIFESTATIONS

Vitamins are the complex organic substances that occur in small amounts in food and are required for normal metabolic activity. Vitamins can be classified as follows.

a. Fat soluble Vitamins—Fat soluble vitamins are A, D, E and K.
b. Water soluble vitamins—Water soluble vitamins are B-complex and C.

Fat-soluble Vitamin

Vitamin A

A major function of vitamin A is to regulate epithelial cell differentiation. Deficiency of vitamin A causes hyperkeratinization of oral epithelium and alteration in tooth development. There may be atrophy of major and minor salivary glands due to vitamin A deficiency which will cause xerostomia and subsequently caries.

Mucosal lesions like leukoplakia can be treated by vitamin A therapy. Dietary sources include liver, kidney, egg, milk and its products and carotenes.

Vitamin D

Vitamin D promotes the absorption of calcium and phosphorus from the intestine. It maintains the level of serum calcium and phosphorus that promotes the calcification of bone.

Oral changes associated with vitamin D deficiency occur during tooth development and calcification due to which there may be hypoplasia of enamel, and the dentin shows poorly calcified spaces, delayed eruption and malalignment of teeth in the jaws.

Vitamin E

Vitamin E deficiency causes (a) disarrangement of teeth, and (b) chalky white teeth.

Vitamin K

Vitamin K deficiency is rare, as 30 days requirement of Vitamin K is stored in liver. Severe hemorrhage can result in acutely ill patients in 7 to 10 days. Vitamin K deficiency results in coagulopathy. Injection of Vitamin K restores the integrity of the clotting mechanisms.

Water Soluble Vitamins

Vitamin B Complex

Thiamine (Vitamin B_1): Thiamine is an important coenzyme essential for glucose metabolism and in the metabolism of branched chain amino acids.

Deficiency of thiamine results in beri-beri. The oral manifestations of thiamine deficiency are hypersensitivity of oral mucosa, burning sensation of tongue and loss of taste. There may be minute vesicles on buccal mucosa, under the tongue and over the palate and diminishing of the taste sensation.

It is found primarily in legumes, whole grains and green leafy vegetables. Daily requirement in diet is 0.5 mg /1000 Kcal.

Riboflavin (Vitamin B_2): It is a heat stable vitamin that functions as a component of FAD and FMN for the reversible transfer of hydrogen and electrons in several enzyme systems. Deficiency of riboflavin may cause angular cheilitis, stomatitis and glossitis. Glossitis is characterized by magenta discoloration of tongue and atrophy of the papillae.

A daily requirement of Riboflavin is about 1.5 mg. Food sources are green leafy vegetables, eggs, liver and milk.

Niacin (Vitamin B_3): Niacin is essential for conversion of fats, proteins and carbohydrates by oxidation–reduction. Deficiency of niacin results in pellagra which is characterized by dermatitis, dementia and diarrhea. Glossitis and generalized stomatitis are the earliest clinical signs of vitamin B_3 deficiency. The entire oral mucosa becomes red and painful. Ulcerations begin at the interdental gingival papillae and spread rapidly. Lean meat, yeast, soyabeans and peanuts are good sources of Niacin.

Pyridoxine (Vitamin B_6): Vitamin B_6 is a group of three chemically related substances: pyridoxine, pyridoxamine and pyridoxal. It helps in conversion of tryptophan to niacin.

The oral manifestations of vitamin B_6 deficiency are angular cheilitis, stomatitis and glossitis.

Recommended dose for children is 0.9 to 1.6 mg/day and for adults is 1.8 to 2.0 mg/day. The main dietary sources are wheat, corn, liver, milk and eggs.

Pantothenic acid: Effects of deficiency are not known in man. In rats deficiency causes ulcerations and hyperkeratosis of oral mucosa, gingival necrosis and resorption of alveolar crest. Sources are liver, egg, wholegrain, cereals and legumes.

Folic acid: Folic acid is necessary for erythropoiesis. Deficiency of folic acid causes megaloblastic or macrocytic anemia. The oral symptoms are burning sensation in mouth and atrophy of lingual papillae. There is generalized stomatitis which may be accompanied by glossitis and cheilitis.

Daily requirement of Folic acid is 0.4 mg/day. Best sources for this vitamin are green leafy vegetables, kidney, liver and yeast.

Vitamin B_{12} (cyancobalamin): It is needed for adequate nerve functioning, protein and carbohydrate metabolism and development of red blood cells. Deficiency of vitamin B_{12} leads to pernicious anemia. The oral manifestations are bright red, smooth and painful tongue.

A daily requirement of 0.003 mg is advised for adults. Liver, kidney, muscles and milk are good sources of vitamin B_{12}.

Vitamin C (Ascorbic Acid)

Vitamin C is necessary for the synthesis of collagen. Collagen is an intercellular constituent of connective tissues. The deficiency of vitamin C leads to scurvy. The peculiar sign of scurvy is an enlargement of marginal gingiva. The gingiva becomes bluish red, spongy and bleeds spontaneously with super-imposed infection. These gingival changes can result in loosening and premature loss of teeth. Scurvy in infants and children may lead to osseous lesions like osteoporosis and defective formation of enamel. Other manifestations of scurvy are poor wound healing, anemia, weakness and hemorrhage under the skin and mucous membrane. A daily requirement of vitamin C is about 50 mg. Dietary sources are citrus fruits, tomatoes, cabbage and other fresh fruits and vegetables.

MINERALS AND TRACE ELEMENTS

There are various minerals and trace elements essential for good oral health. Important among them are as follows.

Calcium

Calcium is found in all the inorganized tissues of the body. It is essential for mineralization of bone and teeth, membrane permeability, neuro-muscular excitability and in the coagulation of blood.

The normal level of calcium in the blood is 9 to 11.5 mg/100 ml. Deficiency of calcium causes reduction in alveolar bone formation, altered calcification of teeth and increased dental caries. Dietary sources are milk, fish, eggs and vegetables.

Phosphorus

Phosphorus is essential for the mineralization of organic matrix of teeth and bone. Normal phosphorus level is 2 to 4 mg/dl. Deficiency of phosphorus can cause osteoporosis of alveolar bone and increased dental caries.

Magnesium

Magnesium is an essential nutritional substance. It takes part in phosphorylation. Deficiency of magnesium may cause degenerative changes in odontoblast, gingival hyperplasia, enamel hypoplasia and widening of periodontal ligament. Dietary sources are vegetables and cereals.

Iodine

Iodine is necessary for the production of thyroxine by the thyroid gland. Deficiency of iodine causes hypothyroidism. Oral manifestations may be gingival hyperplasia, slow eruption of teeth and root resorption. Sources of iodine are seafoods, cod-liver oil, milk and meat.

Iron

Iron is necessary for the formation of hemoglobin. Deficiency of iron can produce oral manifestations like delayed healing of wound, gingivitis, glossitis and stomatitis. Dietary sources are green leafy vegetables, legumes, meat, fish. Supplementary sources of iron are syrup, paste and malt (Fig. 4.1).

Fluoride

Fluoride is an important trace element. Optimal ingestion of fluoride during tooth mineralization produces the tooth which will resist caries.

Fluorides are important for prevention of initiation of dental caries by making tooth surface resistant to acid.

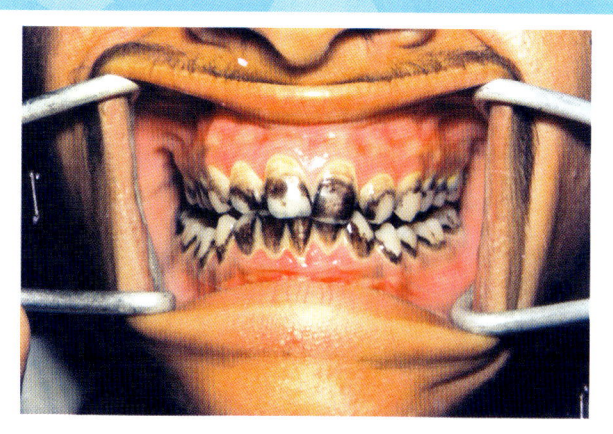

Fig. 4.1: Black stains on teeth are due to consumption of iron preparation in syrup, paste and malt form

Fluoride is also given in the management of Paget's disease. The optimum water fluoride level is 1ppm. If it exceeds 2 to 3 ppm, the fluoride gets precipitated in the teeth and bones, this is called fluorosis or mottling.

BIBLIOGRAPHY

1. Brown JP, Bibby BG. Effects on caries of sugars administered before tooth eruption. Caries Res 1970;4:56.
2. Caldwell RC. Physical properties and their caries-producing potential. J Dent Res 1970;49:1293.
3. Critchley P. Effects of foods on bacterial metabolic processes. J Dent Res 1970;49:1283.
4. Dawes C. Effects of diet on salivary secretion and composition. J Dent Res 1970;49:1263.
5. Giorgio AJ. Current concepts of iron metabolism and the iron deficiency anemias. Med Clin N Amer 1970;541:399.
6. Henkin RI. The role of taste in disease and nutrition. Borden Rev Nutr Res 1967;28(4).
7. Huenemann RL, Shapiro LR, Hampton MC, Mitchell BW. Food and eating practices of teenagers. J Amer Diet Ass 1968;53:17.
8. Navia JM. Effects of minerals on dental caries. In: Gould, RF (ed.). Dietary Chemicals vs. Dental Caries. Advances in Chemistry. Washington DC, American Chemical Society 1970;(94).
9. Neuman WF, Neuman MW. Recent advances in bone growth and nutrition. Borden's Rev Nutr Res 21 (No. 4), July-Aug, 1960.
10. Nizel AE. Amino acids, proteins and dental caries. In: Harris RS (ed.): Dietary Chemicals vs. Dental Caries. Advances in Chemistry Series 1970;(94):23.
11. Stewart, Ray E, Barber TK, Troutman KC, Wei SHY. Pediatric Dentistry. Scientific foundations and clinical practice: 2nd ed., CV Mosby Co., 1982;561-75.
12. Wei SHY. Nutritional aspects of dental caries. Infant Nutrition. (2nd edn.) Philadelphia, WB Sauders Co. 1947.

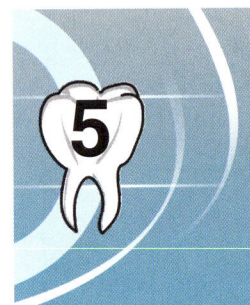

Pathology Related to Oral Medicine

Dorland Medical dictionary has defined pathology as the study of changes in the tissues and organs caused by disease. Taber's Medical Dictionary has defined pathology as the study of the nature and cause of disease which involve changes in structure and function. Stedman's Medical dictionary has defined pathology as the medical, and specialty practice, concerned with all aspects of disease, but with special reference to the essential nature, causes, and development of abnormal conditions, as well as the structural and functional changes that result from the disease processes.

In other words pathology is the study that is concerned with all aspects of disease like nature, cause and development of abnormal conditions as well as structural and functional changes due to disease process. A knowledge of pathology helps in diagnosis, treatment and prevention of disease. A clinician may obtain pathologic information by theoretical and technical procedures of microbiology, parasitology, immunology and hematology.

INFLAMMATION

Dorland Medical dictionary has defined inflammation as a protective tissue response to injury or destruction of tissues, which serves to destroy, dilute, or walloff both the injurious agent and the injured tissues. However, in other words inflammation can be defined as the local response of cellular and vascular tissues to injury due to any agent. It is a protective reaction, since it tends to eliminate or limit the spread of injurious agent.

The cause of injury leading to inflammation may be physical, chemical, traumatic, infective or immunologic in nature.

Signs of Inflammation

The following are the clinical signs of inflammation:

Swelling

The swelling in the area results from congestion, edema, or an exudate in the local tissues.

Heat

The sensation of heat is caused by an increased local blood flow.

Redness

Redness is due to dilatation of small blood vessels within an area of injury.

Pain

Pain is produced due to increase in tissue tension within the inflamed area which becomes tense due to accumulation of exudates.

Loss of Function

Function is lost due to restricted muscular movements as a result of pain and swelling of the inflamed area.

Types of Inflammation

There are four types of inflammation that are tissue responses to injury and disease:

Acute Inflammation

It lasts from several days to several weeks and mainly involves the polymorphonuclear leukocyte.

Chronic Inflammation

It is low grade type of inflammation and extends over a period of months. It is characterized by involvement of lymphocytes, plasma cells and fibroblastic proliferation.

Subacute Inflammation

It extends for a period of weeks or months and has characteristics of both the acute and chronic types.

Chronic Granulomatous Inflammation

It is a response to a specific disease such as syphilis, tuberculosis, fungal infection or foreign body reaction.

It is manifested by the mobilization of giant cells, lymphocytes, plasma cells, and histiocytes that form diffuse or circumscribed masses.

Acute Inflammation

Changes that takes place in acute inflammation can be studied under following headings:

Changes in Vascular Calibre and Flow

Due to injury the earliest response is transient vasoconstriction of arterioles which is re-established in few minutes. Next is vasodilatation which elevates the local hydrostatic pressure resulting in transudation of fluid into extracellular space. Due to increase in hydrostatic pressure there is an increased permeability of blood vessels which causes slowing of blood flow.

Increased Vascular Permeability

After injury, inflammatory exudate accumulates rapidly within the injured area due to increase in the rate of escape of water and proteins from small blood vessels i.e. increased vascular permeability. Increase in vascular permeability depends upon the type and severity of the injury.

Emigration of Leukocytes

The accumulation of leukocytes in an area of injured tissue is most important feature of inflammatory response. Migration of leukocytes takes place in three distinct stages.
  i. *Pavementing and margination of leukocytes:* In the early stages of inflammation there is slowing or stasis of blood stream due to which central stream of cells widens and peripheral plasma zone becomes narrower because of loss of plasma by exudation, this process is known as margination. As a result, neutrophils of the central column come close to the vessel wall, this is known as pavementing.
  ii. *Leukocytic emigration:* The peripherally marginated and pavemented neutrophils move along the endothelial surface, penetrate the basement membrane and escape into the extravascular space, known as emigration.
  iii. *Chemotaxis:* Leukocytes in the extravascular tissue migrate towards a specific chemical substance by a process known as chemotaxis.

Phagocytosis

Phagocytosis is the process of ingesting foreign particles, microorganisms, dead tissues and degenerated cells. This process is carried out by phagocytes which are of two types.
  i. *Microphages:* Microphages appear early in acute inflammatory response, e.g. Microphages polymorphonuclear neutrophils.
  ii. *Macrophages:* Macrophages arise from circulating monocytes. They are activated by the factors present in inflammatory exudate. Phagocytes engulf a wider range of microorganisms, kill them by antibacterial substances and then degrade them by hydrolytic enzymes.

Chronic Inflammation

Chronic inflammation is a prolonged process in which tissue destruction and inflammation occur at the same time. Chronic inflammation can be caused by following three ways.
  a. Prolonged acute inflammation progressing into chronic inflammation.
  b. Repeated attacks of acute inflammation.
  c. Chronic inflammation with no initial acute phase.

Characteristics of Chronic Inflammation

  i. Mononuclear cell infiltration: Chronic inflammation is infiltrated by mononuclear inflammatory cells like circulating monocytes, tissue macrophages and multinucleated giant cells.
  ii. Necrosis and tissue destruction: Destruction of tissue and necrosis is common in many chronic inflammatory lesions.
  iii. Proliferative changes: Tissue destruction or necrosis causes proliferation of small blood vessels and fibroblasts which results in the formation of inflammatory granulation tissue.

HYPERTROPHY

Hypertrophy is an increase in the size of parenchymal cells due to which there is enlargement of the organ or tissue. Hypertrophy can be divided into physiologic, compensatory and pathologic.

Physiologic Hypertrophy

It is caused either by increased functional demand or by hormonal stimulation. Examples are as follows.

a. Enlarged size of uterus in pregnancy.
b. Hypertrophied muscles in manual laborers and athletes.

Compensatory Hypertrophy

It may occur in survivor of a pair of organs, when one is removed. Examples are as follows.
a. Hypertrophy of the nephrons of remaining kidney, when other one is removed.
b. Removal of one adrenal gland leads to hypertrophy of opposite adrenal gland.

Pathologic Hypertrophy

In pathologic hypertrophy affected organ becomes enlarged and heavy.
a. Left ventricular hypertrophy in aortic valve diseases.
b. Hypertrophy of smooth muscles of stomach in pyloric stenosis.

HYPERPLASIA

Hyperplasia is an increase in number of parenchymal cells resulting in enlargement of organ or tissue. Hyperplasia can be divided into, physiologic, pathologic and compensatory.

Physiologic Hyperplasia

Physiologic hyperplasia occurs under the influence of hormonal changes. The examples are as follows.
a. Hyperplasia of female breast at puberty and during pregnancy.
b. Prostatic hyperplasia in old age in males.

Pathologic Hyperplasia

It is caused due to excessive stimulation of hormones. The examples are as follows.
a. Hyperplasia of endometrium following excess of oestrogen.
b. Formation of skin warts from hyperplasia of epidermis due to papilloma virus.

Compensatory Hyperplasia

Increase in number of cells after removal of part of an organ. The examples are as follows.
a. Regeneration of epidermis following skin abrasion.
b. Regeneration of liver after partial hepatectomy.

INFECTION

Infection is an invasion of the tissues of the body by disease-producing microorganisms and the reaction of these tissues to the microorganisms and their toxins. These microorganisms cause infective diseases in human beings. Most infective diseases depend upon the inter-relationship between disease-producing properties of microorganisms and defence capacity of host against invading microorganisms. The host and microorganism relationship is determined by following factors.

Factors in Relation to Microorganisms

Route of Entry

Microorganisms gain entry into the body by various routes. For example through inhalation (respiration), ingestion, inoculation (parenteral), transplacental and by direct contact (contagious infection).

Spread of Infection

The microorganisms after entering the body spread further through the blood vessels, lymphatics and phagocytic cells.

Production of Toxins

Microorganisms release two types of toxins, exotoxins and endotoxins. Exotoxins are secreted by living bacteria and have effect at distant sites. Endotoxins are constituents of the cell wall of gram-negative bacteria and are released on the lysis of bacteria. These toxins damage cell membrane and kill neutrophils, polymorphs and macrophages.

Factors Relating to Host

Barrier Against Invasion

The keratinized layer of the epidermis is an excellent mechanical barrier to microbial invasion, a break in continuity of skin and mucous membrane allows microorganisms to enter the body. The secretions of glands opening on the skin provide an environment in which many bacteria do not survive. Mucus secretions of oral cavity and acids in stomach prevent bacterial colonization.

Immune Defence Mechanisms

When microorganisms invade the body, the defensive reactions of body limit the multiplication and spread of microorganisms and bring about their destruction. These reactions are as follows.
  i. The inflammatory reaction
 ii. Phagocytosis and destruction of microorganisms.
iii. The immune system.

SHOCK

Shock is defined as state of collapse of the body which results from an acute fall in cardiac output. The principal effects of shock are reduction in effective circulatory blood volume and inadequate perfusion of cells and tissues. Shock is of two types, primary and secondary.

Primary Shock

Primary shock is neurogenic in nature in which pain and anxiety result in sudden reduction of venous return to the heart. It occurs immediately after an injury, severe pain and emotional state like fear or surprise.

Secondary Shock

Secondary shock occurs due to hemodynamic disorders in which there is change in capillary permeability and loss of plasma into tissue spaces. It occurs some time after the injury.

Etiology and Types of Shock

Shock can be classified under three headings according to the etiology.
a. *Hypovolemic shock:* Hypovolemic shock is caused by reduction in blood volume due to severe hemorrhage and fluid loss. For example, in trauma, hemorrhagic disorders, severe burns and diarrhea.
b. *Cardiogenic shock:* Cardiogenic shock results from severe fall in cardiac output secondary to acute diseases of heart. The commonest cause is myocardial infarction. Other conditions include rupture of valve, cardiac arrhythmias, and pulmonary embolism.
c. *Septic shock:* Septic shock is associated with severe bacterial infection that releases toxins, vasoactive substances and cytokines that causes hypotension. Septic shock is common complication of gram-negative infection. It is induced by endotoxins. Gram-positive septicemia is less common and is induced by exotoxins.

Biochemical Mechanism of Shock

Reduced circulating blood volume
↓
Decreased venous return to heart
↓
Fall in cardiac output
↓
Reduced blood flow
↓
Reduced supply of oxygen
↓
Tissue anoxia
↓
Shock

HEALING OF ORAL WOUND

Healing is the process of return to health or closure of wound and ulcers. Healing is the ability of damaged tissue to repair itself and is considered one of the primary survival mechanisms.

Factors Affecting the Healing of Oral Wounds

Healing of oral wounds is influenced by the number of factors which are as follows.

Site of Wound

Wound present in an area having good vascular supply heals more rapidly as compared to wound in area which is less vascular.

Movement of Wound Area

If the wound is in an area which is immobilized, the healing is rapid whereas the wound present in an area of constant movements heals slowly due to the repeated disruption of formation of connective tissue by the movements.

Temperature

Local temperature at the site of wound also influences rate of healing. When the temperature at the site of wound is slightly higher than body temperature, wound healing is accelerated, while in hypothermia and in excessive hyperthermia wound healing is delayed.

Nutritional Factors

Protein is an essential constituent that influences the rate of healing. It is necessary for fibroblastic proliferation in wounds. Vitamin C is necessary for regulation of collagen formation and intercellular ground substance of the connective tissue. Deficiency of vitamin C delays the healing process.

Age of Patient

Wounds in younger person heal more rapidly than wounds in older persons.

Infection

Wounds which are protected from bacterial irritation heal faster as compared to wounds that are subjected to physical or bacterial irritation.

BIBLIOGRAPHY

1. Kardachi BJ, Newcomb GM. A clinical study of gingival inflammation and renal transplant recipients taking immuno-suppressive drugs. J Periodontol 1978;49:307.
2. Page RC, Schroeder HE. Pathogenesis of inflammatory periodontal disease. A summary of current work. Lab Invest 1976;33:32-5.
3. Slots J. The microflora of black stain on human primary teeth. Scand. J Dent Res 1974;82:484.
4. World Health Organization. Epidemiology, etiology and prevention of periodontal diseases. Technical Report Series No. 621, Geneva, WHO 1978.

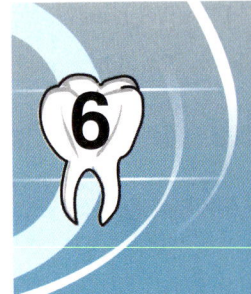

Oral Examination and Diagnosis

INTRODUCTION

According to Stedman's Medical Dictionary 'Diagnosis is the determination of the nature of a disease, injury or congenital defect'. Mosby's dental dictionary has defined diagnosis as 'the translation of data gathered by clinical and radiographic examination into an organized, classified definition of the condition present'. According to Taber's Medical Dictionary 'Diagnosis is the use of scientific and skillful methods to establish the cause and nature of the patient's illness. However, diagnosis is the process of identification of diseases by evaluating the history of disease process, signs and symptoms and laboratory investigations. Oral diagnosis is an identification of oral diseases, abnormalities, congenital and developmental defects in oral cavity by history, clinical examination, radiological and laboratory investigations.

PROCEDURE OF ORAL DIAGNOSIS

The diagnostic procedure may be divided as follows:
1. History taking
2. Examination of the patient
3. Specialized examination procedures, radiological and laboratory investigations.
4. Establishing a diagnosis through differential diagnosis
5. Treatment planning.

1. History Taking and Recording

The patient history is the description of the patient's symptoms conveyed to the clinician in his or her own words or by attendant if patient is unable to communicate. History taking is essential for establishing a correct diagnosis. It very much depends upon the clinician and patient relationship. Listening attentively with interest and compassion encourages the patients to reveal their problems to the dental surgeon.

Constituents of Patient History

A. *Routine information:* It includes the patient's name, address, age, sex, marital status and the name and address of the referring physician or dentist.
B. *Chief complaint:* Chief complaint is the description of the chief problem of the patient for which he or she has visited dental clinic for seeking treatment. It must be recorded in patient's own words.
C. *History of present illness:* It includes the events from the onset of problem till the time of history taking. Additional information like, whether, the patient has consulted any other clinician or taken some other treatment for the same complaint, also constitute the history of present illness.
D. *Past dental history:* Past dental history includes the information about the previous restorative, endodontic, periodontic or surgical treatment and any complication of previous dental treatment. It also gives an idea about the patient's consciousness towards the dental care.
E. *Past medical history:* In past medical history the patient is interrogated for serious conditions that can be of concern to the dental surgeon like cardiac, pulmonary, renal or liver diseases, diabetes mellitus, drug allergy, immunological disorders, infectious diseases, radiation therapy, transfusion, medications, hematological disorders, psychiatric problems and pregnancy.
F. *Family history:* Family history collects the information about the diseases that are running in the family members like cardiovascular disease (hypertension), tuberculosis, infectious diseases like hepatitis B, bleeding disorders, diabetes mellitus and hereditary and congenital disorders which have significance in dental treatment.
G. *Social history:* Social history provides the facts about the patient's personality, tobacco and alcohol use and his awareness of oral hygiene measures.

Proforma for history recording should be filled by patient/guardian.

2. Examination of the Patient

The examination of the patient is the second step of diagnosis procedure. It includes general examination and examination of head, neck, oral cavity and individual teeth.

General Examination

The general examination starts from the moment the patient enters the dental clinic. The clinician should observe the build, gait or any physical deformity in the patient before seating him on the dental chair. He should record the temperature, pulse rate and blood pressure of the patient as it can indicate the presence of any systemic disease. The normal range of these vital signs are as follows.

Vital sign	Normal range
Temperature	98.6°F or 37°C
Pulse rate	65 to 80 beats per minute in adults
	100 beats per minute in children.
	55 to 65 beats per minute in persons above about 70 years of age
Blood pressure	Systolic 100 to 120 mm Hg, diastolic 80 mm Hg.

Examination of Head, Neck and Oral Cavity

A complete physical examination of the structure of the head, neck and oral cavity is essential for diagnosing and treating oral diseases.

Extraoral Examination

Face
   i. *Skin:* Inspect the patient's skin for pigmentation, abnormalities, moles, swelling, scars and lacerations.
   ii. *Eyes:* Examine the eyes for conjunctival lesions or any abnormality in pupils and sclera.
   iii. *Nose:* Any deformity or obstruction in the nose should be noted.

Temporomandibular joint: Palpate the joints for swelling, pain and tenderness, clicking and grinding sounds on opening and chewing; deviation in the path of the mandible during protrusive and lateral movements.

Neck: Examination of the neck includes the examination of submandibular and cervical lymph nodes. These lymph nodes get enlarged due to infection, inflammation and as a result of metastatic spread of a malignant tumor. Midline structures like hyoid bone and thyroid gland should be palpated for any tenderness, nodules or masses.

Intraoral Examination

Oral mucosa: Oral mucosa should be examined for any alteration in texture and elasticity, ulcers, vesicles, abnormal growth and red, white and pigmented lesions.

Lips: Carefully observe the mucosal surface of the lips for ulcers, nodules and keratotic lesions; note cracking or fissuring at angles and palpate the lips gently for any swelling.

Tongue: Examine the tongue for developmental and congenital anomalies like ankyloglossia; and macroglossia; coating, ulcer, lesions and traumatic injuries.

Gingiva: Observe color, contour, consistency, texture, enlargement, nodules, swellings, fistulae inflammation and lesions of the gingiva.

Salivary glands: In examination of salivary glands, note the dryness of mucosa or excessive flow of saliva; any swelling in the mouth due to enlargement of salivary glands; palpate for any obstruction in salivary duct.

Teeth: Note mobile and carious teeth, root stumps, fractured teeth, missing and supernumerary teeth, occlusal discrepancies, discolored teeth and plaque and calculus deposition.

Hard palate and soft palate: Inspect the palate for swellings, fistulae, tori, ulcers, papillary hyperplasia, leukoplakia and asymmetry of structure or function.

Floor of the mouth: Observe openings of Whartson's ducts, any swellings, the salivary collection, ulcers, red and white patches.

3. Specialized Examination Procedures and Laboratory Investigations

Specialized examination procedures and laboratory investigations are carried out to confirm or rule out a diagnosis. Various supplementary examination procedures which can provide visible evidence of suspected physical abnormalities are as follows:

a. Teeth: Dental pulp vitality test, radiographs, radio-visiography (RVG) (Fig. 6.1)
b. Tongue: Ultrasonic imaging of base of tongue and electromyography
c. Taste: Electrogustometry
d. Salivary glands: Sialography
e. Thyroid-Isotopic scanning techniques
f. Temporomandibular joint: Arthrography and arthroscopy
g. Head: MRI and CT scan

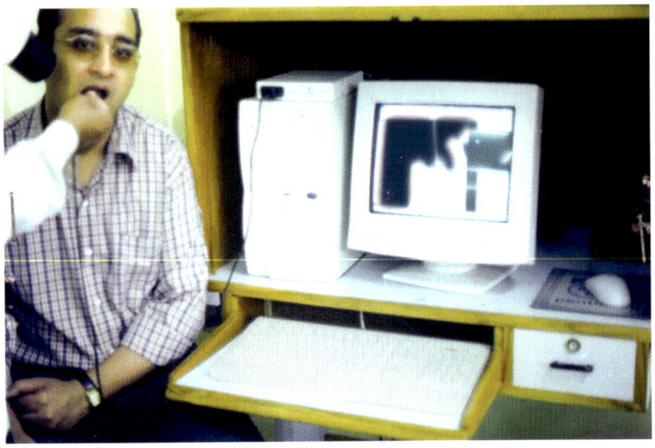

Fig. 6.1: Radiovisiography (RVG) (*Courtesy* Deptt. of Periodontology CSMMU, Lucknow)

Laboratory Investigations

In laboratory investigations tissue, blood, urine and other specimens are taken from the patient for biochemical, microscopic, immunologic and microbiologic investigations.

Specimens are obtained from the oral cavity by different techniques like scraping the cells as in exfoliative cytology, aspirating the tissues as in fine needle aspiration cytology and by tissue biopsy. The specimens of blood tissue, tissue discharge, tissue fluid, urine and pus are sent for laboratory investigations and thus assist in diagnosis of oral lesions like periodontal abscess, candidiasis, lesions of jaw bones and oral mucosa.

4. Establishing the Diagnosis

Usually the diagnosis is self-estimated, but in some conditions when the clinical data is complicated, the diagnosis is made by reconsidering the patient's history, clinical and laboratory examinations. The symptoms and complaints of the patient should be arranged in sequence of severity and according to it diagnosis of disease should be established.

The diagnosis should be entered in patient's record for insurance and medicolegal purpose. If more than one diagnosis is made, the diagnosis for the main complaint should be written first.

5. Treatment Planning

The procedure of diagnosis like history taking, clinical examination and laboratory investigations helps the dental surgeon to decide a plan of treatment for the complaint or disease for which the patient is seeking help. The plan of treatment includes the procedures for control and treatment of current disease as well as preventive and maintenance measures.

BIBLIOGRAPHY

1. DeNucci DJ, Chen CC, Sobiski C, Meehan S. The use of SPECT bone scans to evaluate patients with idiopathic jaw pain. Oral Surg Oral Med Oral Pathol Oral Radiol Endod 2000;90:750-7.
2. De Rossi SS, Glick M. Lupus erythematosus: considerations for dentistry. J Am Dent Assoc 1998;129:330.
3. Khan O, Archibald A, Thomson E, Maharaja P. The role of quantitative single photon emission computerized tomography (SPECT) in the osseous integration process of dental implants. Oral Surg Oral Med Oral Pathol Oral Radiol Endod 2000;90:228-32.
4. Larheim TA, Westesson PL, Hicks DG, et al. Osteonecrosis of the temporomandibular joint correlation of magnetic resonance imaging and histology. J Oral Maxillofac Surg 1999;57:888-98.
5. Orient JM. Sapira's art & science of bedside diagnosis. 3rd edn. Philadelphia: Lippincott Williams & Wilkins 2000.
6. Patton LL, Shugars DC. Immunologic and viral markers of HIV–I disease progression, implications for dentistry, J Am Dent Assoc 2000;131-345.
7. Paurazas SB, Geist JR, Pink FE, et al. Comparison of diagnostic accuracy of digital imaging by using CCD and CMOS-APS sensors with E-speed film in the detection of periapical bony lesions. Oral Surg Oral Med Oral Pathol Oral Radiol Endod 2000;89:356-62.
8. Terakado M, Hashimoto K, Arai Y, et al. Diagnostic imaging with newly developed orthocubic super-high resolution computed tomography (Ortho-CT). Oral Surg Oral Med Oral Pathol Oral Radiol Endod 2000;89:509-18.
9. White SC, Heslop EW, Hollender LG, et al. Parameters of radiologic care. An official report of the American Academy of Oral and Maxillofacial Radiology. Oral Surg Oral Med Oral Pathol Oral Radiol Endod 2001;91:498-511.

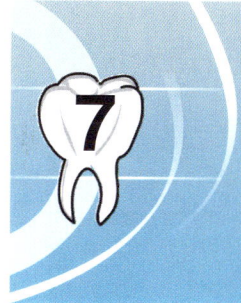

7
Developmental Disorders Affecting Oral and Para Oral Structures

Developmental disorders are the anomalies that are present from birth and persist either throughout life or may manifest only for few years. These developmental disturbances may be hereditary or congenital. Congenital anomaly exists at birth, but is not necessarily inherited, it is caused due to an influence occurring during gestation upto the birth, where as hereditary diseases are transmitted through genes of parental germ cell.

DEVELOPMENTAL DISORDERS OF THE TEETH

Disorders in Size of Teeth

Microdontia

Microdontia is a condition in which teeth appear smaller in size or are actually smaller in size than normal. It may involve single tooth, pair of teeth or the whole dentition. Single tooth may be peg shaped (Fig. 7.1). In true generalized microdontia the teeth are smaller than normal size, whereas in relative generalized microdontia the normal sized teeth appear smaller when they are present in jaws that are larger than normal. Microdontia is commonly seen in the case of pituitary dwarfism and ectodermal dysplasia.

Macrodontia

Macrodontia refers to the teeth that are abnormally large in size. In true generalized macrodontia, all the teeth are larger than normal as in the case of pituitary gigantism and facial hemihypertrophy. Relative generalized macrodontia is a condition in which normal teeth appear larger as they are present in smaller jaws.

Disorders in Number of Teeth

Anodontia

The term anodontia refers to congenital absence of teeth due to lack of tooth germ development. In total anodontia all the teeth either deciduous or permanent are missing.

Partial anodontia or oligodontia or hypodontia involves single tooth or group of teeth. False anodontia is a condition in which teeth are missing in oral cavity due to their impaction or extraction.

Supernumerary Teeth

A supernumerary tooth is an additional tooth exceeding the normal number of dentition. It may resemble the teeth with which it is associated. A supernumerary tooth develops either due to splitting of the permanent tooth bud or from an extra tooth bud arising from the dental lamina. Common supernumerary teeth are mesiodens (between the maxillary central incisors), paramolars (placed buccally or lingually to the molars) and distomolars (distal to third molars).

Accessory Teeth

Accessory teeth are also supernumerary teeth but do not resemble normal teeth in shape, size or location.

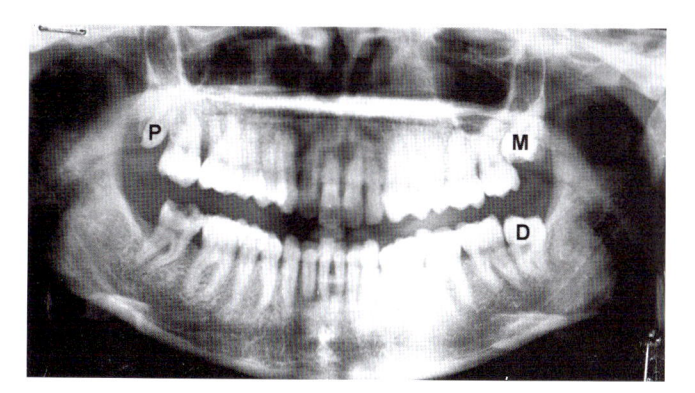

Fig. 7.1: Orthopantograph showing maxillary left third molar peg shaped (shown by P), right third molar in mesioangular impaction (shown by M) Mandibular left third molar missing and right third molar in slight distoangular impaction (shown by D)

Predeciduous Teeth

Predeciduous dentition is a rare condition in which ill-formed teeth occur on gingiva over the crest of ridge prior to deciduous dentition and can be easily removed without forceful extraction. These are hornified epithelial structures without roots and usually found in mandibular incisor area. These teeth arise either from the bud of an accessory dental lamina or from an accessory bud of the dental lamina.

Disorders in Shape of Teeth

Fusion

Fusion is the condition in which two teeth get united during the development by the union of their tooth bud to form a single tooth. Fusion may be either complete or incomplete. Complete fusion occurs when two developing tooth germs are fused together before the calcification process. This results in the formation of single large tooth. If the contact of the teeth occurs after the formation of the portion of tooth crown, there is fusion of roots only.

It may occur between two normal teeth or a normal tooth with a supernumerary tooth.

Concrescence

Concrescence refers to the condition in which there is union of the roots of two adjacent teeth by cementum only after the eruption or after the root formation has been completed. It occurs as a result of trauma or crowding of teeth due to which there is resorption of interdental bone, so that the two adjacent roots come close to each other and get fused due to deposition of cementum.

Gemination

Gemination arises from division of a single tooth germ during development, resulting in incomplete formation of two teeth. Normally it occurs as a bifid crown upon a single root.

Dilaceration

Dilaceration is an angular distortion or bend or curve in the root of the tooth or at the junction of the root and crown. It results from trauma during development of tooth. (Fig. 7.2).

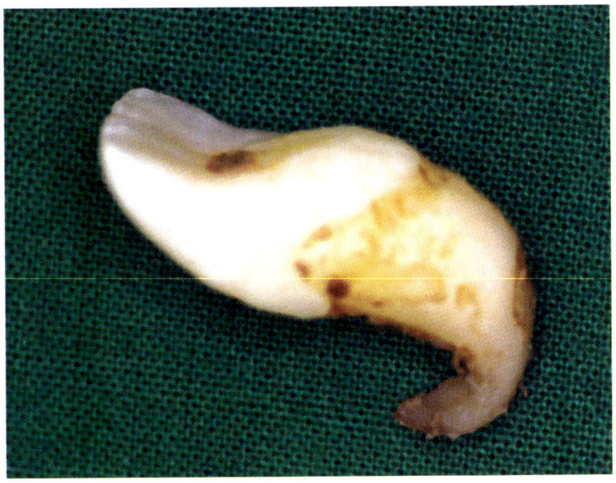

Dens Evaginatus

Dens evaginatus is a condition in which there is appearance of protuberance or globule of enamel on the occlusal surface of premolars. It is caused due to evagination and proliferation of the inner enamel epithelium and odontogenic mesenchyme into the dental organ during early tooth development. It is also known as occlusal enamel pearl, occlusal tuberculated premolar, evaginated odontome and Leong's premolar.

Fig. 7.2: Dilaceration (*Courtesy* Dr Mithilesh Chandra, Noida)

Dens-in-Dente (Dens Invaginatus; Dilated Composite Odontome)

It is an anomaly of the tooth found mainly in permanent maxillary lateral incisors. It can affect the crown in which there is invagination of the enamel organ into the dental papilla. It occasionally occurs in the roots of teeth due to invagination of the root sheath of Hertwig.

Taurodontism

Taurodontism is a dental anomaly in which crown of the tooth is large in size with elongated and enlarged pulp chamber which extends deeply into the root. Taurodontism may occur due to genetic disorders or failure of Hertwig's epithelial sheath to invaginate at the proper level. Taurodontism affects both the deciduous and permanent dentitions and most commonly occurs in molars.

Disorders in Structure of Teeth

Amelogenesis Imperfecta

Amelogenesis imperfecta is an ectodermal disorder in which enamel is defective in structure. The affected teeth show discoloration due to enamel wear following dentin exposure. Three basic types of amelogenesis imperfecta are as follows.

i. Hypoplastic type: in which there is defective enamel matrix deposition but normal mineralization.

ii. **Hypocalcification:** characterized by defective mineralization but normal matrix.
iii. **Hypomaturation:** in which there is immaturation of enamel crystals.

Dentinogenesis Imperfecta

Dentinogenesis imperfecta is characterized by opalescent or grey-colored teeth involving both primary and permanent dentition. It may be hereditary or associated with osteogenesis imperfecta. There is early loss of enamel exposing the dentin which undergoes rapid attrition. Radiograph shows obliteration of the pulp chamber and root canals and roots are short and blunt.

Enamel Hypoplasia

It is a developmental disorder of teeth characterized by defective enamel matrix formation resulting in reduction in thickness of enamel. It may be hereditary or acquired. Hereditary enamel hypoplasia involves both deciduous and permanent dentition and only the enamel is affected. Acquired enamel hypoplasia is caused by various local or systemic factors, in which both enamel and dentin are affected. Various environmental factors responsible for enamel hypoplasia are local trauma or infection, congenital syphilis, dental fluorosis (mottling), nutritional deficiency and exanthematous fever. (Figs 7.3 and 7.4)

Dentinal Dysplasia

Dentinal dysplasia is a hereditary disorder involving both deciduous and permanent dentition. There is normal enamel formation but atypical dentin formation. The roots are short, blunt and malformed. There is obliteration of pulp chamber and root canals in deciduous teeth. Teeth become mobile and get exfoliated prematurely because of abnormally short roots.

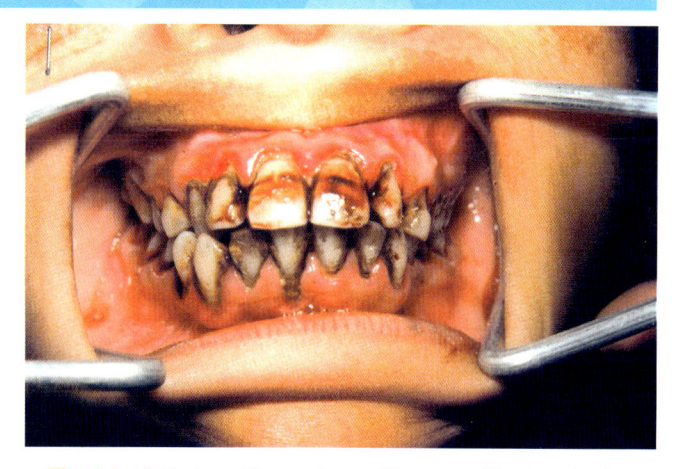

Fig. 7.4: Mottled maxillary incisors with poor oral hygiene having calculus, plaque and materia alba

Regional Odontodysplasia

It is a developmental disorder of the teeth of unknown etiology, characterized by defective formation of dentin and enamel. Most frequently affected teeth are maxillary permanent incisors and cuspids. It may involve both the deciduous and permanent teeth; and the affected teeth exhibit either delay or failure in eruption. This condition may arise due to somatic mutation.

Radiograph reveals large pulp chamber with very thin enamel and dentin which give them ghost like appearance.

Periapical Cementoma

Presence of excessive cementum at the root apex is called periapical cementoma (Fig. 7.5).

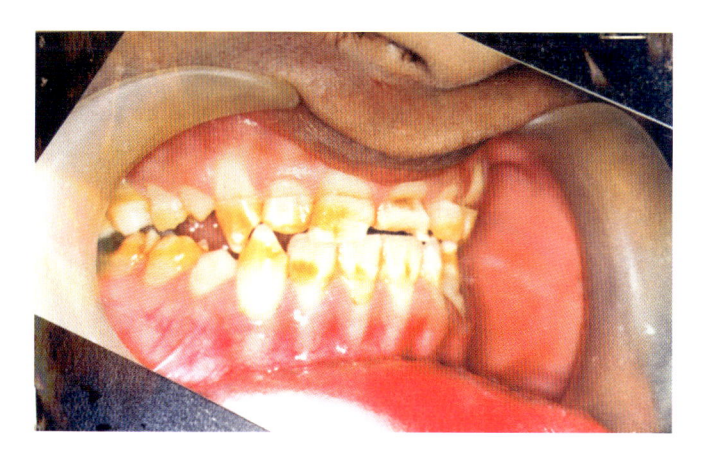

Fig. 7.3: Hypoplastic abraded and mottled teeth

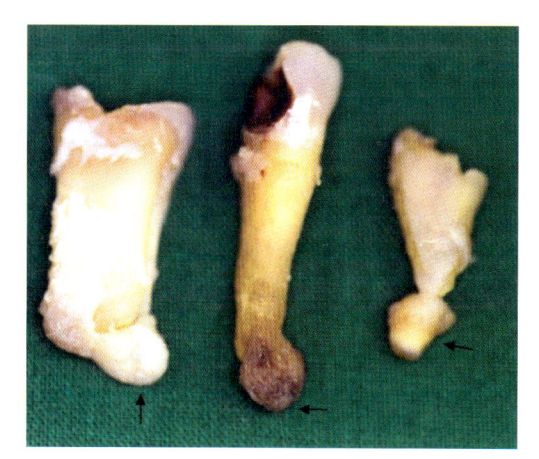

Fig. 7.5: Periapical cementoma attached to root apices of teeth (shown by arrows) (*Courtesy* Dr Mithilesh Chandra, Noida)

24 Oral Medicine

Disorders in Tooth Eruption

Premature Eruption

Occasionally the deciduous teeth (usually mandibular incisors) get erupted into the oral cavity of infants at birth. These teeth are called natal teeth. In these teeth there is almost no root present. (Fig. 7.6) Neonatal teeth are the deciduous teeth that erupted prematurely in the oral cavity within 30 days of birth. These conditions of premature eruption may be due to endocrine disturbance.

For uncomplicated eruption of adjacent teeth, as far possible, natal and neonatel teeth should not be extracted. They may be extracted only if they are hypermobile and there is a danger of their avulsion and swallowing by the child. In breastfeeding such child, the mother may feel some problem. It has been abserved that gradually the child becomes conditioned so as not to bite during sucking. Mother can use breast pump if she cannot bear the discomfort.

Delayed Eruption

Delayed eruption of deciduous and permanent teeth is associated with local factors like fibromatosis gingiva, in which dense connective tissue does not allow the eruption of the tooth. Systemic conditions like hypothyroidism, rickets, cleidocranial dysplasia and cretinism are also responsible for delayed eruption.

Ectopic, Impacted and Embedded Teeth

Eruption of tooth at an abnormal place is called ectopic eruption. Impacted or embedded tooth refers to a tooth which fails to erupt in oral cavity due to lack of eruption force. An impacted tooth is an unerupted or partially erupted tooth positioned against the physical barrier like bone, dense connective tissue and another tooth. The maxillary and mandibular third molars and the maxillary canines are the most common impacted teeth (Figs 7.7 to 7.10).

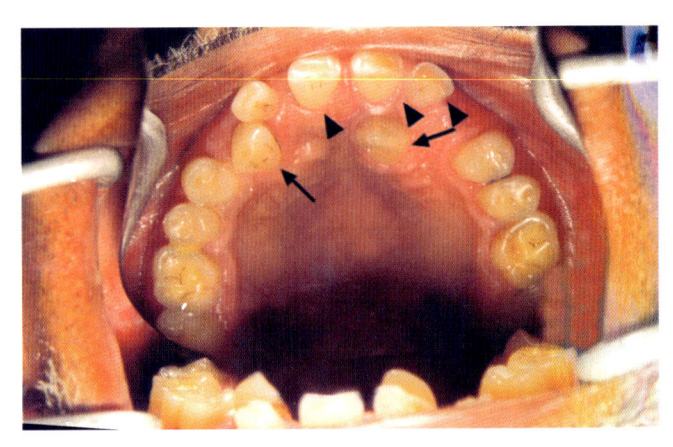

Fig. 7.7: Ectopically placed maxillary canines (shown by arrows) and attrited incisors (shown by arrowheads)

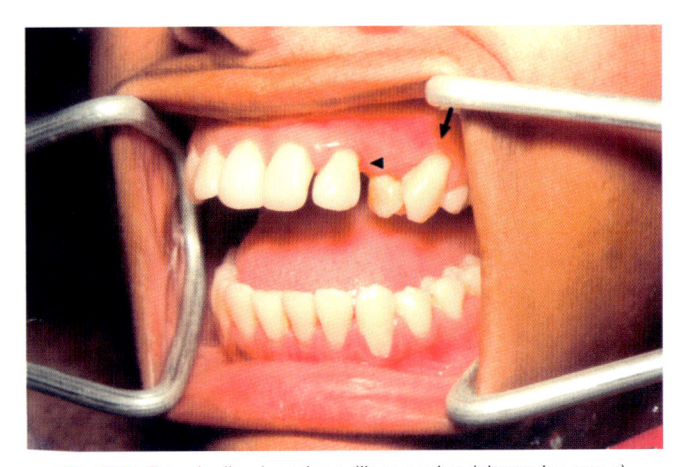

Fig. 7.8: Ectopically placed maxillary canine (shown by arrow) and premolar (shown by arrowhead)

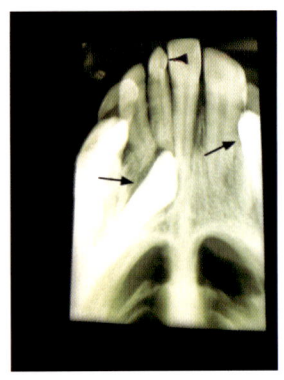

Fig. 7.9: Occlusal X-ray showing bilateral impacted canines (shown by arrows) and peg shaped lateral incisor (shown by arrowhead)

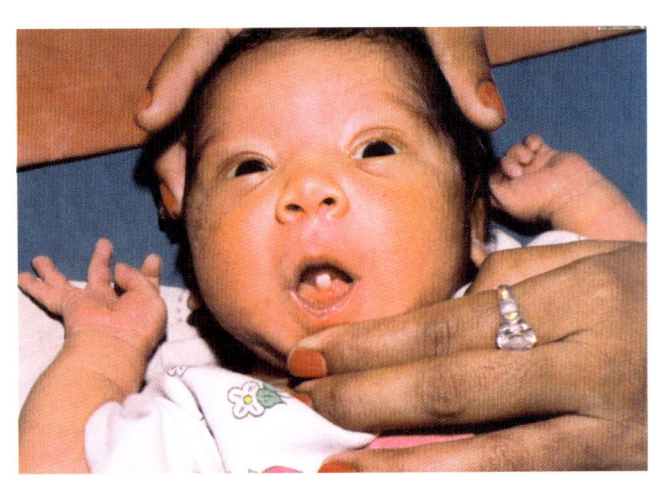

Fig. 7.6: Natal mandibular incisor

Developmental Disorders Affecting Oral and Para Oral Structures

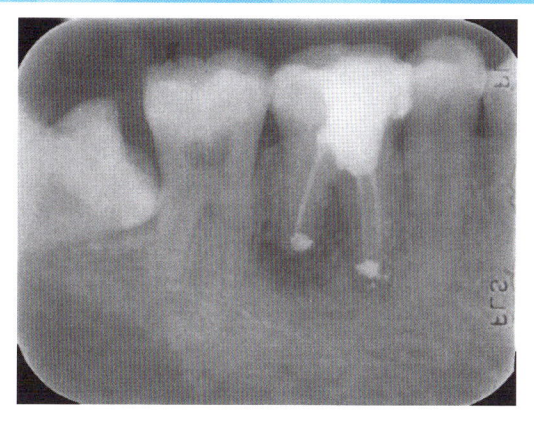

Fig. 7.10: Impacted mandibular third molar and replanted first molar with apical seal done with silver amalgam

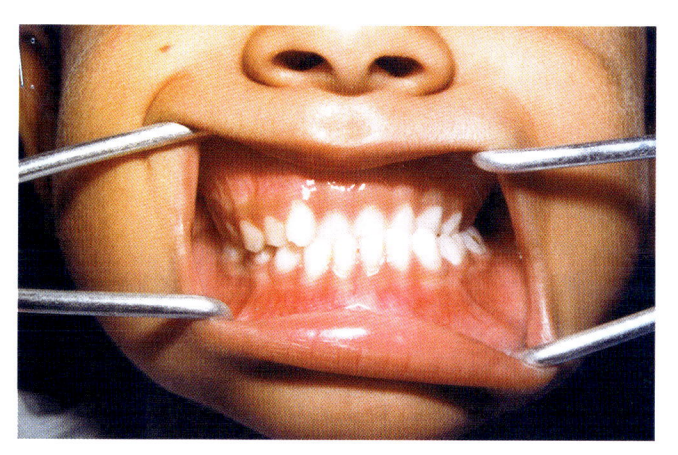

Fig. 7.11: Deciduous teeth in cross bite (maxillary incisors are placed lingually to mandibular incisors)

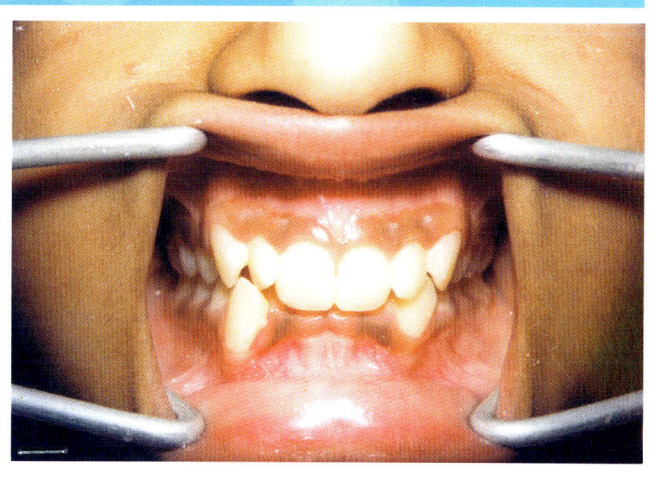

Fig. 7.12: Centpercent deep overbite, maxillary incisors completely covering crowns of mandibular incisors

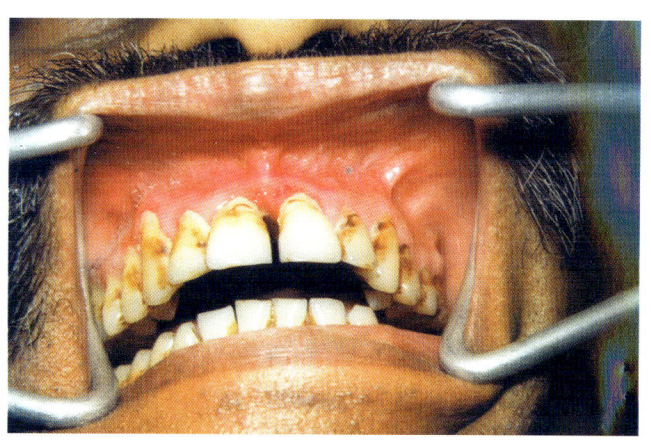

Fig. 7.13: Diastema with injured interdental gingival papilla and calculus, plaque and materia alba on teeth

Cross Bite

Normally maxillary anterior teeth are placed labially to the mandibular anterior teeth. When the maxillary anterior teeth are placed lingually they are called in cross bite (Fig. 7.11).

Deep Overbite

On occluding the teeth normally maxillary anterior teeth vertically cover the mandibular anterior teeth by 1 to 2 mm. When maxillary teeth completely cover the crowns of mandibular teeth it is called cent percent deep bite (Fig. 7.12). When half crowns are covered it is called fifty percent deep bite.

Diastema

Abnormal spacing between the two adjacent teeth in the same arch is called diastema. Due to diastema interdental gingival papilla is prone to trauma (Fig. 7.13).

DEVELOPMENTAL DISORDERS OF THE JAWS

Agnathia

Agnathia is a rare congenital anomaly characterized by the absence of maxilla or mandible. In this condition usually a part of jaw is missing. In mandible either ramus or condyle or one side of mandible may be missing. Likewise in maxilla one maxillary process or premaxilla may be missing.

Micrognathia

The term micrognathia means a small jaw, it can affect either the maxilla or mandible. Micrognathia is of congenital or acquired type. Acquired type of micrognathia is caused due to ankylosis or injury in the area of temporomandibular joint and trauma and infection of the middle ear.

Congenital micrognathia is seen in congenital heart disease and Pierre-Robin syndrome. Micrognathia of maxilla is due to deficiency in premaxillary region; characterized by retracted middle third of the face. The patient with mandibular micrognathia shows retrusion of chin, in which the condyle is placed posteriorly in relation to the skull.

Macrognathia

Macrognathia refers to the condition in which the jaws becomes abnormally large. It may involve both upper and lower jaws but usually the mandible is affected. Macrognathia may be hereditary or associated with other conditions like Paget's disease, acromegaly, pituitary gigantism and *leontiasis ossea*.

Facial Hemiatrophy

In facial hemiatrophy there is progressive atrophy of one side of the face. The defect starts in first or second decade of life and appears as a white line or furrow which gradually progresses into atrophy of skin, muscles and bone. There is reduced growth of jaw on affected side and eruption of teeth is also delayed. Facial hemiatrophy may be caused by trauma, infection, trigeminal neuritis and malfunction of the cervical sympathetic nervous system.

Facial Hemihypertrophy

Facial hemihypertrophy is a condition that exhibits enlargement of one side of face and related structures like bone of maxilla and mandible, teeth and tongue. It may be caused by chromosomal abnormalities, hormonal imbalance, alteration in the intrauterine life, incomplete twinning and vascular and neural abnormalities. The oral manifestations of facial hemihypertrophy are increase in the size of crown and root of teeth and increase in their rate of development. The tongue on the side of hypertrophy becomes larger.

DEVELOPMENTAL DISORDERS OF THE TONGUE

Microglossia

Microglossia is a rare developmental anomaly characterized by the presence of small tongue.

Macroglossia

Macroglossia refers to enlargement of the tongue. It may be congenital or secondary. In congenital macroglossia, there is over development of tongue musculature whereas secondary macroglossia occurs due to various factors like Hurler's syndrome, hemangioma, lymphangioma, neurofibromatosis, cretinism and acromegaly. Macroglossia produces displacement of teeth and leads to malocclusion.

Ankyloglossia (Tongue Tie)

Ankyloglossia is a partial or complete fusion of the tongue to the floor of the mouth. It is due to the presence of abnormally short lingual frenum that limits the movement of the tongue or when the frenum is attached near to the tip of the tongue. It causes difficulty in speech and can be treated surgically.

Median Rhomboid Glossitis

It is a congenital anomaly of the tongue, characterized by red, smooth and slightly raised patch of papillae-free mucosa located behind the circumvallate papillae. It is caused by disturbance in the embryonic development of the tongue and is also associated with chronic candidal infection.

Fissured or Scrotal Tongue

It is a painless condition of tongue characterized by presence of numerous grooves on the dorsal surface. It is mostly seen in the patients older than 50 years of age, and may be caused by genetic defects, chronic trauma or vitamin deficiency (Fig. 7.14).

There may be pain or irritation due to accumulation of food debris in the grooves.

Cleft or Bifid Tongue

Cleft or bifid tongue is a rare congenital anomaly in which tongue is divided in the midline for a greater or lesser distance. It occurs due to failure of union between the two lateral lingual swellings during early development of tongue. It is found in oral-facial digital syndrome and Meckel's syndrome.

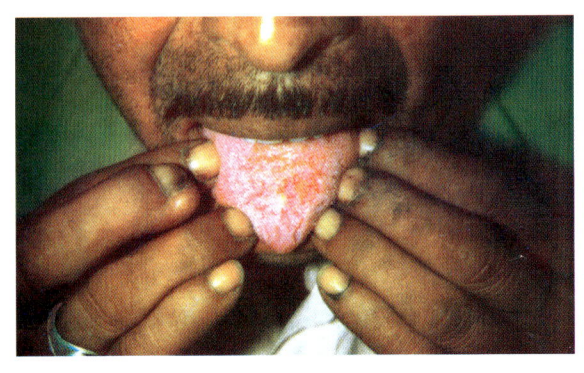

Fig. 7.14: Fissured tongue (Scrotal tongue)

Lingual Thyroid Nodule

The lingual thyroid nodule is an anomalous condition in which a portion of the thyroid gland persists within the tongue. It occurs due to failure of thyroid anlage to migrate at its normal position during development. It appears as a nodular mass near the base of the tongue causing dysphonia, dysphagia and hemorrhage with pain.

DEVELOPMENTAL DISORDERS OF LIPS AND PALATE

Cleft Palate

Cleft palate is a congenital anomaly caused due to disturbance in the fusion of embryonic palatal shelves. The cleft may involve both hard and soft palates. The causes of cleft palate may be as follows:
1. Hereditary factors
2. Nutritional deficiency during pregnancy
3. Inadequate vascular supply
4. Lack of developmental forces
5. Steroid therapy during pregnancy
6. Infections

Cleft palate represents a fissure in the roof of the palate which opens in the nasal cavity. The patient has difficulty in eating and drinking due to regurgitation of food and liquid through the nose. Cleft palate can be treated by surgical procedure which is carried out at the age of 18 months (Figs 7.15 and 7.16).

Cleft Lip

It is a congenital facial abnormality usually of upper lip. It is caused due to failure of union of medial and lateral nasal prominences and maxillary process. Cleft lip can be classified as follows:
a. Unilateral incomplete cleft lip
b. Unilateral complete cleft lip
c. Bilateral incomplete cleft lip
d. Bilateral complete cleft lip

The incomplete cleft extends for a short distance towards the nostril whereas, the complete cleft extends into the nostrils and commonly involves the palate (Fig. 7.16).

Congenital Lip Pits

Congenital lip pits are depressions, usually placed bilateral and symmetrical on the vermilion surface of the lower lip. It is caused by failure of union of the embryonic lateral sulci of the lip or by notching of the lip at an early stage of development.

Double Lip

Double lip is characterized by an excess fold of tissue on the inner aspect of the lip. It usually occurs on the upper lip. It may be the manifestation of Ascher's syndrome.

Cheilitis Glandularis

It is a developmental anomaly characterized by enlargement of the lower lip. Due to hereditary factors, exposure to sun, and dust and use of tobacco; the labial salivary glands become enlarged and nodular with dilation and inflammation of the orifices of the secretory ducts. This causes swelling, ulceration, enlargement and aversion of the lower lip.

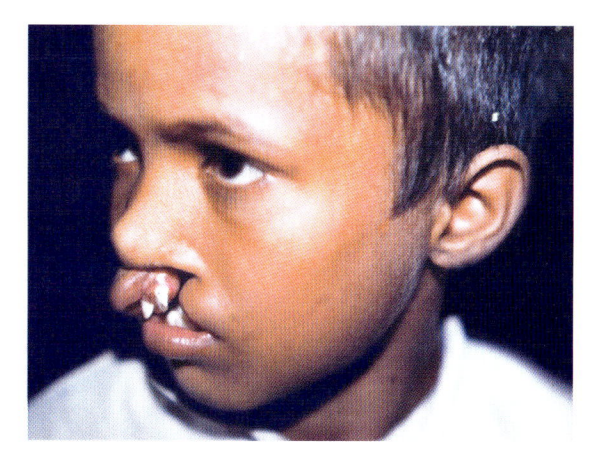

Fig. 7.15: Unilateral complete cleft of lip, alveolus and palate (*Courtesy* Dr S C Pandey, Lucknow)

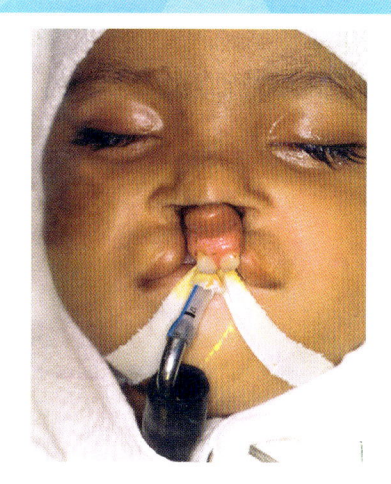

Fig. 7.16: Bilateral complete cleft of lip, alveolus and palate separating out premaxilla with two deciduous central incisor (preoperative photograph) (*Courtesy* Dr SC Pandey, Lucknow)

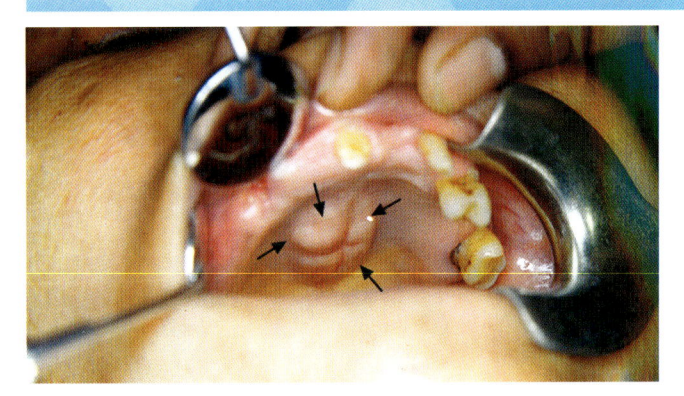

Fig. 7.17: Torus palatinus, (shown by arrows) severely attrited teeth and partial anodontia

Torus Palatinus

Torus palatinus is a bony enlargement (hyperostosis) occurring in the midline of the hard palate. (Fig. 7.17)

DEVELOPMENTAL DISORDERS OF THE ORAL MUCOSA

Fordyce's Granules (Spots)

Fordyce's granules is a developmental anomaly marked by the presence of numerous small, slightly raised, yellowish-white granules on the mucosa of the cheeks and inner surface of lips. They appear more in males, usually during puberty and increase in number with age.

Histologically they are identical to sebaceous glands. (Fig. 7.18).

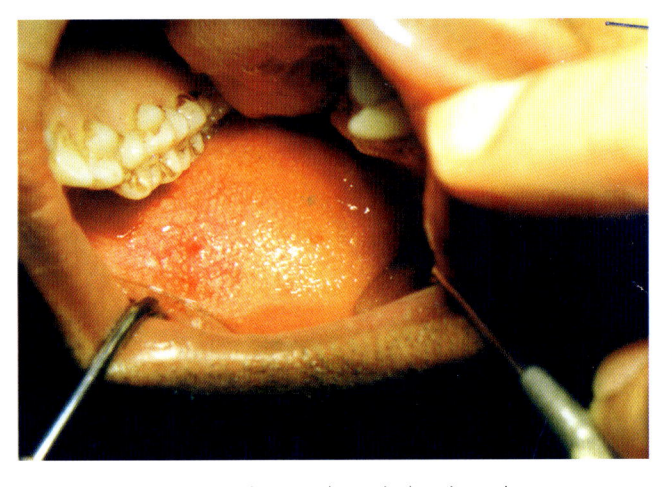

Fig. 7.18: Fordyce's spots (granules) on buccal mucosa

White Sponge Nevus

It is an autosomal dominant condition that usually affects only the oral mucosa. It is characterized by white, raised and spongy patches. White sponge nevus may either be confined to small area or extends to larger area. The affected mucosa is white or gray, folded, thickened and spongy.

Focal Epithelial Hyperplasia

Focal epithelial hyperplasia is characterized by numerous nodular lesions, with a sessile base distributed throughout the oral mucosa. It occurs most commonly on the lower lip and is absent in palate and floor of mouth. The condition usually occurs in children between 3 to 18 years of age, and regresses itself in 4 to 6 months.

Peutz-Jegher's Syndrome (Hereditary Intestinal Polyposis with Melanin Syndrome)

Peutz-Jegher's syndrome is characterized by numerous, focal, melanotic spots on the lips and oral mucosa. Pigmentation is also seen around the mouth which fades away after the puberty. This syndrome is also associated with multiple intestinal polyps which sometimes get transformed into malignancy. Peutz-Jegher's syndrome is an autosomal dominant inheritance, caused by mutation in genes.

Epidermolysis Bullosa Dystrophica

It is an inherited chronic non-inflammatory disease which involves skin and oral cavity.

The condition is characterized by the formation of bullae and erosion due to slight trauma. Oral mucosa appears gray, smooth, thick and elastic. There is immobility of the lips and microstomia because the lingual and buccal sulci get closed due to scarring. It may get transformed into oral carcinoma and thus can be fatal.

Fibromatosis Gingivae (Hereditary Gingival Fibromatosis, Elephantosis Gingivae, Congenital Macrogingival)

Fibromatosis gingivae is a generalized diffused overgrowth of the gingival tissues due to fibrous hyperplasia. It appears as a dense diffuse, smooth or nodular overgrowth of the gingival tissues of one or both arches at the age of eruption of incisors.

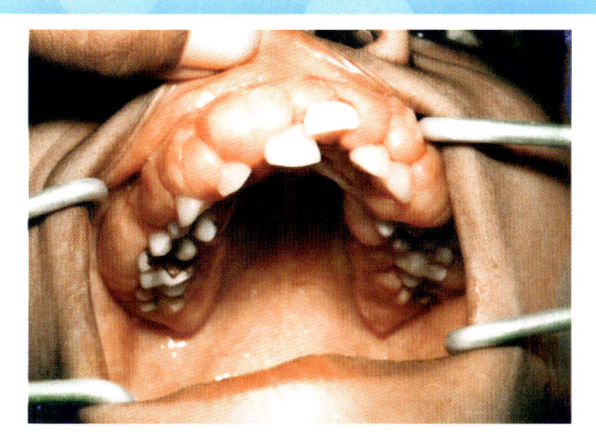

Fig. 7.19: Fibromatosis gingivae (occlusal view)

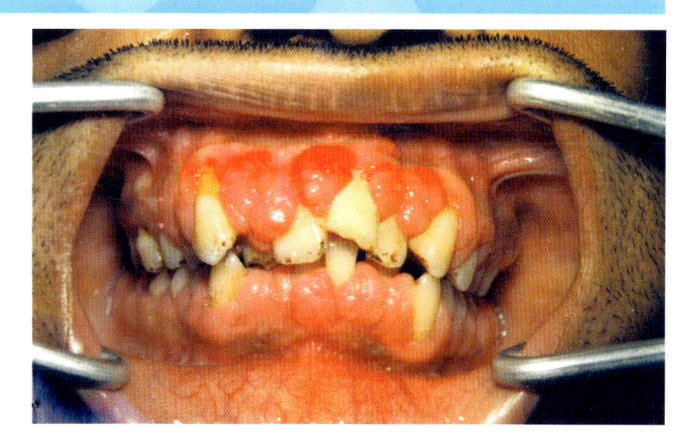

Fig. 7.20: Fibromatosis gingivae (facial view)

Treatment

Surgical removal of the excessive hyperplastic tissue. Repeated reappearance has been observed which stops after the extraction of the involved teeth (Figs 7.19 and 7.20).

BIBLIOGRAPHY

1. Baughman RA, Heidrich PD Jr. The oral hair: An extremely rare phenomenon. Oral Surg 1980;49:530.
2. Buchner A, Hansen LS. Lymphoepithelial cysts of the oral cavity. Oral Surg 1980;50:441.
3. Connor MS. Anterior lingual mandibular bone concavity. Oral Surg 1979;48:413.
4. Correll RW, Jensen JL, Rhyne RR. Lingual cortical mandibular defects. Oral Surg 1980;50:287.
5. Eveson JW, Lucas RB. Angiolymphoid hyperplasia with eosinophilia. J Oral Path 1979;8:103.
6. Graber, LW: Congenital absence of teeth: a review with emphasis on inheritance patterns. J Am Dent Assoc 1978;96:266.
7. Melnick M, Eastman JR, Goldblatt LI, Michaud M, Bixler D. Dentin dysplasia, type II: A rare autosomal dominant disorder. Oral Surg 1977;44:592.

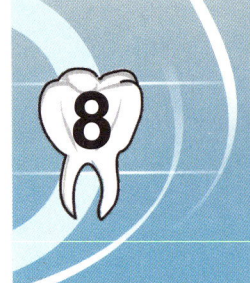

Diseases of Teeth and Supporting Tissues

The common diseases that affect the teeth and supporting tissues (periodontium and gingiva) are dental caries, gingivitis and periodontitis. These are the most prevalent diseases in the world. The prevalence of these diseases has greatly increased in modern times probably because of changes in dietary habits. These diseases may be caused by local factors or systemic factors.

DENTAL CARIES

Mosby's dental dictionary has defined caries as "an infectious disease with progressive destruction of tooth substance, beginning on the external surface by demineralization of enamel or exposed cementum". Taber's Medical dictionary has defined dental caries as progressive decalcification of enamel and dentin of a tooth'. Stedman's Medical dictionary has defined dental caries as a localized, progressively destructive disease of teeth, which starts at the external surface with the apparent dissolution of inorganic components by organic acids. In other words dental caries is an infectious microbiologic disease of the teeth characterized by localized demineralization of the inorganic portion and destruction of the organic portion of the teeth.

Etiology of Dental Caries

Number of theories has been proposed to explain the etiology of dental caries, which are as follows:
a. Acidogenic theory
b. Proteolytic theory
c. Sucrose chelation theory
d. Autoimmune theory
e. Proteolytic chelation theory

Out of these theories, the most accepted one is acidogenic theory which was proposed by WD Miller in the year 1882. According to this theory, dental caries is a chemico-parasitic process which takes place in two stages. In primary stage, bacteria present in the plaque produce acids by fermentation of carbohydrates. In second stage, this acid decalcifies the enamel and dentin and causes their destruction, leading to caries formation.

The process of tooth destruction by caries is influenced by following four factors:
a. Carbohydrates
b. Microorganisms
c. Dental Plaque
d. Acids

Types and Classification of Dental Caries

Pit and Fissure Caries

Pit and fissure caries develops in the occlusal surfaces of molars and premolars, lingual surfaces of maxillary anterior teeth and buccal and lingual surfaces of molars.

Smooth Surface Caries (Proximal Caries)

Smooth surface caries originate on the smooth surfaces of teeth. It is usually seen in the proximal surface of the teeth below the contact-point, which are not accessible to the toothbrush and cleansing effect of tongue, buccal mucosa and fibrous food.

Root Caries (Senile Caries)

These carious lesions are located on the cementum of the exposed root surfaces of the teeth. As this area is not properly accessible to oral hygiene measures, the rough surface of the cementum influence the plaque accumulation, which initiates the caries process. These caries are associated with aging, so are called "senile caries".

Rampant Caries

Rampant caries are of sudden onset, wide spread, rapidly burrowing, which involves multiple surfaces in multiple number of teeth at the same time. In rampant caries involvements of new caries lesions is 10 or more on healthy teeth surfaces per year. These caries involve the pulp within a short span of time and affect those surfaces of teeth which are considered immune to the dental caries. It occurs both in adults and children.

Nursing Bottle Rampant Caries

Nursing bottle caries is a rampant type of caries that affects the deciduous dentition. It commonly involves the maxillary incisors, followed by first molars and then canines. These caries occur in those children, who are fed milk or other form of carbohydrates like fruit juice, honey etc. by a nursing bottle for a longer duration, specially at the bed time or other than normal feeding time (Fig. 8.1).

Recurrent Caries

Recurrent caries occurs around the margin of the restoration. It is due to inadequate extension of the restoration and poor adaptability of the restorative material to the cavity, which influence the retention and entrance of the carbohydrates and bacteria, between the filling and the tooth structure.

Arrested Caries

In arrested dental caries, the carious lesion after initiation and destruction of some tooth surface, stop progressing and becomes inactive as the area becomes self cleansing. The lesion appears hard, black or brownish in color. It occurs in both deciduous and permanent dentition. The arrested caries occurs on occlusal surfaces having large open cavity which does not retain food. The open cavity gets exposed to cleansing action of saliva and tooth brushing and gradually burnished until it takes a polished and shiny surface.

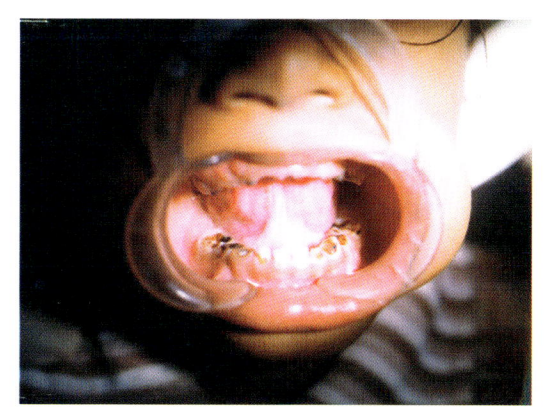

Fig 8.1: Nursing bottle rampant caries involving all deciduous teeth except mandibular central incisors. (*Courtesy* Dr VK Gopinath, Chennai)

Chronic Caries

Chronic dental caries progresses at a slower rate and involves the pulp much later, as the pulp gets enough time to recede and be protected by reparative dentin. Usually the lesions of chronic dental caries are very large, and wide open therefore, less food is retained and the acids produced by the microorganisms are neutralized by saliva. It commonly occurs in adults.

Radiation Caries

Radiation caries is a type of acute and rampant caries induced by radiation therapy used in the treatment of oral and maxillofacial malignancies. It occurs mostly on the cervical regions of the teeth, and rarely on the incisal edges and on the tips of the cusp. It may be due to reduction in salivary secretion which is a side effect of radiotherapy.

DISCOLORATION OF TEETH

Discoloration of teeth can be divided into extrinsic and intrinsic discoloration.

Extrinsic Discoloration

Extrinsic discoloration is found on the outer surface of the teeth. It is caused due to surface staining by tobacco, tea, chromogenic bacteria and chemical substances such as strong iodine and chlorhexidine mouthwashes and silver nitrate.

Intrinsic Discoloration

Intrinsic discoloration of teeth is due to deposition of various substances within the enamel and dentin. It may be due to local or systemic factors or drug induced.

Local Causes

i. Pulp hemorrhage due to trauma
ii. Hemorrhage during pulp extirpation
iii. Medicaments
iv. Necrosis of pulp tissue
v. Restorative material
vi. Internal resorption

Systemic Causes

i. Hereditary opalescent dentin (violet or bluish purple)
ii. Congenital porphyria (red or purple)
iii. Endemic fluorosis (mottled brown)
iv. Jaundice (yellow or brown)
v. Erythroblastosis fetalis (grayish brown)

Drug Induced

Tetracycline (yellow to gray or brown).

Common Internal Discolorations

The most common cause of internal tooth discoloration is decomposition of traumatized and necrosed pulp. Decomposition of necrosed pulp results in formation of color-producing compounds which enter the dentinal tubules and cause discoloration. Traumatic injury to the tooth results in rupture of blood vessels in the pulp due to which blood diffuses into the dentinal tubules and gives pinkish brown color to the tooth.

Discoloration of tooth may also occur due to hemorrhage during extirpation of pulp. Tetracycline discoloration is the permanent discoloration of dentin but it can be removed by bleaching. Administration of tetracycline during dentin formation forms chelate compounds with organic and inorganic substances of the teeth. This compound is very stable and gives the teeth gray-brown to dark-brown color.

Treatment of Discolored Tooth

The extrinsic stains of tobacco, chemical substances and calculus can be removed by scaling and polishing. The intrinsic discoloration of teeth can be removed by the process of bleaching. Bleaching of tooth can be done by superoxol and sodium perborate.

Bleaching of discolored teeth due to endemic fluorosis and tetracycline is done by the solution of anesthetic ether, hydrochloric acid and superoxol.

ABRASION OF THE TEETH

Abrasion is the grinding or wearing away of the teeth by a mechanical process. It usually occurs on enamel and cementum and dentin of an exposed root on the buccal surface. The most commonly affected teeth are the maxillary anterior teeth and first molars and maxillary and mandibular premolars. Abrasion causes opening-up of the dentinal tubules, due to which patient complains of sensitivity to hot and cold. On anterior teeth abrasion produces saucer shaped depression (Figs 8.2 and 8.3).

Abrasion may appear as a V-shaped, polished furrow at the cementoenamel junction with gingival recession.

Etiology of Abrasion

The following are the causes of abrasion:
a. Excessive use of abrasive containing dentrifice.

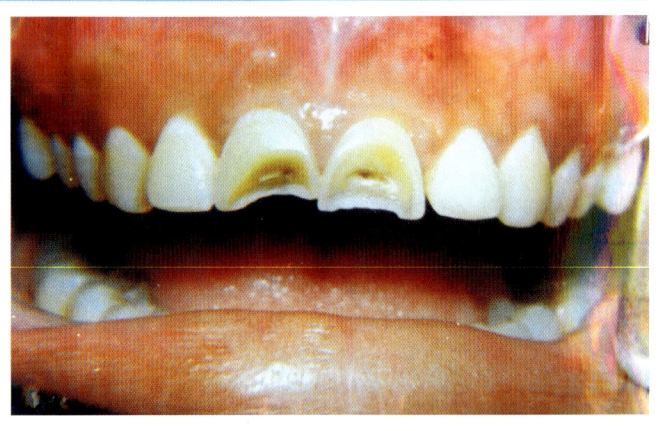

Fig. 8.2: Tooth powder abrasion of maxillary central incisors

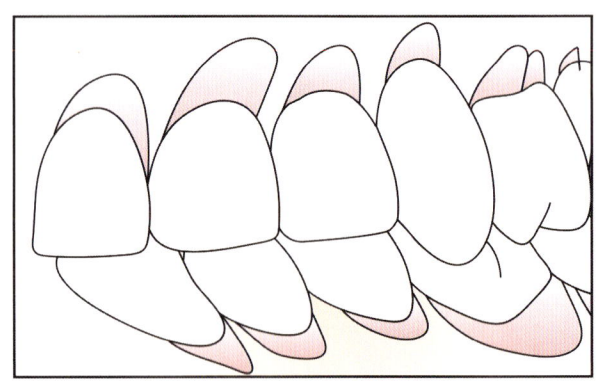

Fig. 8.3: Cervical abrasion of cementum and dentin in exposed root portion due to wrong tooth brushing

b. Faulty tooth brushing techniques (Brushing strokes in horizontal direction rather than vertical direction).
c. Improper use of dental floss and tooth picks.
d. Habitual opening of bobby pins and holding of nails and pins between the teeth results in notching of the incisal edges.
e. Pipe smoking.

ATTRITION OF THE TEETH

Attrition is the loss of tooth substance resulting from friction caused by tooth-to-tooth contact. Attrition occurs on the incisal, occlusal and proximal surfaces of the teeth. Attrition is associated with the process of aging, as the person becomes older, he or she exhibits more attrition as compared to young individuals. The severity and rate of attrition depends upon the quality of diet, habits like bruxism and

Diseases of Teeth and Supporting Tissues

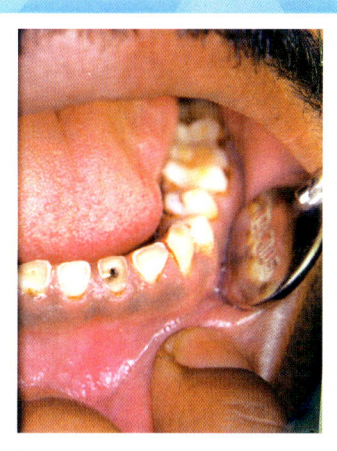

Fig. 8.4: Attrition of mandibular teeth

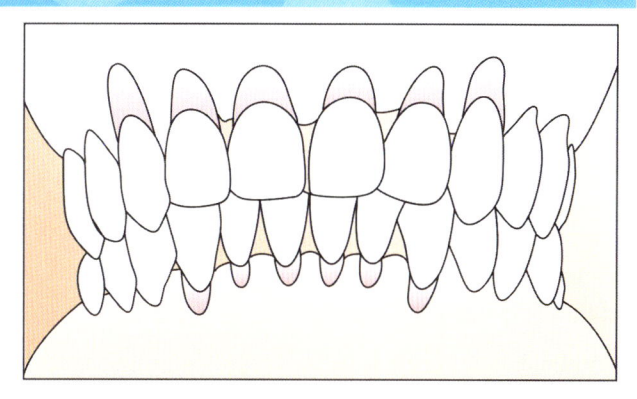

Fig. 8.5: Generalized erosion on the surface of teeth

tobacco chewing, and force and strength of masticatory muscles. In case of advanced attrition there is flattening of incisal and occlusal surfaces of the teeth which results in reduction in the cusp height. (Fig. 8.4)

EROSION OF THE TEETH

Erosion refers to chemical destruction of the tooth substance, without the involvement of any bacterial process. Erosion occurs frequently on the gingival third of labial or buccal surfaces of teeth. Sometimes there may be generalized erosion which may involve all surfaces of the teeth. Erosion occurs as a result of decalcification of teeth, and this decalcification is because of some acids which come either from the internal or external sources. Gastric hydrochloric acid is the important internal source of acid which causes erosion of the teeth. The erosion of teeth due to gastric acid is found commonly in patients of bulimia nervosa, which is characterized by induced chronic vomiting. Due to chronic vomiting, there is erosion of the lingual surface of maxillary teeth.

External sources of acids come from consumption of acidic cold drinks, citrus fruits and acidic fruit juices. The workers in various industries where acid is utilized (e.g. galvanizing factories, ammunition factories or battery manufacturing factories) exhibit dental erosion.

Erosion appears as a shallow, polished depressions on the enamel surface and unpolished depressions on the surface of cementum and dentin (Fig. 8.5).

Abfraction

Abfraction are very thin wedge shaped defects due to minute cracks in the cervical region of the tooth. These are due to tensile stress concentration in the cervical area of the crown

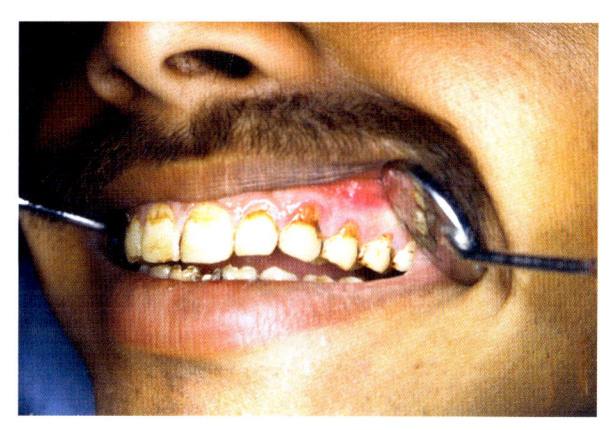

Fig. 8.6: Abfraction in the maxillary teeth. In the canine abfraction has been superimposed by caries

as a result of occlusal forces in some other area of the same tooth (Fig. 8.6).

GINGIVITIS AND GINGIVAL ABSCESS

Gingivitis refers to inflammation of the gingiva. It is the most common gingival disease. According to severity and duration of inflammation, gingivitis can be classified into acute, sub-acute and chronic gingivitis.

Etiological Factors

Local Factors

Local factors are as follows:
a. Local irritants like plaque and calculus.
b. Impaction of food due to improper proximal contacts.
c. Faulty oral hygiene measures.
d. Malposed teeth which are not accessible to cleansing action of toothbrush.
e. Overhanging margins of restorations.
f. Overcontoured crowns.

g. Mouth breathing habits which cause drying of gingival surface.
h. Use of tobacco.
i. Ill-fitting clasp of removable partial dentures or orthodontic appliances.
j. Local oral infections.
k. Use of drugs or chemicals.

Systemic Factors

Systemic factors are as follows:
a. Nutritional deficiency diseases such as scurvy.
b. Hormonal changes during pregnancy, puberty and menopause.
c. Diabetes and endocrine dysfunctions.
d. Immunological disorders.
e. Hematological disorders such as leukemia.
f. Allergy.
g. Metal intoxications.
h. Psychosomatic disorders.

Clinical Features

a. In inflammation the normal "coral pink" color of gingiva changes into red or bluish red.
b. Bleeding occurs from gingival sulcus even on mild provocation as during tooth brushing or probing.
c. The surface of gingiva becomes smooth and shiny with loss of stippling.
d. There is increase in the rate of production of gingival fluid.
e. Edematous and fibrotic changes appear in gingiva due to inflammation. (Fig. 8.7 to 8.10)

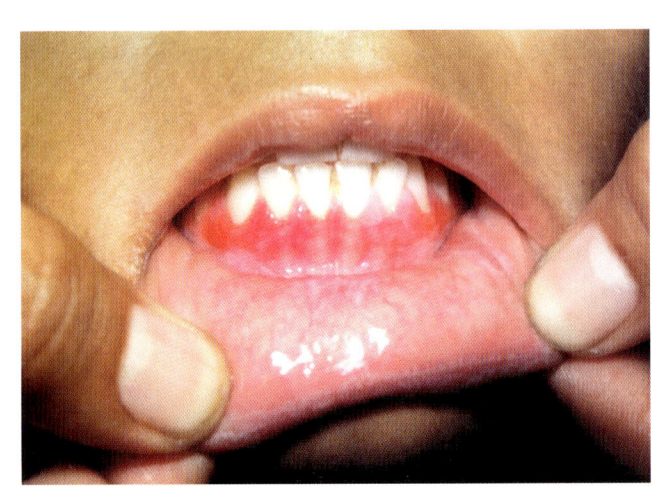

Fig. 8.7: Mild gingivitis

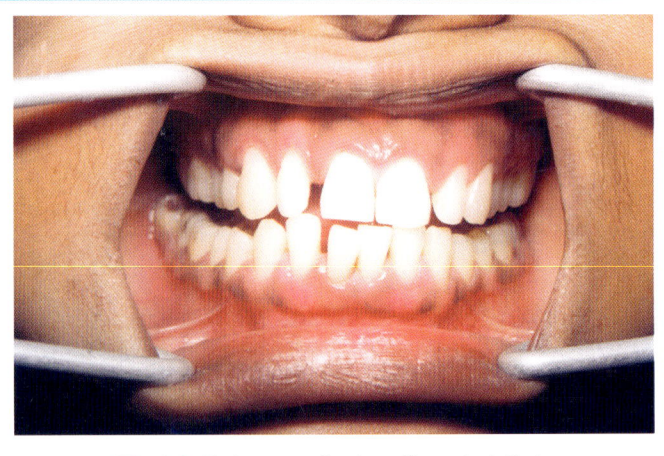

Fig. 8.8: Early generalized papillary gingivitis in mandibular anterior teeth

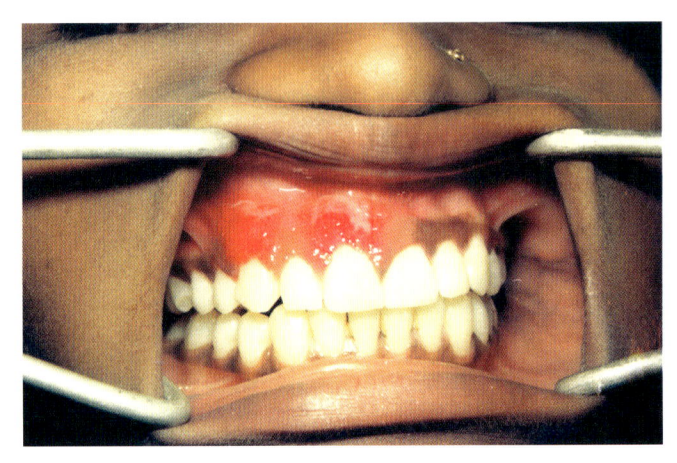

Fig. 8.9: Desquamative gingivitis

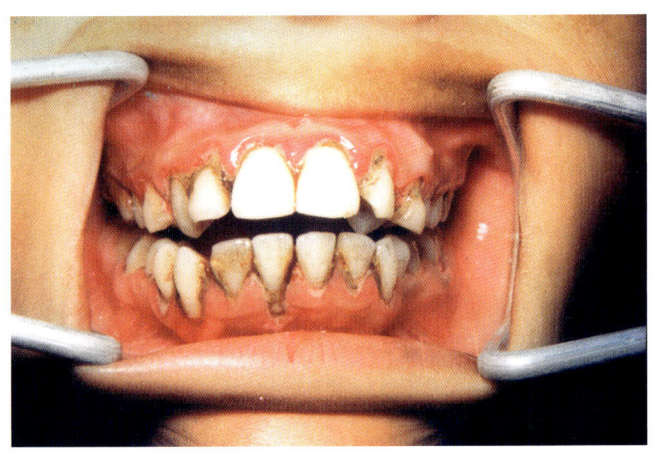

Fig. 8.10: Gingivitis due to calculus

Treatment

Treatment of gingivitis starts with removal and control of plaque. The teeth are scaled and cleaned to remove all the deposits and are polished with a fine pumice. Polishing smoothens the surface of the tooth and resists the formation of calculus. Other sources of local irritation should also be eliminated. Oral irrigation or rinsing by 0.12 to 0.2% chlorhexidine daily is most effective in treatment of gingivitis.

GINGIVAL ENLARGEMENT

Gingival enlargement refers to overgrowth of the gingival tissues. Gingival enlargement can be classified as follows:
1. Inflammatory gingival enlargement.
2. Fibrotic gingival enlargement (drug induced).
3. Gingival enlargement associated with systemic conditions.

Inflammatory Gingival Enlargement

Inflammatory gingival enlargement starts as a slight ballooning of interdental papilla or marginal gingiva which gradually increases in size and covers a part of the crown. The gingiva appears smooth, shiny and edematous which bleeds spontaneously (Fig. 8.11).

Inflammatory gingival enlargement is caused due to prolonged exposure to dental plaque. Factors responsible for plaque accumulation are poor oral hygiene, cervical caries, food impaction, malposed teeth, traumatogenic teeth, faulty restorations, irritation from clasp of removable partial denture, orthodontic appliances and mouth breathing habits (Fig. 8.12).

Fibrotic Gingival Enlargement (Drug-induced)

It is non-inflammatory type of gingival enlargement which is mostly associated with administration of various drugs

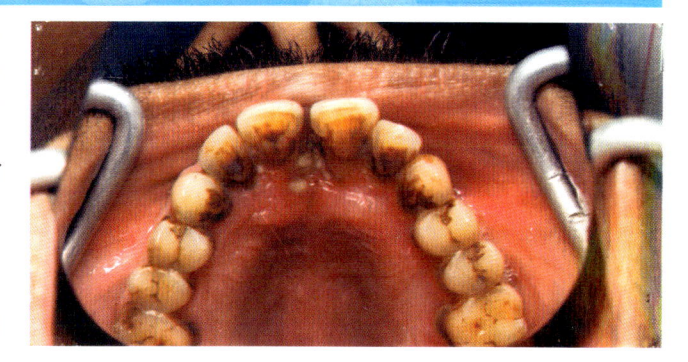

Fig. 8.12: Infected traumatic ulcers of incisive palatal papilla due to traumatogenic mandibular incisors

like phenytoin, nifedipine and cyclosporine. Enlargement of gingiva induced by phenytoin, an anticonvulsant drug, occurs in 40 to 50% of the patients who use the drug for more than 3 months. The lesion starts as a bead like enlargement of gingival margin and interdental papillae which gradually covers the portion of the crown of the teeth. The lesion is mulberry shaped, firm and resilient with no tendency of bleeding.

Cyclosporine is an immunosuppressive agent used in the treatment of autoimmune disease and is given after organ transplantation. The dosage of more than 500 mg per day induces gingival overgrowth and affects more than 30% of the patients receiving the drug. The enlarged gingiva appears pink, dense, resilient with a little bleeding tendency.

Nifedipine is a calcium channel blocker and the dose of more than 48 mg per day may produce gingival hyperplasia in about 20 percent of the patients receiving the drug. These drugs alone do not cause gingival enlargement, local irritation from plaque and calculus or faulty restorations and appliances contribute in the enlargement of gingiva.

Treatment of these drug-induced gingival hyperplasia includes proper oral hygiene measures, elimination of local gingival irritants and discontinuation of the drug. Gingivectomy may be carried out to reduce the tissue bulk.

Gingival Enlargement Associated with Systemic Conditions

Gingival enlargement may occur in systemic conditions like pregnancy, puberty, and vitamin C deficiency.

Enlargement in Pregnancy

In pregnancy, gingival enlargement may be either marginal or generalized. The hormonal changes during pregnancy influence the aggravation of previous inflammation caused from local irritation. The enlarged gingiva appears bright

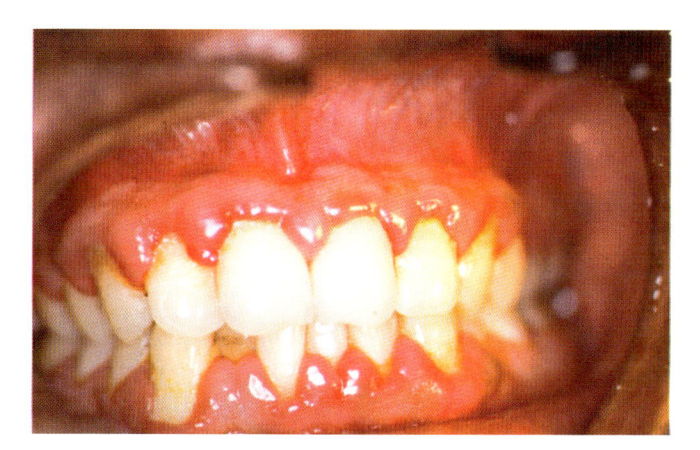

Fig. 8.11: Gingival enlargment of interdental papillae

red, soft and friable with smooth-shiny surface. Gingival enlargement during pregnancy can be prevented by the removal of local irritants and maintenance of proper oral hygiene.

Enlargement in Puberty (Puberty Gingivitis)

Enlargement of gingiva may be seen in both male and female adolescents during puberty. The enlargement is marginal and interdental and is mainly confined to facial gingiva. Pubertal gingival enlargement occurs due to massive recurrence of the inflammatory gingiva in presence of local irritants, which reduces itself after puberty but does not disappear until local irritants are removed. (Fig. 8.13)

Enlargement in Nutritional Deficiency

Enlargement of gingiva in nutritional deficiency is mainly due to deficiency of vitamin C. Deficiency of vitamin C, directly itself does not cause enlargement of gingiva, but it causes hemorrhage, degeneration and edema of the gingival connective tissue which exaggerate the inflammation. Inflammation along with scurvy produces massive gingival enlargement. The gingiva appears bluish red, soft and friable with smooth-shiny surface. Hemorrhage also occurs on slight provocation like palpating with the side of the probe.

Systemic diseases like leukemia and Wegener's granulomatosis result in gingival enlargement. In leukemia, the gingiva appears bluish red with shiny surface. The enlargement may be diffused or marginal, localized or generalized. Gingiva is of firm consistency but bleeds spontaneously or on slight provocation. Wegener's granulomatosis and sarcoidosis are the granulomatous diseases characterized by oral mucosal ulceration, red and smooth gingival enlargement, tooth mobility and exfoliation of teeth.

PERIODONTITIS

Periodontitis refers to inflammation of the periodontium. When inflammation extends from marginal gingiva to the supported periodontium there is transition from gingivitis to periodontitis, microbial plaque, calculus, food impaction and overhanging margins of restorations are the most important factors in the development of periodontal diseases. Periodontitis begins as a simple marginal gingivitis. If the gingivitis is not treated, the gingiva becomes more inflamed and swollen with ulceration in subcular epithelium. There is formation of deep periodontal pocket, which favours the growth and multiplication of various microorganisms. These microorganisms contribute in osteoclastic activity of the alveolar bone.

In severe periodontitis, gingiva appears enlarged and edematous and teeth become mobile. The patient complains of a bad taste, bleeding gums and hypersensitivity of teeth due to exposure of cementum.

Treatment

Treatment involves removal of local irritants by scaling and curettage, elimination of pockets by gingivectomy, and recontouring the supporting tissues to normal physiologic architecture by periodontal surgery.

JUVENILE PERIODONTITIS

Juvenile periodontitis is characterized by rapid destruction of alveolar bone with premature loss of tooth in children and young adults. It occurs in adolescence, between puberty and 20 years of age. In early juvenile periodontitis there is no apparent inflammation but deep periodontal pockets are present. There is mobility and migration of the first molars and the incisors. Root surfaces become sensitive to hot and tactile stimuli. Dull and radiating pain may occur during mastication (Fig. 8.14).

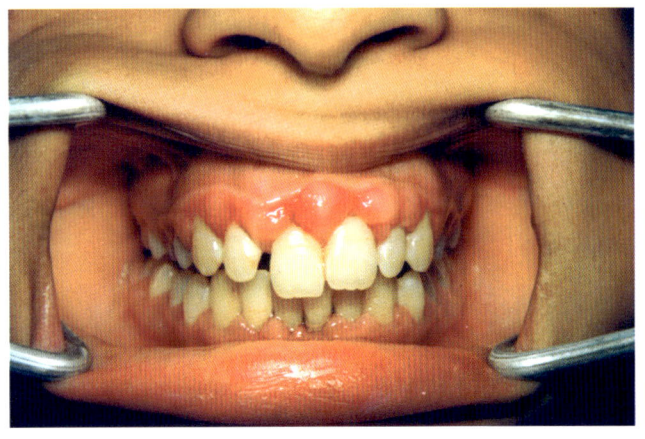

Fig. 8.13: Puberty gingivitis

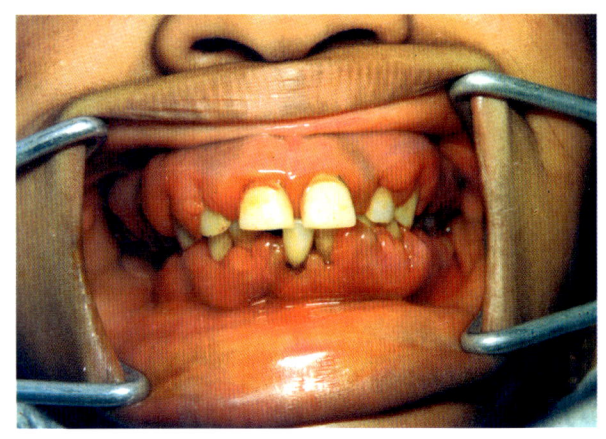

Fig. 8.14: Juvenile periodontitis

Treatment

Treatment of juvenile periodontitis may involve extraction of the affected teeth with very poor prognosis, standard periodontal treatment (Scaling, root planing, curettage and flap surgery), and antibiotic therapy.

BIBLIOGRAPHY

1. Bez C, Demarosi F, Sardella A, et al. GM-CSF mouth rinses in the treatment of severe oral mucositis: A pilot study. Oral Surg Oral Med Oral Pathol Oral Radiol Endod 1999;88:311-5.
2. Danilenko DM. Preclinical and early clinical development of keratinocyte growth factor: An epithelial-specific tissue growth factor. Toxicol Pathol 1999;27:64-71.
3. Enwonwu CO, Falker WA, Idigbe EO, Savage KO. Noma (Cancrum oris) questions and answers. Oral Dis 1999;5:144.
4. Farrell CL, Rex KL, Kaufman SA, et al. Effects of keratinocyte growth factor in the squamous epithelium of the upper aerodigestive tract of normal and irradiated mice. Int J Radiat Biol 1999;75:609-20.
5. Hospers GA, Eisenhauer EA, de Vries EG. The sulfhydryl containing compounds WR-2721 and glutathione as radio-and chemoprotective agents. A review, indications for use and prospects. Br J Cancer 1999;80:629-38.

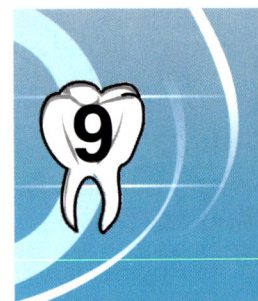

Diseases of the Pulp and Periapical Tissues

INTRODUCTION

The dental pulp is a vascular connective tissue within rigid dentinal walls. It consists of tiny blood vessels, nerves, collagen fibers, undifferentiated mesenchymal cells and cellular elements like fibroblasts and odontoblasts. It forms the primary dentin during the development of tooth, secondary dentin after tooth eruption and reparative dentin in response to any stimuli. Pulp reacts to bacterial infection or to any other stimuli by an inflammatory response which is perceived only as pain. Most of the diseases of pulp are the sequelae of dental caries, but various mechanical, thermal and chemical injuries are also responsible for inflammatory changes in the pulp.

ETIOLOGY OF PULP DISEASES

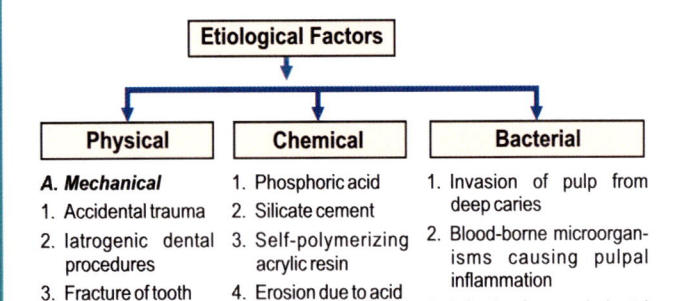

Etiological Factors

Physical

A. Mechanical
1. Accidental trauma
2. Iatrogenic dental procedures
3. Fracture of tooth
4. Pathologic wear (attrition, abrasion)

B. Thermal
1. Heat from cavity preparation
2. Heat conduction through deep filling without base
3. Frictional heat during polishing of the filling

C. Electrical
1. Galvanic current from dissimilar metallic fillings

Chemical
1. Phosphoric acid
2. Silicate cement
3. Self-polymerizing acrylic resin
4. Erosion due to acid

Bacterial
1. Invasion of pulp from deep caries
2. Blood-borne microorganisms causing pulpal inflammation
3. Infection from periodontal ligament space

DISEASES OF THE PULP

Reversible Pulpitis (Pulpal Arterial Hyperemia)

Reversible pulpitis or pulpal arterial hyperemia is a localized mild inflammatory condition of the pulp. It is characterized by sharp pain of short duration associated with thermal changes, especially by cold food and exposure of tooth to cold air and sweets; but usually disappears on the removal of thermal irritant. This condition exists in the tooth with deep carious lesion, inadequately insulated restoration and exposed dentin at the neck of the tooth. The treatment of reversible pulpitis is directed towards the removal of the cause. Early restoration of developing carious lesion, use of cavity varnish or cement base before placing a restorative material and desensitization of cervical region of teeth having gingival recession are recommended to prevent reversible pulpitis.

Acute Irreversible Pulpitis

Irreversible pulpitis is an acute inflammatory condition of the pulp, characterized by severe lancinating longer lasting type of pain in the affected tooth.

Clinical Features

The pain is usually caused by hot or cold stimuli, sweets and packing of food into cavity which persists for a longer duration even after the removal of stimuli. The pain may also increase when the patient is in supine position, which occurs due to changes in intrapulpal pressure.

In acute pulpitis, there is accumulation of inflammatory exudate in the pulp which does not escape from the solid confinement of the dentin due to which there is increase in the intrapulpal pressure, resulting in excruciating pain. The most common cause of irreversible pulpitis is bacterial involvement of pulp through dental caries. The affected tooth discloses a deep cavity extending to the pulp or secondary caries under a filling.

Treatment

Treatment of irreversible pulpitis consists of complete removal of pulp and root canal treatment. In early cases of acute pulpitis, pulpotomy (removal of coronal pulp) and placement of dressing material over the radicular pulp can be done for the survival of the tooth. Extraction can be considered if the tooth cannot be restored.

Chronic Pulpitis

Chronic pulpitis may arise from a dormant acute pulpitis or as a chronic type of disease from onset. Chronic pulpitis is characterized by mild, dull and throbbing pain which mostly occurs at the intervals, rather than continuous. The affected tooth is less sensitive to hot and cold stimuli. Even in the case of chronic pulpitis with large open cavity and exposure of the pulp, there is relatively less pain. Chronic pulpitis is treated by root canal treatment or extraction of the tooth.

Chronic Hyperplastic Pulpitis (Pulp Polyp)

Chronic hyperplastic pulpitis or "pulp polyp" is a chronic pulpal inflammation due to an extensive carious exposure, characterized by proliferation of granulation tissue of the pulp.

Clinical Features

Chronic hyperplastic pulpitis is commonly seen in the teeth of children and young adults. The teeth most commonly involved are the deciduous molars and the first permanent molars. The affected tooth exhibits a large carious lesion, through which a fleshy, reddish pulpal mass protrudes out and fills the entire cavity. The pulp polyp is usually painless but may cause discomfort during mastication due to transmission of pressure to the apical region. The polypoid tissue may bleed easily because of rich vascular supply. Pulp polyp results from slow, progressive carious exposure of a young and resistant pulp subjected to chronic low grade stimulus.

Treatment

Treatment of pulp polyp involves removal of hyperplastic pulpal mass by curettage or excavation, then removal of pulp tissue by root canal treatment followed by restoration of the tooth. The affected tooth that cannot be restored and made servicable should be removed.

Necrosis of the Pulp

Necrosis refers to the death of pulp. Necrosis mostly results from untreated pulpitis, either acute or chronic, but it can also occur after a traumatic injury in which pulp gets destroyed. Necrosis may be partial, involving only the coronal pulp or complete necrosis which involves radicular pulp also. The first indication of the necrosis of the pulp is discoloration of the tooth. Tooth with necrotic pulp usually causes no pain. It may respond to hot stimuli due to presence of vital nerve fibers passing through the adjacent inflamed tissue.

Treatment of pulpal necrosis consists of root canal treatment of the affected tooth.

Internal Resorption

Internal resorption is an idiopathic resorptive process which begins from internal dentinal surface of the teeth. It is caused due to trauma or persistent chronic pulpitis which results in the formation of odontoclasts by activating reserve undifferentiated connective tissue cells of the pulp.

Clinical Features

When the resorption begins in the root, the tooth is asymptomatic. Internal resorption in the crown of the tooth appears as a reddish area called "pink spot" which represents the granulation tissue filling the resorbed dentinal area showing through the remaining overlying tooth substance. If left untreated, internal resorption may lead to perforation of tooth surface, pain and fracture of tooth.

Treatment

If the internal resorption is discovered early before the perforation of root or crown; root canal treatment is the treatment of choice. Root canal is sealed with calcium hydroxide paste and is renewed periodically until the defect is repaired.

Pulp Calcification

In pulp calcification, portion of the pulp tissue is replaced by calcific material. The chief morphologic forms of pulp calcification are localized pulp stones or denticles and diffuse calcifications. These calcific masses may be either present in the pulp chamber or root canal. Pulp stones or denticles are further classified according to the structure as true or false denticles and according to the location as free, attached or embedded pulp stones.

True Pulp Stones (Denticles)

True pulp stones are composed of dentin and formed by detached odontoblasts or Hertwig's root sheath. They resemble secondary dentin and are commonly found in pulp chamber.

False Pulp Stones (Denticles)

False denticles are made up of concentric layers of calcified tissue deposited around a central nidus.

Diffuse Calcification

These are the amorphous, unorganized linear strands of calcified masses, mostly found in the radicular pulp. They lie parallel to the blood vessels or nerve fibers of the pulp tissue.

Etiology

Pulp calcification may occur due to local metabolic dysfunction or trauma leading to tissue hyalinization or vascular damage respectively. The fibrosed hyalinized tissue undergoes mineralization and thrombosis due to vascular damage and with time transforms into pulp stone.

Clinical Significance

Pulp stones do not produce any symptoms but occasionally may cause referred pain which may be rarely of neuralgic type. They may produce obstruction in pulp extirpation during root canal treatment. (Fig. 9.1)

DISEASES OF PERIAPICAL TISSUES

There is an interrelationship between the pulp and periapical tissues, so once the infection gets established in the pulp, the inflammation spreads into the periodontal ligament. The products of tissue necrosis, microorganisms and their toxins and tissue debris reach the periapical area through the various accessory canals and give rise to periapical diseases.

Acute Apical Periodontitis

Acute apical periodontitis is an acute inflammatory condition of the periodontium. It may be associated with both vital and nonvital teeth. It may occur in vital teeth due to occlusal trauma caused by high restoration, abnormal occlusal contacts and wedging of foreign objects between the teeth. In nonvital teeth it may be caused due to spread of infection from the necrotic pulp through the root canal, over instrumentation or forcing of bacteria and excessive medicaments through the apical foramen into the periapical tissues and by perforation of root during cleaning and shaping of root canals.

Clinical Features

The patient complains of pain in the tooth especially during mastication. Sometimes the tooth may be slightly extruded due to accumulation of the inflammatory exudate. The tooth shows tenderness on percussion.

Treatment

Acute apical periodontitis is treated by determining the cause and relieving the symptoms. After removal of the cause, the affected tooth should be treated endodontically if pulp is having irreversible hyperemia or pulpitis.

Periapical Abscess

In periapical abscess, there is localized accumulation of pus in the alveolar bone at the apex of the root. It is caused due to spread of infection from the necrosed pulp through the apical foramen into the periapical region. It may arise as a result of irritation of periapical tissue either by mechanical manipulation or by the application of chemicals, but the most common cause is bacterial invasion of dead pulp tissue.

Clinical Features

The earliest symptom of periapical abscess is tenderness of the tooth and its slight extrusion from the alveolus. There is severe throbbing pain and swelling in adjacent tissue close to the affected tooth. The swelling increases with progression of infection and the tooth becomes mobile and more painful. In untreated case, the infection may progress

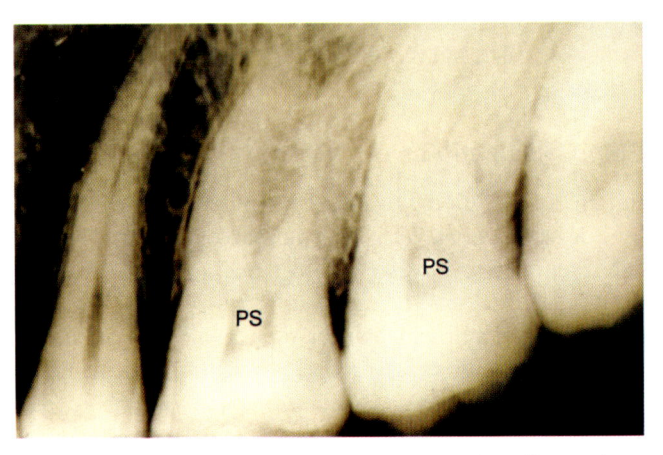

Fig. 9.1: Pulp stones (PS) in the pulp chambers of maxillary molars

to periostitis, osteitis and cellulitis. As the disease progresses there is more and more accumulation of pus. The surface tissue get distended from pressure of pus and opens intraorally or extraorally through a tiny opening or sinus tract. The patient looks pale and weakened and may complain of headache, malaise and foul breath. There may be elevation of body temperature and localized lymphadenitis.

Treatment

The initial step of the treatment is establishing drainage of pus and controlling systemic reactions by antibiotic and analgesic therapy. In the second step the root canal treatment of the affected tooth should be carried out.

Alveolar Abscess

The infection and the toxins may reach the alveolar bone, giving rise to acute alveolar abscess. There may be toxins and infection left in the alveolar bone which results in the chronic alveolar abscess which is a chronic infection in the periapical alveolar bone. The infection is of long-standing and is of low grade. It is caused due to spread of infection from the necrosed pulp to the periapical region or may be the sequela of acute alveolar abscess.

Clinical Features

A tooth associated with acute alveolar abscess is painful and there will be swelling on the face (Fig. 9.2). By the treatment and drainage the swelling may disappear.

A tooth associated with chronic alveolar abscess is usually asymptomatic. There may be presence of sinus tract on labial and buccal aspect of an involved tooth which provides drainage of the pus and prevents swelling in the affected region. In infected extraction wound in patient with poor oral hygiene maggots may appear (Figs 9.3 and 9.4). If the affected tooth is grossly carious the drainage may occur through the root canal. In case of absence of sinus tract, the bacterial products and cellular debris are phagocytized by macrophages.

Treatment

Chronic alveolar abscess is treated by eliminating infected pulp from the root canal. After proper cleaning, shaping and obturation of root canal, the periradicular tissue repairs itself.

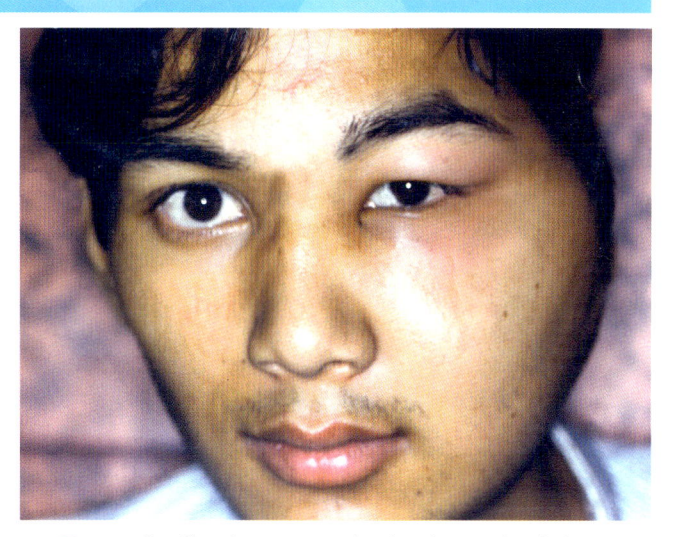

Fig. 9.2: Swelling due to acute alveolar abscess in relation to left maxillary first molar

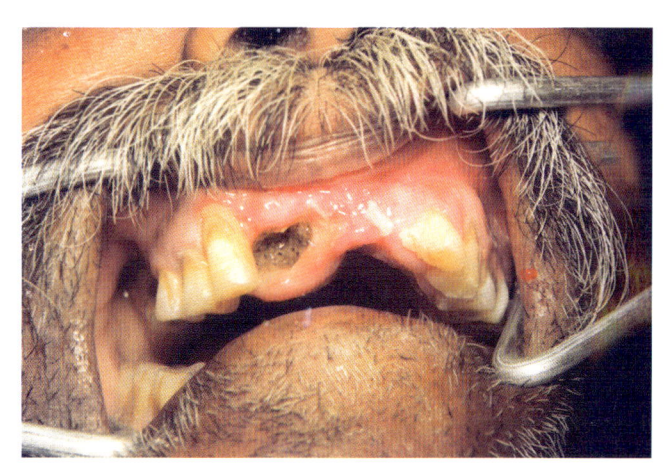

Fig. 9.3: Maggots (appearing as black dots) in the infected socket of a maxillary lateral incisor

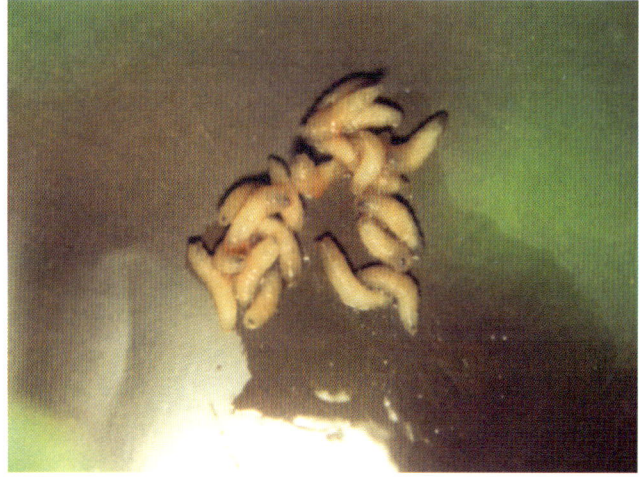

Fig. 9.4: Appearance of maggots removed from socket

Periapical Granuloma

A periapical granuloma is a mass of granulomatous tissue surrounded by a fibrous capsule at the apex of the tooth. It is associated with nonvital tooth and is caused due to diffusion of bacterial toxins from necrosed pulp into periradicular tissues through apical and lateral foramina. The formation of granulation tissue is a defensive reaction of the alveolar bone to mild infection or continuous irritation from an infected tooth.

Clinical Features

Most of the cases of periapical granuloma are asymptomatic. The involved tooth is usually not tender on percussion. In few cases, the associated tooth may produce sensitivity to percussion or mild pain during mastication. The involved tooth may look slightly elongated from its socket. Rarely, it may break down to form a fistulas tract and undergo suppuration.

Treatment

Periapical granuloma is treated by root canal treatment, with or without subsequent apicoectomy. When the cause of inflammation is removed, the granulomatous tissue gets resorbed with repair of trabeculated bone. The untreatable tooth requires extraction.

Radicular Cyst (Periapical Cyst)

Radicular cyst is an odontogenic cystic lesion which involves the apex of the tooth. It is caused due to physical, chemical or bacterial injury that results in necrosis of pulp followed by proliferation of epithelial cell rests of Malassez, present in periodontal ligament.

Clinical Features

The involved tooth is usually carious, fractured or discolored. The cyst manifests itself as extraoral or intraoral swelling. The pressure of the cyst causes expansion and distortion of the cortical plates which leads to disturbance in occlusion. Teeth may also become mobile. Pain may occur, if the cyst is infected. If left untreated, the cyst continues to grow and the cortical plate become thinned or perforated and may lead to pathologic fracture.

Treatment

The radicular cyst can be treated by following methods:
 i. Root canal treatment in case of small cyst.
 ii. Surgical enucleation is done when cyst is of medium size.
 iii. Marsupialization is done when the cyst is of very large size.

External Root Resorption

External root resorption is the process of destruction of the cementum and/or dentin of the root of tooth which begins from the outer surface of the tooth.

Etiology

The important causes and situations in which external resorption may occur are as follows:
a. Periradicular inflammation.
b. Pressure of cysts or tumor.
c. Reimplantation of tooth.
d. Excessive force during orthodontic treatment.
e. Pressure of impacted teeth.
f. Systemic diseases.

Clinical Features

External root resorption is generally asymptomatic. When the root is completely resorbed, the tooth becomes mobile. When the resorbed root is replaced by bone, the tooth becomes immobile; this type of resorption is known as Replacement Resorption or Ankylosis. Radiographically, external resorption appears as raggedness or blunting of the root apex.

Treatment

The treatment of external resorption depends upon its etiological factors. If it is caused due to periapical disease of pulpal origin, root canal treatment stops the resorption. In case of reimplantation of teeth, root resorption can be ceased by preparation of root canal and obturation with calcium hydroxide paste. External resorption due to excessive orthodontic force can be stopped by reducing these forces.

DISEASES OF PERIODONTAL TISSUES

Periodontal Abscess

Periodontal abscess is a localized purulent inflammation of the periodontal tissues. It is caused due to extension of infection from the periodontal pocket into the supporting periodontal tissues.

Clinical Features

In acute stage there will be painful swelling in the gingiva. The adjacent tooth may also be painful with loss of function (Fig. 9.5).

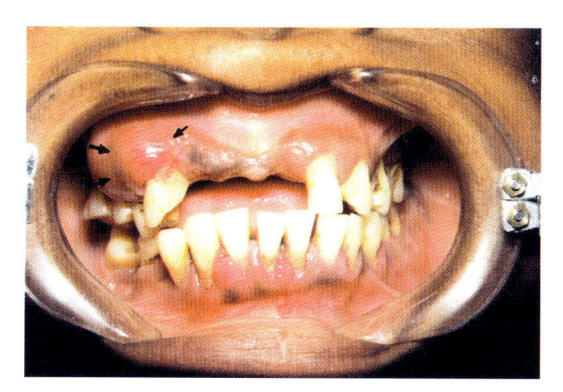

Fig. 9.5: Swelling due to acute periodontal abscess in relation of right maxillary canine and premolars (shown by arrows)

Treatment

The periodontal abscess can be acute or chronic. In acute abscess drainage is established under antibiotic cover through the deep pocket or external incision. Premature contact of the tooth with its antagonists should be removed by grinding. In chronic periodontal abscess flap operation is carried out under antibiotic cover.

Gingival Abscess

The gingival abscess is a small lesion of the marginal or interdental gingiva which is usually produced by an impacted foreign object.

Treatment

Drainage is established by incising the fluctuant area of the lesion. After drainage if the residual lesion is large then it must be surgically removed.

BIBLIOGRAPHY

1. Chen SY, Fantasia JE, Miller AS. Hyaline bodies in the connective tissue wall of odontogenic cysts. J Oral Path 1981;10:147.
2. Mincer HH, McCoy JM, Turner JE. Pulse granuloma of the alveolar ridge. Oral Surg 1979;48:126.
3. McMillan MD, Kardos TB, Edwards JL, Thorburn DN, Adams DB, Palmer DK. Giant cell hyaline angiopathy or pulse granuloma. Oral Surg 1981;52:178.
4. Robertson PB, Luscher B, Spangberg LS, Levy BM. Pulpal and periodontal effects of electrosurgery involving cervical metallic restoration. Oral Surg 1978;46:702.
5. Stern MH, Dreizen S, Mackler BF, Levy BM. Antibody-producing cells in human periapical granulomas and cysts. J Endod 1981;7:447.
6. Stern MH, Dreizen S, Mackler BF, Levy BM. Isolation and characterization of inflammatory cells from the human periapical granuloma. J Dent Res 1982;61:1408.

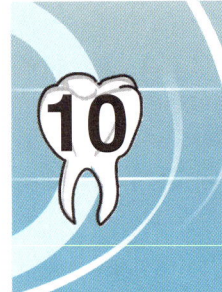

10
Ulcerative and Vesiculobullous Lesions of the Oral Cavity

INTRODUCTION

Ulcer as described by Dorland Medical dictionary is a local defect or excavation of the surface of an organ or tissue. Stedman's Medical dictionary has described ulcer as a lesion through the skin or mucous membrane resulting from loss of tissue usually with inflammation. Taber's Medical dictionary has defined an ulcer as an open sore or lesion of the skin or mucous membrane accompanied by sloughing of inflamed necrotic tissue. However, in other words ulcer is a well circumscribed depressed lesion in the epithelium of skin and mucous membrane, over which the epidermal layer has been lost. Vesicle is a small elevated blister of less than 1 cm in diameter containing clear fluid. Bullae is a fluid filled blister of more than one cm in diameter and appears as a circumscribed area of separation of the epidermis from subepidermal structures.

These ulcerative and vesiculobullous lesions are caused due to various factors like trauma, infections, immunologic disorders or manifestations of systemic diseases. The mucosa of oral cavity is very thin due to which vesicles and bullae break easily into ulcers. These ulcers are traumatized by teeth and food and become infected by oral microbial flora. Ulcerative and vesiculobullous lesions of the oral mucous membrane have almost similar clinical appearance. So, in making diagnosis of ulcerative and vesiculobullous diseases, detailed history of present illness and thorough clinical examination of exposed mucosal surface is necessary.

These oral mucosal lesions can be categorized as follows: (1) According to duration (a) acute (b) chronic lesions (2) According to number (a) single (b) multiple lesions, and (3) According to their occurrence in the oral cavity. (a) primary, (b) secondary and (c) recurrent lesions.

ACUTE MULTIPLE LESIONS (ULCERS AND BLISTERS)

Acute multiple ulcers and blisters in the oral cavity are mostly caused by viral infections. The main viruses causing infections are (a) *Herpes simplex* virus (b) Coxsackievirus and (c) *Varicella-zoster* virus. Cytomegalovirus may cause oral ulceration in immuno-compromised patients.

Herpes Virus Infection

Eight out of eighty herpesviruses cause infection in humans. These are herpes simplex virus (HSV) 1 and 2, *Varicella-zoster* virus, Cytomegalovirus, Epstein-Barr virus, and human herpesvirus 6(HHV6). They all contain a DNA nucleic acid. They remain latent in host neural cells hence evade the host immune response. Normally among all the herpes viruses only HSV1, HSV2 and *varicella-zoster* cause oral mucosal disease. In HIV patients sometimes cytomegalovirus cause oral ulceration.

Herpes Simplex Virus (HSV) Infection

The commonest cause for ulcerations in oral cavity is infection by *Herpes simplex* virus (HSV) which is of two types—*Herpes simplex* virus 1 and 2 (HSV1 and HSV2). HSV1 causes oral and pharyngeal infection and skin diseases above the waist whereas HSV2 affects mostly the genital area and causes infection below the waist, but with changing sexual habits both the types can cause infection of either oral or genital area. (Fig.10.1)

Primary Herpes Simplex Virus Infection

It is an initial exposure of the patient to *herpes simplex* virus. Virus gets transmitted during intimate personal contact. Fingers of clinician may also get infected on contact with saliva or lesions of the mouth of patient who is asymptomatic carrier of HSV, so all clinicians should wear gloves in order to avoid direct contact with lesion.

Clinical features: HSV infection usually occurs during adolescence or early adulthood. The incubation period is commonly 5 to 7 days. The patient gives the history of systemic symptoms occurring 1 or 2 days before the appearance of lesions on the oral mucosa. These prodromal symptoms (early symptoms before appearance of the disease itself) are fever, malaise, nausea, headache and anorexia.

One or two days after generalized symptoms appear, small vesicles surrounded by inflammatory base appear on the oral mucosa. These vesicles soon rupture due to oral functions to form shallow and round ulcers (Figs 10.1 and 10.2). Another important oral manifestation of HSV infection is appearance of acute marginal gingivitis. There may be inflammation of pharynx and enlargement of cervical and submandibular lymph nodes.

Diagnosis: HSV infection is easily diagnosed by the history of prodromal symptoms before the eruption of oral vesicles, round and shallow ulcers and acute marginal gingivitis. Appearance of prodromal symptoms differentiate it from other viral infections in which both systemic and local symptoms appear at the same time. Diagnosis can be made positive by various laboratory investigations like cytologic examination, HSV isolation and antibody titer.

Treatment: The most effective drug in the treatment of HSV infection is acyclovir, an antiviral drug. Acyclovir controls *herpes simplex* infections by inhibiting DNA replication in HSV infected cells. Other antiviral drugs for HSV infection are idoxuridine, vidarabine, trifluridine and ganciclovir. Acyclovir reduces the duration of fever, pain, lesions and viral shedding. New antiherpes drugs, famciclovir and valacyclovir are more effective in less dose. Therefore new drugs are more useful in treatment of immunosuppressed patients. The systemic symptoms are managed by administration of antipyretic drugs. Topical anesthetic agents like dyclonine hydrochloride 0.5% can be used to relieve pain from ulcers. Antibiotics are not helpful in the treatment of primary herpes infection and use of corticosteroids is contraindicated.

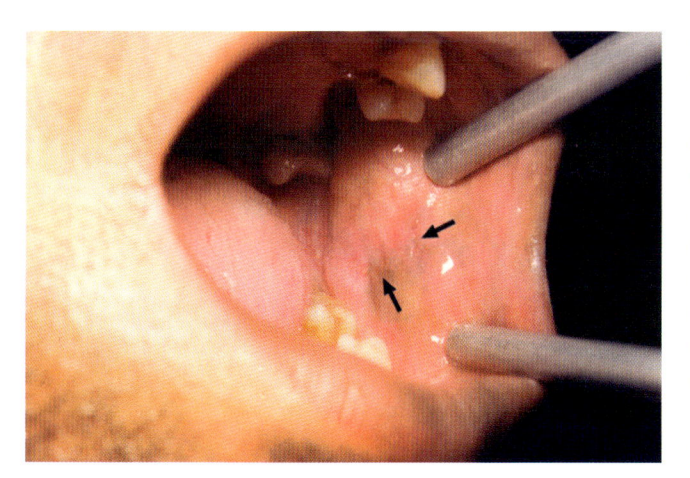

Fig. 10.1: Primary oral herpes simplex virus infection of buccal mucosa (shown by arrows)

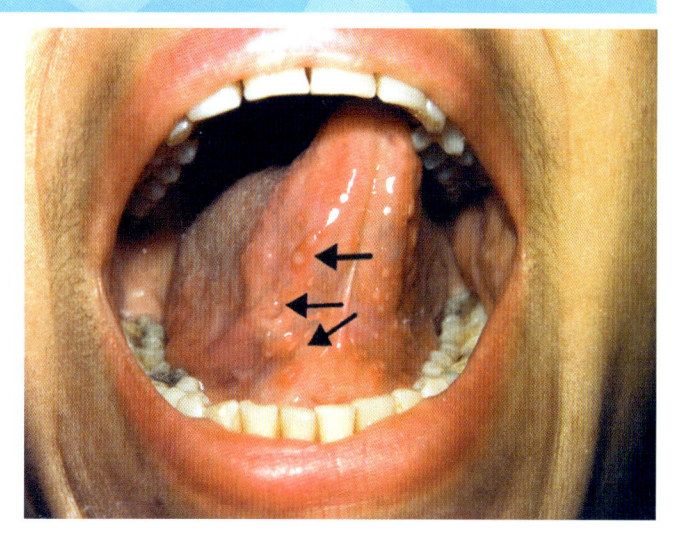

Fig. 10.2: Herpetic stomatitis of ventral surface of tongue (shown by arrows)

Varicella-Zoster Virus Infection

Varicella-zoster virus (VZV) causes two types of infections in man (a) chicken pox (varicella) and (b) shingles (herpes zoster). Primary infection with this virus causes chicken pox. After the healing of primary disease VZV becomes dormant in dorsal root ganglia of spinal nerves or extramedullary ganglia of cranial nerves. This dormant virus sometimes becomes reactivated and causes lesions of *herpes zoster* (shingles).

Clinical Features

Chicken pox is characterized by mild systemic symptoms and generalized eruptions. These eruptions are maculopapular lesions which are extremely pruritic and develop into vesicles with an erythematous base. It may also affect the spinal and cranial nerves. The nerves most commonly affected are C3, T5, L1, L2 and first division of trigeminal nerve.

The systemic symptoms persist for 2 to 4 days which manifest as severe pain, paresthesia and tenderness along the course of affected nerve. Clusters of unilateral vesicles also appear along the course of nerve, which appear as involvement of single dermatomic area. These vesicles turn to scab in 1 to 7 days and heal in 2 to 3 weeks. The oral and facial lesions due to *herpes zoster* virus are mostly due to involvement of first, second and third division of trigeminal nerve (Fig. 10.3).

The oral lesions associated with *herpes zoster* are severe scarring of facial skin, pulpal necrosis and internal root resorption. In immuno-suppressed patients *herpes zoster* lesions may lead to necrosis of underlying bone and

Oral Medicine

exfoliation of teeth. Other complications may be postherpetic neuralgia, corneal scarring and blindness.

Diagnosis: During prodromal period, when only pain is present without lesions diagnosis is difficult. Diagnosis is very easy when the full clinical picture pain and unilateral vesicles are present. Lesions of *herpes zoster*, can be easily differentiated from other multiple lesions of the mouth, which are bilateral and not present along the course of branch of trigeminal nerve as compared to unilateral lesions of *herpes zoster*, which are accompanied by pain along the course of affected nerve. Laboratory investigations like cytology and viral isolation can be carried out to confirm the diagnosis.

Treatment

The aims of the treatment are the following.
a. To shorten duration of the disease.
b. To prevent postherpetic neuralgia in patients above fifty years of age.
c. To prevent spreading in immunocompromised patients.

The mild cases of *Varicella-zoster* virus infection in young individual can be treated by acyclovir, or newer antiherpes drugs such as valacyclovir or famciclovir. The recommended oral dose of acyclovir is 800 mg five times a day. About 20% of oral dose of acyclovir is absorbed. New drugs have greater bioavailability, hence are more effective. Intralesional use of a combination of steroids and local anesthetics to decrease healing time and prevent postherpetic neuralgia has been recommended by some workers. Postherpetic neuralgia is treated by prolonged use of topical application of capsaicin. Capsaicin is extracted from hot chilli peppers. It may cause burning sensation of skin. For treatment of postherpetic neuralgia gabapentin or tricyclic antidepressant is used.

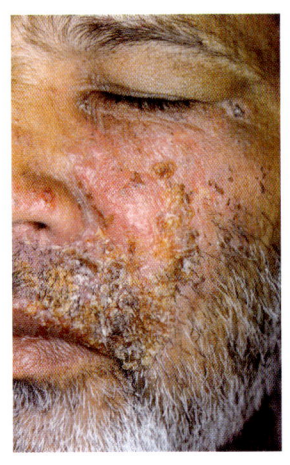

Fig. 10.3: Herpes zoster infection of left side of the face involving maxillary branch of trigeminal nerve

Coxsackievirus Infections

Coxsackieviruses are RNA enteroviruses that have been categorized into two groups, A and B containing twenty four and six types of viruses respectively. Most of the infections of the oral region are caused by group A coxsackie virus which are herpangina, acute lymphonodular pharyngitis and hand-foot-and-mouth disease.

Herpangina

Majority of cases of herpangina are caused by coxsackie virus A4. It occurs in epidemics having highest incidence from June to October. It mostly affects children between 3 to 10 years of age but can also affect adults (Fig.10.4).

Clinical features: The incubation period of infection is 2 to 10 days. Initial clinical features are fever, chills, sore throat, anorexia and dysphagia. Lesions start as pitted or dotted macules which develop into papules and vesicles involving posterior pharynx, tonsils, tongue and soft palate. These vesicles rupture within 1 or 2 days into small ulcers.

Diagnosis: Herpangina can be clinically differentiated from other infections of primary HSV by the fact that the herpangina occurs in epidemics, whereas HSV infection occurs at constant rate. Lesions of herpangina usually involve posterior part of oral cavity as compared to HSV infection, which affects anterior portion of the mouth. The laboratory study does not show ballooning degeneration or multinucleated giant cell as in the case of *herpes simplex* and *herpes zoster*.

Treatment

Herpangina is a mild self-limiting disease which usually heals without specific antiviral treatment in 1 week. There is no specific medicine for this virus. Supportive treatment like proper fluid intake, analgesic and topical anesthesia to facilitate eating and swallowing can be administered. Antibiotic therapy is useless.

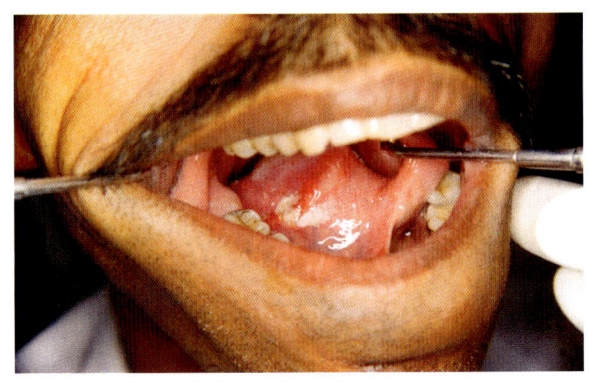

Fig. 10.4: Coxsackie virus infection- Herpangina involving lower border of tongue

Acute Lymphonodular Pharyngitis

Acute lymphonodular pharyngitis is a variant of herpangina and caused by coxsackievirus A10. The lesions are distributed as in herpangina but yellow-white nodules appear which do not develop into vesicles and ulcers. Only supportive treatment is required as it is self-limiting.

Hand-Foot-and-Mouth Disease

Hand-foot-and-mouth disease is a rare infection mostly caused by coxsackievirus A 16. Rarely A5, A7, A9, A10, B2 or B5 enterovirus 71 also have been isolated. The clinical features of this disease are low grade fever, sore mouth, pearl-gray vesicles on the fingers, toes, palms and soles accompanied by vesicles and ulcerations on hard palate, tongue and buccal mucosa. The disease mostly affects children from 8 months to 4 years of age. The oral lesions are more extensive than observed in herpangina. Although it may affect adults upto the age of 33 years. Treatment is only supportive as the clinical manifestations usually subsides within 5 to 14 days.

Contact Allergic Stomatitis

Allergic stomatitis is an inflammatory alteration of the oral mucosa associated with allergic reactions. Allergic reactions may cause erythema, vesicles, ulcerations and angioneurotic edema of the oral mucosa. These reactions may result from contact allergy or systemic administration of drugs.

Contact allergy is the result of delayed-type hypersensitivity reactions to topical antigens. When it occurs on skin it is known as Dermatitis Venenata and on oral mucosa it is referred as stomatitis venenata. The lesions due to allergens are less frequent on oral mucosa than skin because oral mucosa has low number of Langerhan's cells which participate in delayed hypersensitivity reactions.

Clinical Features

Contact allergy of oral mucosa can be caused by various substances like constituents of dental amalgam, acrylic dentures, chrome-cobalt dentures, toothpaste, other oral hygiene products (peppermint or cinnamon) impression materials and benzocaine. Allergy to acrylic is mostly caused by free monomer and is characterized by angular cheilitis and inflammation. Allergy due to dental amalgam is usually caused by mercury. Lesions consist of mucosal erythema, edema and ulcerations. Toothpaste may rarely cause contact allergy which is characterized by cracking, swelling and fissuring of lips; angular cheilitis, gingival swelling and ulcerations. Other manifestation of allergic stomatitis is plasma cell gingivitis characterized by generalized erythema and edema of attached gingiva.

Treatment

The lesions gradually disappear when cause (allergen) is removed. Allergic stomatitis is managed on the basis of severity of the lesions. If contact allergy is of mild type, removal of the allergen is sufficient. In case of severe allergic stomatitis, treatment includes topical application of corticosteroids.

Erythema Multiforme (EM)

Erythema multiforme is an inflammatory disease of skin and mucous membrane. It is characterized by eruption of various types of skin lesions like macules, papules, vesicles and bullae which soon rupture into ulcers and erosions, giving it a multiform appearance, hence it is called 'Multiforme'. Erythema multiforme is a cell mediated immune disease. It is mostly initiated by microorganisms and drugs. Microorganisms that causes EM are *herpes simple virus* and *mycoplasma pneumoniae*. The drugs associated with EM are sulphonamides, phenobarbitol, trimethoprim and penicillin. It is also called as Erythema multiforme Exudativum and Ectodermosis Erosiva pheriorificialis.

Clinical Features

Erythema multiforme mostly affects children and young adults. It has an acute onset with extensive lesions on the skin and mucosa. The commonly involved cutaneous areas are hands, feet, face and neck. The characteristic lesion of the EM is target lesion which consists of centrally located bulla, surrounded by edema and bands of erythema.

The oral lesion in the EM starts as bullae on an erythematous base which rapidly breaks into irregular, large and deep ulcers which may often bleed. Lesions mostly involve the lips resulting in severe erosion. The patient faces difficulty in eating and swallowing of food (Fig.10.5).The more severe form of disease are Steven-Johnson syndrome and toxic epidermal necrolysis.

Treatment

There is no specific treatment. Erythema multiforme of mild type can be treated by supportive measures, which include

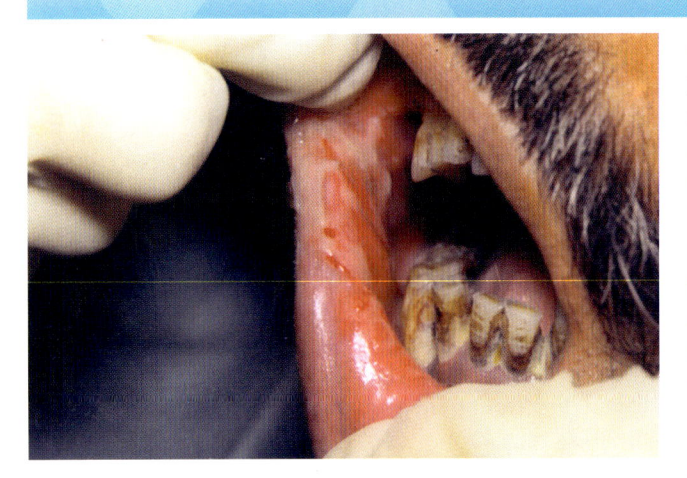

Fig. 10.5: Extensive ulceration of buccal mucosa in erythema multiforme

soft and liquid diet and topical anesthetizing agent for symptomatic relief. Severe type of EM is treated by administration of chlorotetracycline and corticosteroids. Severe cases of recurrent EM should be treated with dapsone, azathioprine, thalidomide and levamisole. Antiherpetic drugs are used to prevent HSV associated with EM.

Acute Necrotising Ulcerative Gingivitis (ANUG)

Acute necrotising ulcerative gingivitis is an inflammatory destructive disease of gingiva characterized by necrosis of the gingiva. It is a fusospirochetal disease and is caused by the fusiform bacilli and spirochete called *Borrelia vincenti*. It is most often found between the individuals of 16 to 30 years of age of both sexes. Etiological factors associated with ANUG are as follows—
  i. Poor oral hygiene with pre-existing marginal gingivitis.
  ii. Change in living habits.
  iii. Prolonged work without adequate rest.
  iv. Smoking.
  v. Psychological stress
  vi. Systemic disorders like leukemia.

Clinical Features

ANUG is characterized by sudden onset, pain, tenderness, increased salivation, metallic taste and bleeding from the gingiva. The teeth may be slightly extruded from the socket and sensitive to pressure. The lesions of ANUG necrotic are punched out, crater like ulcerations commonly at the crest of interdental papillae and marginal gingiva. In severe cases interdental papilla and marginal gingiva may be necrosed and disappear. Ulceration may also develop on pharyngeal area. In HIV infected patients ulceration develop rapidly. These ulcerations may also develop on the lips, cheeks, palate and tongue. In severe case lesions progress to involve the alveolar bone. The mouth odor is offensive.

Treatment: Necrotic areas are debrided along with irrigation and periodontal curettage in the subsequent visits. Hydrogen peroxide (1.5% to 2%) and chlorhexidine (0.12 to 0.2%) can be used as mouthwash. Metronidazole, tinadizole and broad spectrum antibiotics are prescribed in severe cases with extensive gingival involvement, lymphadenopathy and systemic symptoms. After acute stage subsides complete periodontal treatment should be done followed by regular home care. More quickly the local adverse factors are removed and oral hygiene is improved, the faster will be disappearance of lesions.

After acute stage subsides complete gingival curettage and root planing should be done. Vigorous rinsing and gentle brushing with soft brush after every meal should be regularly done at home by the patient.

Rarely serious sequelae may be gangrenous stomatitis or noma, septicemia and toxemia and very rarely even death.

ORAL ULCERS SECONDARY TO CANCER CHEMOTHERAPY

In the management of tumors, hematologic malignancies and bone marrow transplantation chemotherapeutic drugs are used. Usual side effect of the anticancer drugs is multiple oral ulcers. Such drugs depress the bone marrow and immune response resulting in bacterial, viral and fungal infections of oral mucosa. Anti-inflammatory drugs reduce the bone marrow related oral ulcerations.

CHRONIC MULTIPLE LESIONS (BLISTERS AND ULCERS)

Chronic multiple blisters and ulcers are characterized by the presence of same type of lesions for a period of weeks to months. The major diseases of this group are pemphigus vulgaris, pemphigus vegetans, cicatricial pemphigoid, bullous pemphigoid, mucous membrane pemphigoid, linear I_gA disease and erosive lichen planus. In immunocompromised patients by HIV infection, cancer chemotherapy, immunosuppressive drugs and herpes simplex infections may cause chronic lesions.

Pemphigus

It is a serious disease in which there is fluid filled vesicles, blisters and bullae of unknown etiology.

Ulcerative and Vesiculobullous Lesions of the Oral Cavity

Pemphigus causes blisters and erosion of the mucous membranes and skin. It is a life-threatening disease. In this there is loss of cell-to-cell adhesion, resulting in the formation of interepithelial bullae.

The important variants of pemphigus are *P. vulgaris*, *P. vegetans*, *P. foliaceus*, *P. erythematosus*, *Paraneoplastic pemphigus* (PNPP) and drug related pemphigus. *P. foliaceous* and *P. erythematosus* do not envolve mucous membrane.

Pemphigus vulgaris (PV)

Pemphigus is an autoimmune bullous disease involving the skin and mucosa. There are four commonly occurring variations of pemphigus; *Pemphigus vulgaris*, *Pemphigus vegetans*, *Pemphigus foliaceous* and *Pemphigus erythematosus*. Among the four, *Pemphigus vulgaris* is the most common form which accounts for the 80% of the cases.

Clinical features: In *Pemphigus vulgaris* there is rapid appearance of vesicles and bullae of varying diameter from few millimeters to several centimeters. Among all the pemphigus lesions *Pemphigus vulgaris* is commonly seen in the adults of 50 to 60 years of age. The lesions of the pemphigus are thin walled bulla on skin or oral mucosa. These bullae lateron ulcerate and continue to progress peripherally leaving large area of detached epithelium. A characteristic feature of the disease is presence of Nikolsky's sign, a phenomenon in which slight pressure or rubbing of normal mucosa results in the formation of a new lesion.

Oral manifestation: In most of the cases of pemphigus vulgaris the oral lesions occur any time during the course of the skin lesions but in about 60% patients much before the skin lesions. Oral lesions begin as bulla on a non-inflamed base which breaks into the shallow irregular ulcers. (1) Epithelial thin layer peels away in an irregular pattern leaving a denuded base. The lesion first appears on the buccal mucosa along the occlusal plane which is exposed to trauma. The other common sites of involvement are palate and gingiva. Usually oral lesions appear upto four months earlier than skin lesions. Sometimes the disease remain confined to the oral mucosa. (Figs 10.6 to 10.10)

Diagnosis: The lesions of the pemphigus are distinguished from the other lesions by several criteria. The lesions of pemphigus continues to progress for a period of weeks to months. The lesions are shallow and irregular with detached epithelium at the periphery.

Laboratory tests: Various laboratory tests like biopsy, cytological examination by Tzanck smear, direct and indirect immunofluorescent antibody test can be carried out to confirm the diagnosis.

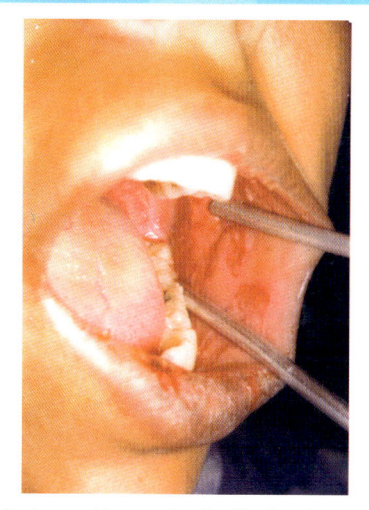

Fig. 10.6: Oral pemphigus vulgaris. Shallow irregular erosions on the buccal mucosa and lips

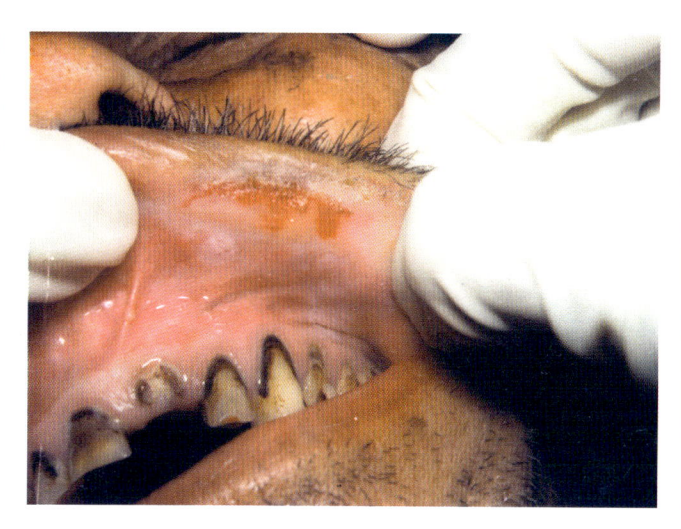

Fig. 10.7: Pemphigus vulgaris on mandibular labial vestibule

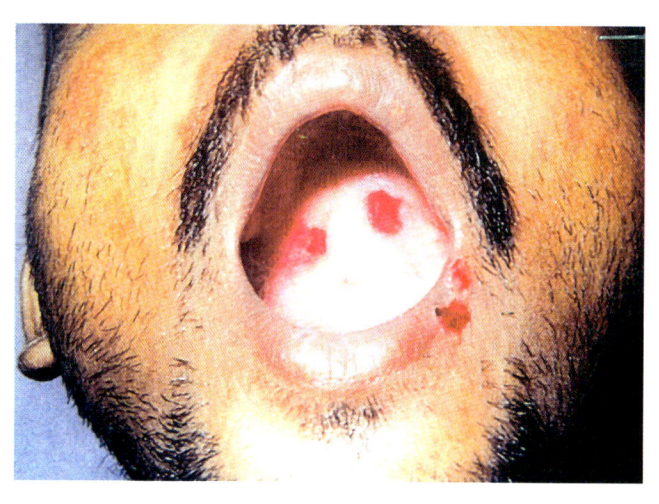

Fig. 10.8: Pemphigus vulgaris, ulcers on tongue and lip

Oral Medicine

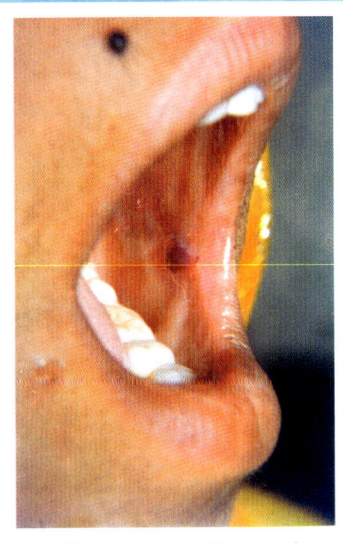

Fig. 10.9: Pemphigus vulgaris. Ulcers on buccal mucosa, one healing ulcer is seen on skin also

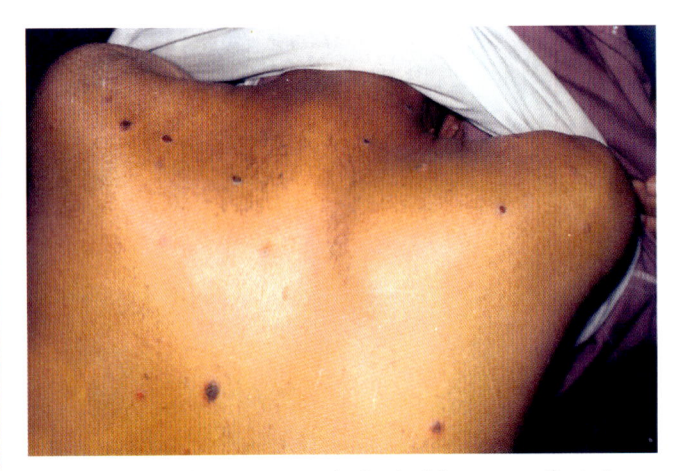

Fig. 10.10: Skin lesions on the back of the same patient of oral pemphigus vulgaris

Treatment: The course of pemphigus vulgaris is variable. The disease terminating in (a) recovery in days to years or (b) death. If the disease is diagnosed at an early stage, when only oral lesions are present; lower doses of medicaments can be used to control the disease. The principal treatment includes high doses (1 to 2 mg/kg/d) of systemic corticosteroids like prednisone, in combination with immunosuppressive drugs such as cyclosporine azathioprine and cyclophosphamide. Immunosuppressive drugs are given to reduce complications of corticosteroids.

Pemphigus Vegetans

Pemphigus vegetans is comparatively benign variant of pemphigus vulgaris because it is self-healing. About 1 to 2% of total pemphigus cases are pemphigus vegetans. It is of following two types:
  i. Neumann type (more common, lesions are like *P.vulgaris*)
  ii. Hallopeau type (less aggressive)

Oral lesions: Oral lesions in both types are common. They are lace-like ulcers with red base and purulent surface. Some authors call it is pyosomatitis vegetans. Treatment is same as *P.vulgaris* (Figs 10.11 and 10.12)

Benign Mucous Membrane Pemphigoid (MMP) or Cicatricial Pemphigoid

Mucous membrane pemphigoid is an autoimmune disease in which antibodies formed against the basement membrane cause separation of the epithelium and connective tissue, forming subepithelial vesicles. It is also known as ocular pemphigus.

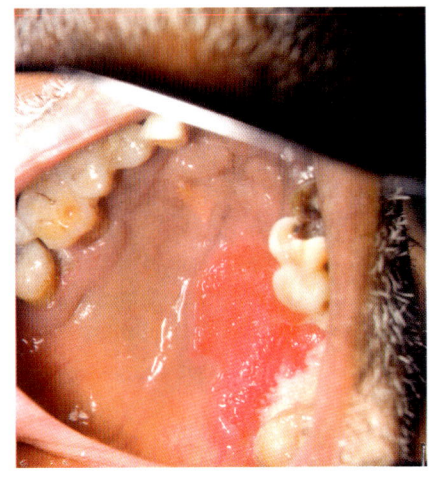

Fig. 10.11: Chronic pemphigus vegetans ulcer on palate with overhanging margins

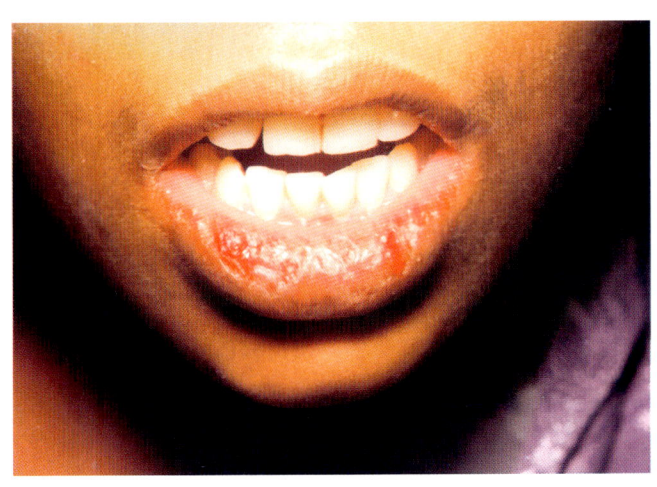

Fig. 10.12: Pemphigus ulcers on lower lip

Ulcerative and Vesiculobullous Lesions of the Oral Cavity

Clinical features: Mucous Membrane Pemphigoid (MMP) is a chronic disease chiefly occurring in patients between 40 to 50 years of age. It is twice as frequent in females as in males. The lesions most commonly occur in oral cavity which are thick-walled and subepithelial in origin (Fig.10.13). It is a slowly developing disease with small-sized lesions. In most of the cases of MMP, the lesions are restricted to gingiva. The initial lesions are vesiculobullous which later on become erosive. Lesions may also occur in conjunctiva and mucosa of palate, lips, esophagus, trachea, larynx and genitals.

Treatment: MMP is not a fatal diseases. Most patients are elderly. Treatment is based on severity of the disease, if the lesions are confined to oral mucosa, systemic corticosteroids are given. The mild cases of MMP can be treated with topical or intralesional steroids. Prolonged use of steroids must be carefully evaluated in chronic cases. If topical and intralesional treatment is unsuccessful, dapsone treatment may be tried. Patients who are resistant to dapsone may be treated with a combination of immunosuppressive drugs and systemic corticosteroids. Some workers have observed success by tetracycline and nicotinamide in controlling the lesions of MMP.

Bullous Pemphigoid (BP) or Parapemphigus

Bullous pemphigoid is a self-limiting chronic disease most commonly observed in old age above 60 years. It is characterized by absence of acantholysis subepithelial vesicles which remain localized and heal spontaneously. Skin lesions are also present which appear as blisters on the inflamed skin. It may last from few months to five years. The split in the basement membrane is accompanied by eosinophil rich inflammatory exudate.

Clinical features: In most of the cases of bullous pemphigoid, oral lesions precede the skin lesions. Oral lesions are found most frequently on the buccal mucosa. The lesions of the oral cavity are smaller, grow at a slower rate and are less painful. The gingiva is also involved and appears as edematous, inflamed and desquamated.

Treatment: Treatment of bullous pemphigoid includes the use of low-dose systemic corticosteroids combined with immunosuppressive drugs and dapsone.

Erosive and Bullous Lichen Planus

Erosive and bullous lichen planus is the severe form of the lichen planus in which there is extensive degeneration of the basal layer of the epithelium due to which it gets separated from the underlying connective tissue. When the disease is characterized by presence of ulcers, it is called Erosive Lichen Planus. If the lesions appear as bullae or vesicles, disease is termed as bullous lichen planus. The erosive lichen planus is associated with drug therapy and systemic diseases. Drugs which initiate the lichenoid reactions are hydrochlorothiazide, NSAIDS, penicillamine and angiotensin converting enzyme inhibitors. The systemic diseases associated with erosive lichen planus are chronic hepatitis and Castleman's tumor.

Clinical features: The disease is characterized by the presence of bullae, vesicles or irregular shallow ulcers on the oral mucosa. The lesions are present for a period of weeks to months. Erosive or bullous lesions are accompanied by typical lichenoid white lesions. Hydropic degeneration of the basal layer epithelium is seen in biopsy. Most of the cases of erosive lichen planus are present along with desquamative gingivitis and are very painful (Figs 10.14 to 10.17).

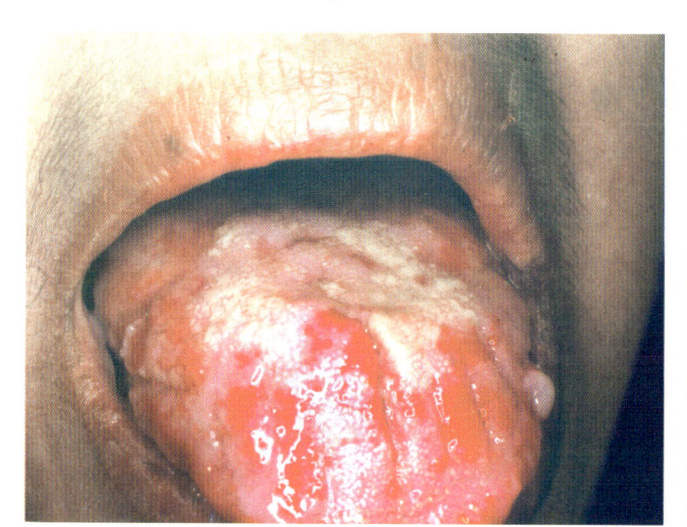

Fig. 10.13: Mucous membrane pemphigoid ulcers on dorsal surface and lateral border of tongue

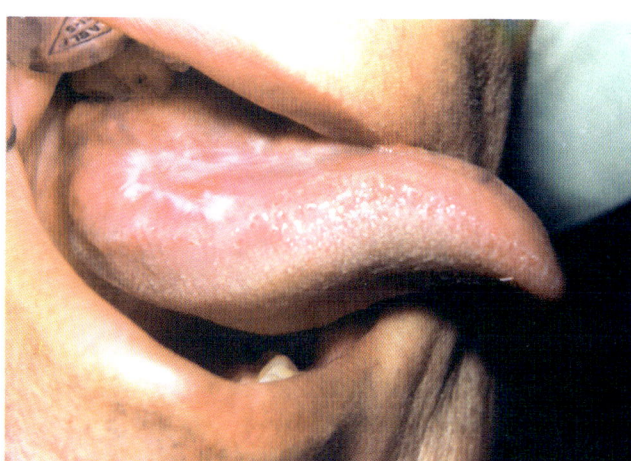

Fig. 10.14: Erosive lichen planus of ventral surface of tongue

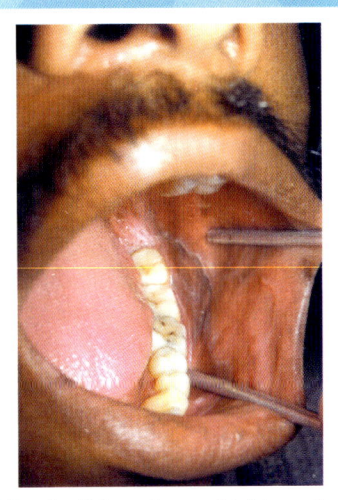

Fig. 10.15: Erosive lichen planus of left buccal mucosa and mandibular retromolar area

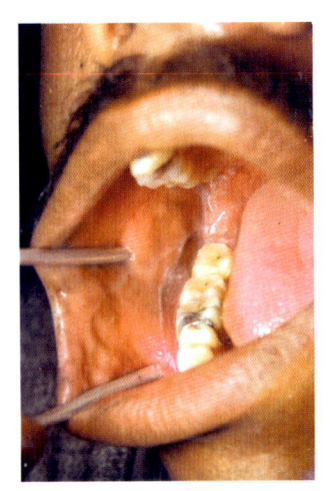

Fig. 10.16: Erosive lichen planus of right buccal mucosa and mandibular retromolar area

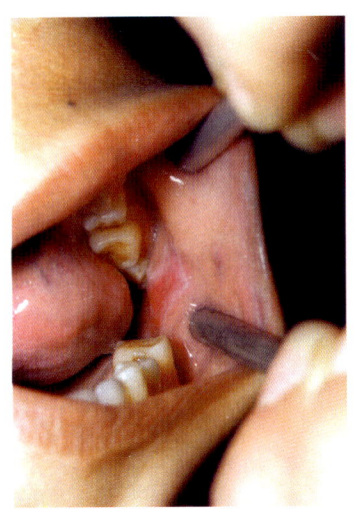

Fig. 10.17: Erosive lichen planus of buccal mucosa

Treatment: The treatment of choice for bullous and erosive lichen planus is topical corticosteroids. The inactive and painless lesions can be treated by intralesional steroids. In the severe cases, systemic corticosteroids for short period of time may also be prescribed. In patients with severe erosions which are resistant to topical steroids cyclosporine rinses are effective. Immunosuppressive drug tacrolimus in topical form are also effective in the treatment of oral erosive lichen planus. In severe resistant cases systemic etretinate, dapsone and photochemotherapy are effective. All the lesions of erosive and bullous lichen planus should be periodically evaluated for changes to squamous cell carcinoma, because these lesions specially in aged patients are prone to malignant changes.

Further details are given in another chapter.

RECURRENT ORAL ULCERS

RECURRENT HERPES SIMPLEX VIRUS INFECTION

Recurrent *herpes simplex virus* infection occurs in those patients who already have been exposed to *herpes simplex* infection and have serum antibodies against another infection. Recurrence of the *herpes simplex* is due to reactivation of virus that remains latent in nerve tissue. It may also occur due to fever, ultraviolet light, trauma to the lips, dental extraction, menstruation and emotional stress.

Clinical Features

The disease starts with the prodromal period of tingling or burning sensation. After the prodromal period the site of the lesion becomes edematous, followed by formation of a cluster of small vesicles, varying in size from 1 to 3 mm in diameter. These lesions break rapidly to form ulcers. Ulcers usually occur on the heavily keratinized mucosa such as palate, gingiva and alveolar ridge.

Treatment

Mild type of recurrent herpes infection in otherwise normal individual can be treated symptomatically. The large, painful and frequent lesions may be treated by acyclovir, which is original safe and effective antiherpes drug. Valacyclovir (250 mg BD), famciclovir (250 mg OD) and penciclovir are new antiviral drugs having greater bioavailability than acyclovir (400 mg BD) are effective in preventing genital recurrences. However these new drugs do not eliminate established latent HSV.

Acyclovir preparations are as follows—
a. Zovirax 200 mg tab. and 250 mg/vial for IV inj.
b. Cyclovir 200 mg tab., 5% skin cream,
c. Herpex 200 mg tab. 3 % eye oint., 5% skin cream.

RECURRENT APHTHOUS STOMATITIS (RAS)

Recurrent aphthous stomatitis is a condition characterized by intermittent episodes of painful ulcers which are limited to oral mucous membrane. The major factors which are responsible for the recurrent aphthous stomatitis are heredity, hematologic deficiency, allergy and immunological disorders. The other etiological factors are - (a) anxiety, (b) trauma, (c) psychologic stress and (d) nutritional deficiency. These ulcers are called (a) Aphthous ulcers, (b) Aphthae and (c) Canker sores.

Clinical Features

Recurrent aphthous stomatitis usually begins during second decade of life. There is burning sensation for 2 to 48 hours before the ulcer appear on the oral mucosa. The lesion starts as a small white papule on an erythematous area which ulcerates and gradually enlarges in next 48 to 72 hours. The ulcers are round, shallow and symmetrical. The most involved site is buccal and labial mucosa, and least commonly involved site is heavily keratinized palate or gingiva. Recurrent aphthous stomatitis can be classified into three types.

Minor Aphthous Ulcers

Minor ulcers are the common form of aphthous ulcers which reach a size of 0.3 to 1.0 cm in diameter. Healing usually completes in 10 to 14 days without leaving a scar (Figs 10.18 and 10.19).

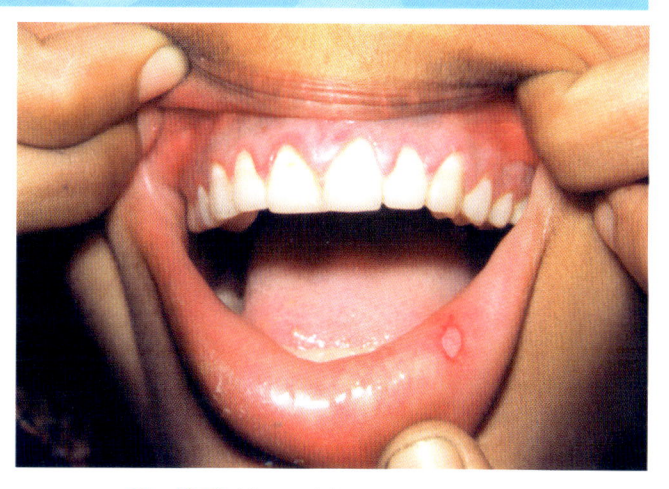

Fig. 10.19: Minor aphthous ulcer on lower lip

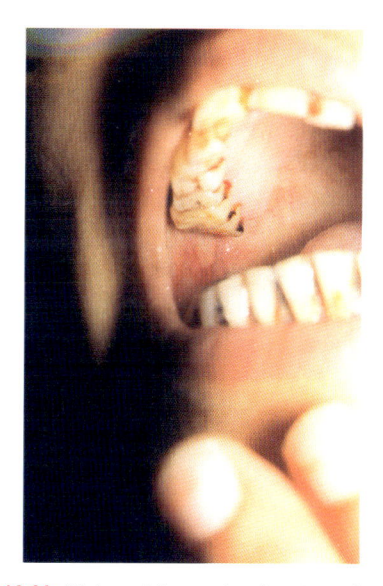

Fig. 10.20: Major aphthous ulcer in retromolar area

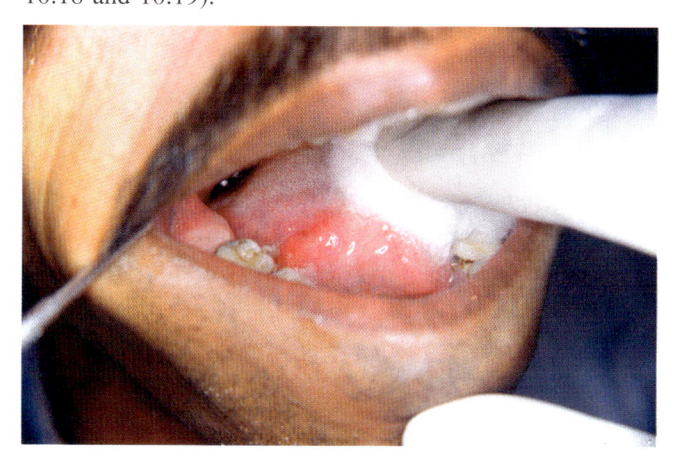

Fig. 10.18: Minor aphthous ulcer on border of tongue

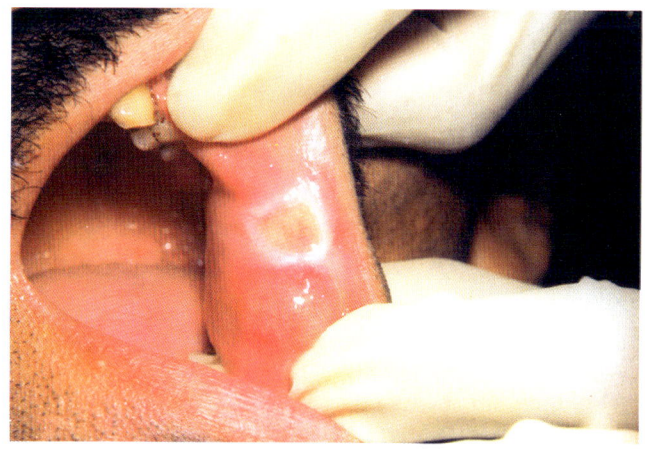

Fig. 10.21: Major aphthous ulcer on buccal mucosa

Major Aphthous Ulcers

Major ulcer is a severe form of aphthae characterized by a numerous, large, deep and frequent ulcers. They are between 1 cm to 5 cm in diameter. The lesions are extremely painful. Healing may take place in 6 weeks and leaves a scar (Figs 10.20 and 10.21).

Herpetiform Ulcers

This is the least common form of recurrent aphthous stomatitis characterized by several number of ulcers, 1 to 2 mm in diameter, scattered over large portion of oral mucosa (Fig. 10.22).

Treatment

The management of recurrent aphthous stomatitis depends upon the severity of the disease. For pain relief topical anesthetic agent and topical diclophenac sodium are used. In mild cases with few ulcers, topical application of emollient (orabase, zilactin) is beneficial. Severe cases can be treated by application of topical corticosteroids preparation like fluocinolone, betamethasone, clobetasol, triamcinolone three or four times daily. The large, inactive and painless ulcers can be treated by intralesional steroid injections, amlexanox topical paste and tetracycline mouth wash and topical paste. If the severe cases which do not respond to local systemic steroids, dapsone, colchicines, pentoxifylline and thalidomide can be prescribed. Before prescribing these drugs their advantages should be evaluated in comparison to their risks. In women of childbearing age, thalidomide should not be used due to risk of severe life threatening and deforming birth defects. The other side effects observed with thalidomide are drowsiness, peripheral neuropathy and gastrointestinal disturbances.

BEHCET'S SYNDROME

Behcet's syndrome is characterized by simultaneously occurring recurrent attacks of oral and genital ulcers and lesions of the eye. Behcet's syndrome is caused by immune complexes that lead to inflammation of small blood vessels and epithelium caused by immunocompetent T-lymphocytes and plasma cells.

Clinical Features

Oral mucosa is the frequent site of involvement of Behcet's syndrome. Recurrent oral ulcers occur in 90% of the patients which are clinically similar to aphthous ulcers. The lesions may be of mild type or deep, large and scarring which can appear anywhere on the oral mucosa. There is occurrence of recurrent genital ulcerations. Eye lesions consist of conjunctivitis, uveitis, keratitis, edema and vascular occlusion.

There may be involvement of joints (arthritis) and central nervous system. Skin lesions are common which are precipitated by trauma. There is appearance of pustule 24 hours after a needle puncture because the patient has cutaneous hyper-reactivity to injection or needlestick.

Treatment

Treatment is mainly symptomatic and depends upon the severity and site of clinical manifestations. The disease is controlled by combination of immunosuppressive drugs and systemic corticosteroids. Oral lesions if not managed by systemic therapy may be treated with topical or intralesional steroids.

Herpes Simplex Virus in Immunosuppressed Patients

Immunosuppressed patients are more prone to an aggressive or chronic herpes infection. Therefore when such patients develop chronic ulceration of oral cavity herpes simplex should also be considered during differential diagnosis. Immunosuppressed patients are the following:

a. AIDS patients
b. Patients
   i. On high doses of corticosteroids,
   ii. On immunosuppressing drug,

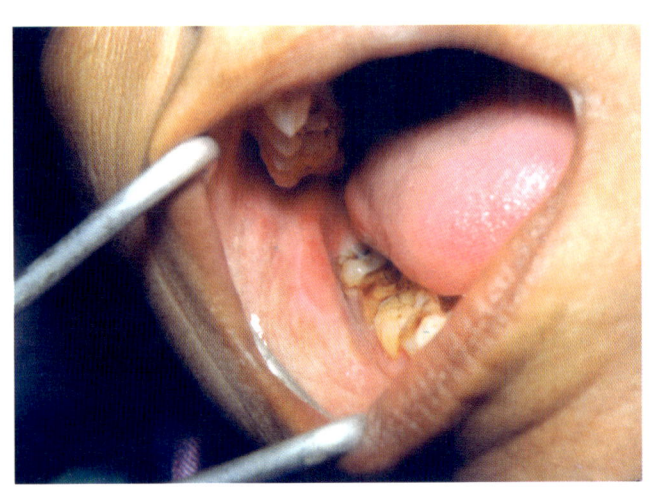

Fig. 10.22: Herpetiform ulcers on cheek and lateral border of tongue with swelling

Ulcerative and Vesiculobullous Lesions of the Oral Cavity

c. Patient with leukemia, lymphoma or other disorders which alter the T-lymphocyte response
d. Transplant patients taking immunosuppressed drug therapy are most susceptible to aggressive HSV infections.

Oral Manifestations

Lesions may appear on the lips and oral mucosa. Aggressive chronic HSV lesions appear in 50% of leukemic and 15% of the transplant patients. The lesions are several centimeters in diameter and lasts for weeks to months. Larger lesions have raised borders composed of white colored vesicles. For confirmation of diagnosis a cytological examination and viral culture should be done.

Treatment

Acyclovir orally or intravenously in immunosuppressed patient with HSV infection. In acyclovir resistant AIDS patients foscarnet has been found effective.

SINGLE ULCERS

TRAUMATIC ULCERS

Etiology for single ulcers is trauma, chemical and infection. Trauma may be due to teeth, dental appliance, food, chemicals, heat and dental treatment. Such ulcers if do not show any healing in one week after removing the etiological factor, then biopsy should be taken to rule out malignancy (Figs 8.12 and 10.23 to 10.26).

A chronic oral ulcer due to infection may be caused by the following:
a. Deep mycosis histoplasmosis
b. Blastomycosis

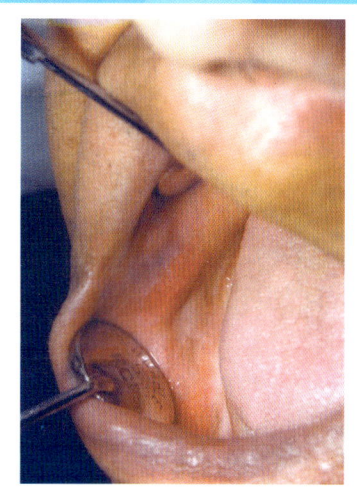

Fig. 10.24: Traumatic ulcer on mandibular ridge due to denture

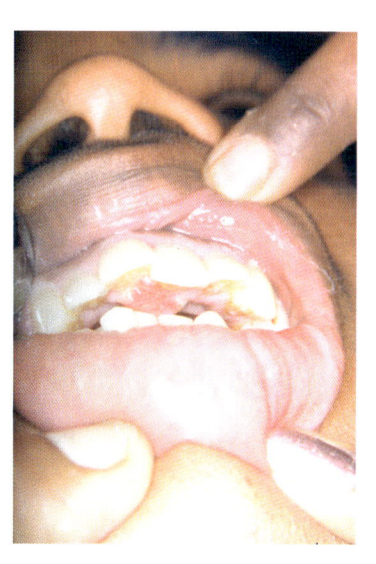

Fig. 10.25: Traumatic ulcer of incisive palatal papilla due to traumatogenic mandibular incisors

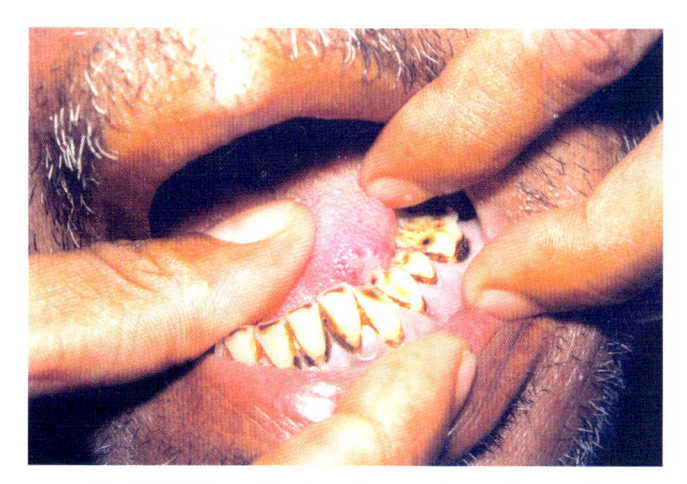

Fig. 10.23: Traumatic ulcer of tongue due to sharp teeth

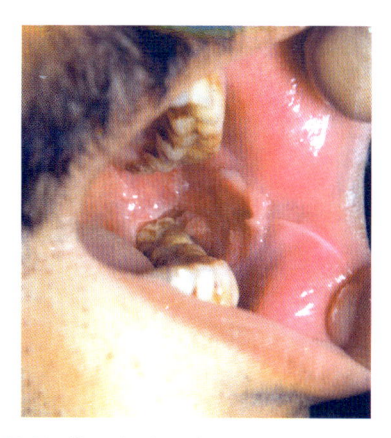

Fig. 10.26: Chronic ulcer due to chronic cheek biting

c. Mucormycosis
d. Aspergillosis
e. Chronic herpes simplex infection
f. Syphilis
g. Cryptococcosis
h. Coccidioidomycosis

FUNGAL ULCERS

Histoplasmosis (Darling's Disease)

Etiological factor is fungus Histoplasma capsulatum. Oral mucosal lesions look like a papule, nodule, vegetation or ulcer. They are present on the buccal mucosa, gingiva, tongue, palate or lips. Low grade fever, productive cough, splenomegaly, hepatomegaly and lymphadenopathy is always present. When single lesion is not treated it may progress from papule to a nodule which enlarges and ulcerate.

Biopsy of infected tissue show small oval yeasts within various types of cells. Treatment is done with ketoconazole or itraconazole for 6 to12 months. Severe disease is treated with intravenous amphotericin B for about 10 week.

Blastomycosis

It is caused by fungus blastomycosis dermatitidis. It is more common in middle aged males. Early signs are mild fever and cough. Infection of the skin, mucosa and bone may occur. Oral manifestation which appear subsequently is nonspecific painless verrucous ulcer with indurated borders. This is often mistaken for squamous cell carcinoma. Beside this hard nodules, radiolucent lesions in the jaw may appear. Radiographs of chest shows pulmonary involvement in all cases.

Different diagnosis of a chronic oral ulcer must include diagnosis of blastomycosis. Treatment is same as histoplasmosis.

Mucormycosis (Phycomycosis)

It is caused by a saprophytic fungus. For healthy person it is nonpathogenic. It can be found in nose, throat and oral cavity. In person with decreased resistance mucormycosis may appear as a pulmonary, gastrointestinal, disseminated and rhinocerebral infection. It may give rise to reddish black nasal turbinate and septum and nasal discharge, fever, swelling of the cheek and facial paresthesia. Early diagnosis is important.

Oral Manifestations

Ulceration of palate, gingiva, lip and alveolar ridge. In patients with decreased resistance mucormycosis should be included in differential diagnosis of large oral ulcers. Diagnosis can be confirmed by biopsy.

Treatment

Surgical debridement of the infected area and systemic amphotericin B for upto 3 months. Blood urea nitrogen and creatinine should be regularly checked as amphotericin B causes renal toxicity.

BIBLIOGRAPHY

1. Balfour HH. Antiviral drugs. N Engl J Med 1999;340:1255-68.
2. Buno IJ, Huff JC, Weston WL, et al. Elevated levels of interferon gamma, tumor necrosis factor alpha, interleukins 2,4,5 but not interleukin 10, are present in recurrent aphthous stomatitis. Arch Dermatol 1998;134:827-31.
3. Calebotta A, Saenz AM, Gonzalez F, et al. Pemphigus vulgaris. Benefits of tetracycline as adjuvant therapy in a series of thirteen patients. Int J Dermatol 1999;38:217-21.
4. Ciarrocca KN, Greenberg MS. A retrospective study of the management of oral mucous membrane pemphigoid with dapsone. Oral Surg Oral Med Oral Pathol Oral Radiol Endod 1999;88: 159-63.
5. Enk AH. Mycophenolate is effective in the treatment pemphigus vulgaris. Arch Dermatol 1999;135:546.
6. Healy CM, Paterson M, Joyston-Bechal S, et al. The effect of sodium lauryl sulfate-free dentifrice on patients with recurrent oral ulceration. Oral Dis 1999;5:39-43.
7. Ho M, Chen ER, Hsu KH, et al. An epidemic of enterovirus 71 infection in Taiwan. N Engl J Med 1999;341:929.
8. Lenz P, Amagai M Volc-Platzer B, et al. Desmoglein 3- ELSA. A pemphigus vulgaris-specific diagnostic tool. Arch Dermatol 1999;135:143-48.
9. Nishikawa T. Desmoglein ELISAs. A novel diagnostic test for pemphigus. Arch Dermatol 1999;135:195-6.
10. Stanley JR. Therapy of pemphigus vulgaris. Arch Dermatol 1999;135:76-7.
11. Tananis R, De Rossi S, Sollecito TP, Greenberg MS. Management of recurrent aphthous stomatitis with colchicine and pentoxifylline. Oral Surg Oral Med Oral Pathol Oral Radiol Endod 2000;89:449.
12. Yiannias JA, el Azhary RA, Hand JH, et al. Relevant contact sensitivities in patients with the diagnosis of oral lichen planus. J Am Acad of Dermatol 2000;42:177.

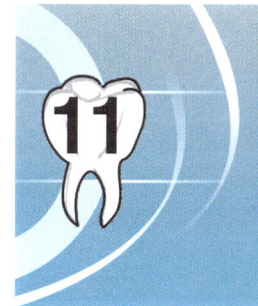

Red and White Lesions of the Oral Mucosa

RED AND WHITE LESIONS

RED LESIONS

Red lesion refers to a portion of the oral mucosa that appears red and may be smooth or granular and velvety in texture. These lesions appear red because the epithelium is thinned out and the underlying blood capillaries get closer to the surface. It may occur alone or with areas of hyperkeratosis (mixed red and white lesions).

WHITE LESIONS

White lesion is an unspecific term describing an abnormal area of the oral mucosa that appears whiter than the surrounding tissue. It is roughened, slightly raised and of different texture from normal tissue. The epithelium of these lesions gets thickened with increased production of keratin (hyperkeratosis), and production of abnormal keratin which imbibes the fluid more readily than normally keratinized oral mucosa, due to which it appears white. White lesions result from traumatic, infectious, chemical or immunological injury to the mucosa or may be due to genetically determined abnormalities of oral mucosa.

White lesions can be again divided into keratotic and non-keratotic white lesions. A white lesion that cannot be removed by rubbing or scraping is referred to as keratotic, and is usually due to increase in thickness of the keratinized layers.

A non-keratotic white lesion is either a debris or a pseudomembrane that can be easily removed by rubbing or scraping.

CLASSIFICATION OF RED AND WHITE LESIONS

ALTERATION IN APPEARANCE AND STRUCTURE OF ORAL MUCOSA

a. Leukoedema
b. Linea alba
c. Fordyce's granules or spots
d. Frictional (Traumatic) keratinization (Keratosis)
e. Lip, tongue and cheek biting
f. Hereditary Benign Intraepithelial Dyskeratosis.

ORAL CANDIDIASIS

a. Acute Candidiasis
   i. Acute pseudomembranous Candidiasis
   ii. Acute atrophic Candidiasis
b. Chronic Candidiasis
   i. Chronic atrophic Candidiasis
   ii. Chronic hyperplastic Candidiasis
   iii. Candidiasis endocrinopathy syndrome

NON-KERATOTIC WHITE LESION

a. Burns of oral mucosa
b. Habitual lip and Cheek-biting
c. Uremic stomatitis
d. Non-keratotic white lesions by infectious agents like Koplik's spot
e. Syphilitic mucous patch

KERATOTIC LESIONS WITHOUT PRECANCEROUS POTENTIAL

a. Traumatic keratosis
b. Focal epithelial hyperplasia
c. Intraoral skin grafts
d. Lesions associated with dental restorations
e. Psoriasiform lesions
f. Keratosis follicularis

RED AND WHITE LESIONS WITH PREMALIGNANT POTENTIAL

a. Stomatitis nicotina palati
b. Erythroplakia

c. Leukoplakia
d. Lichen planus
e. Oral submucous fibrosis (OSMF)
f. Lesions associated with smokeless tobacco or alcohol use
g. Oral lesion associated with reverse smoking
h. Lupus erythematosus (Systemic and Discoid)
i. Dyskeratosis congenita

ALTERATIONS IN APPEARANCE AND STRUCTURE OF NORMAL ORAL MUCOSA

Leukoedema

Leukoedema is an abnormality of the buccal mucosa characterized by greyish white, wrinkled and opalescent appearance. In majority of cases it occurs bilaterally and involves the buccal mucosa, but sometimes may extend up to the lip mucosa. It is most noticeable along the occlusal line in the bicuspid and molar region. (Figs 11.1 and 11.2).

This alteration disappears on stretching or scraping the mucosa, but reappears itself when mucosa returns to its normal condition. Leukoedema occurs most often in the individuals of 15 to 35 years of age and mostly affects males.

The etiology of leukoedema is unknown but is closely correlated with tobacco use and amount of smoking. Sometimes ulcerative changes take place in leukoedema. Leukoedema is simply a variation of normal mucosa and is harmless, so no treatment is required. Histologically it does not show keratinization. It never shows malignant changes but may undergo ulcerative change (Fig. 11.3).

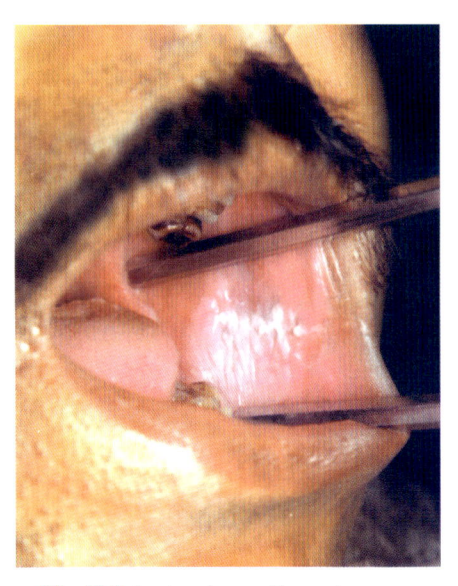

Fig. 11.1: Leukoedema of buccal mucosa

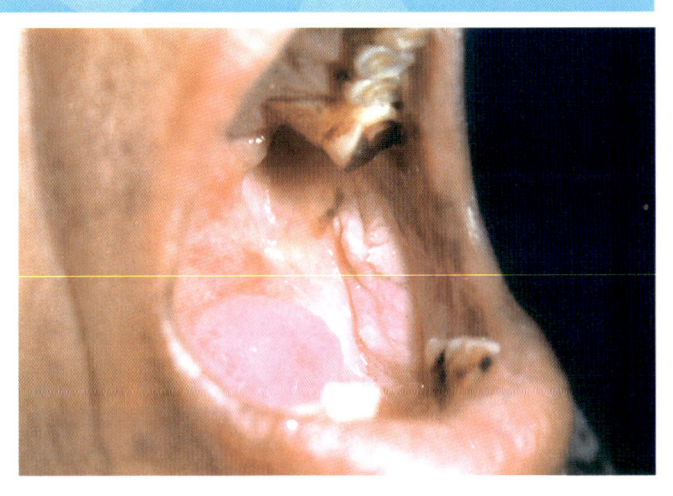

Fig. 11.2: Leukoedema (advanced stage) of posterior area of mandibular ridge

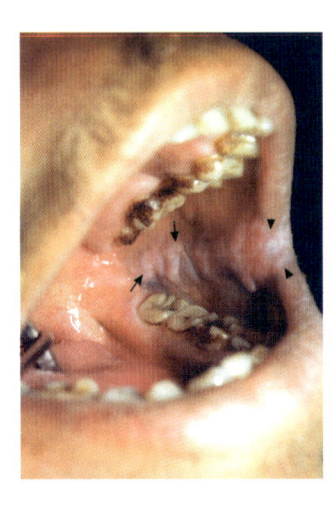

Fig. 11.3: Ulcerative changes in leukoedema (advanced stage) of buccal mucosa (shown with arrows) with angular cheilitis (shown by arrow heads)

Linea Alba

The mucosa that does not cover the bone as in cheeks, floor of mouth and soft palate is generally non-keratinized with few rete processes and non-collagenous lamina propria. But sometimes a line of keratinization can be found on buccal mucosa parallel to the line of occlusion, which is referred to as linea alba. It may result due to chronic irritation of the buccal mucosa resulting from contact with the teeth. No treatment of linea alba is required in most of the patients as gradually it disappears by itself. If it persists smoothing of the buccal edges of the adjacent teeth may be required (Fig. 11.4).

Red and White Lesions of the Oral Mucosa

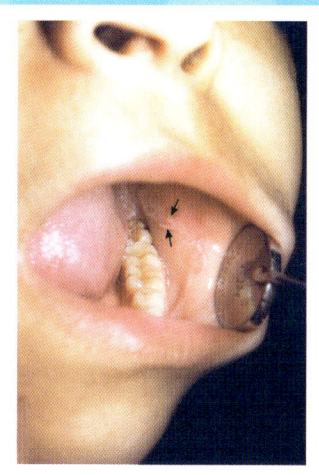

Fig. 11.4: Linea alba on buccal mucosa (shown by arrows)

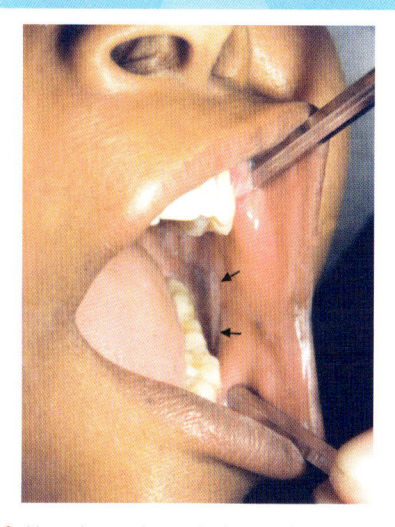

Fig. 11.6: Hyperkeratotic patch due to chronic cheek biting (shown by arrows)

Fordyce's Granules

Fordyce's granules have been discussed in chapter 7.

Frictional (Traumatic) Keratinization or Frictional Keratosis (FK)

Frictional keratosis (FK) or traumatic keratinization is defined as a white patch having rough surface, which is usually related to a source of mechanical irritation and usually disappear after elimination of the irritation.

The other areas of the oral mucosa may also show increased keratinization due to constant irritation from smoking, food texture, dental appliances and other oral environmental irritants. Usually it gradually disappears on removal of the irritant within two weeks. If it persists for more than two weeks even after removing the etiological factors biopsy should be performed to rule out dysplastic changes. Although traumatic keratosis if not associated with other factors usually does not undergo malignant changes (Figs 11.5 and 11.6).

Lip, Tongue and Cheek Biting

When oral mucosa gets impinged between the margins of the maxillary and mandibular teeth it may give rise to cheek, tongue or lip biting. If it continues for weeks it is called chronic biting. The acute biting is only once a while and may give rise to blister or hemangioma. The chronic biting may give rise to ulcers at the place where mucosa gets impinged. Where tooth is missing, pointed and elevated buccal mucosa may appear adjacent to missing tooth. The blister contains serous fluid and the hemangioma contains blood. Rarely hemangioma can occur due to the impinging of denture border (Figs 11.7 to 11.11).

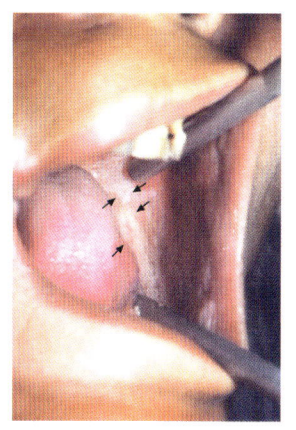

Fig. 11.5: Hyperkeratotic patch on the alveolar ridge due to ill fitting dentures (shown by arrows)

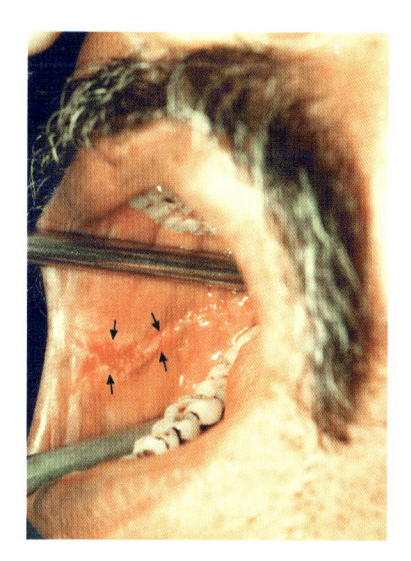

Fig. 11.7: Chronic cheek biting from canine to third molar giving rise to ulceration (shown by arrows)

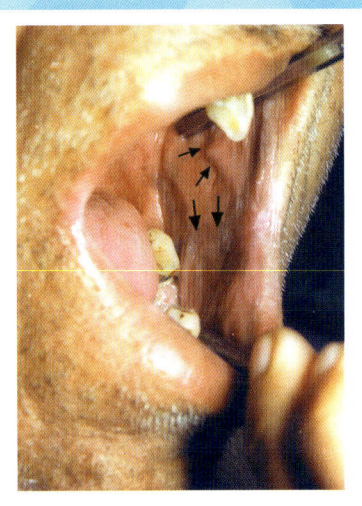

Fig. 11.8: Cheek biting (shown by arrows). Pointed elevated buccal mucosa appear adjacent to the missing tooth (shown by arrow heads)

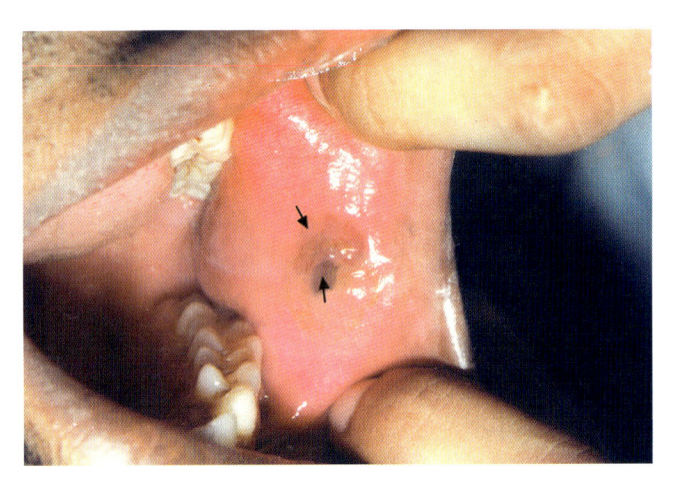

Fig. 11.9: A blister on buccal mucosa due to cheek biting (shown by arrows)

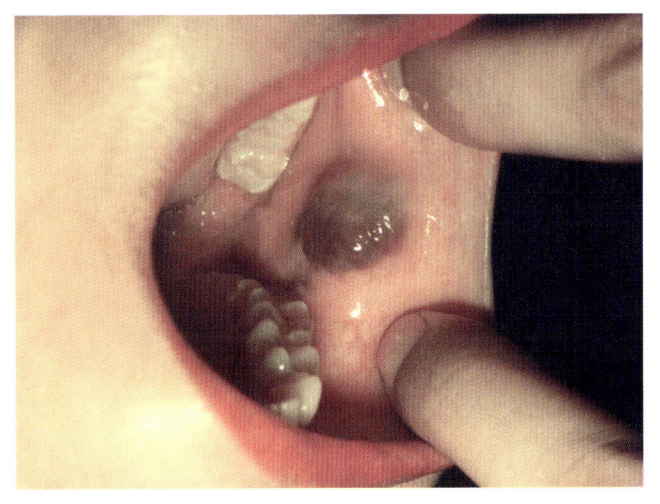

Fig. 11.10: Hemangioma of buccal mucosa due to cheek biting

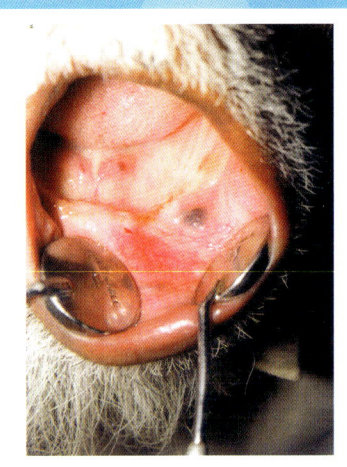

Fig. 11.11: Hemangioma of labial mucosa due to impinging denture border

Hereditary Benign Intraepithelial Dyskeratosis (HBID) (Witkop's Disease)

Its oral lesion appear as white, spongy, macerated lesions of the buccal mucosa. On cytologic examination, white epithelial pearl 'or' cells within cells 'or' tobacco cells are visible. Treatment—HBID is a benign condition and does not bother patient, hence no treatment is required.

Oral Candidiasis

Candidiasis is a disease caused by infection with a fungus candida. Candida species are the normal inhabitant of the microbial flora of the oral cavity. Though most of the species of candida are involved in causing infection, candida albicans is more pathogenic than other candida species. Candidiasis is related with both keratotic and non-keratotic white lesions. Candida may be a carcinogen or promoting agent.

Oral candidiasis can be classified into acute or chronic candidiasis.

Acute Candidiasis

Acute Pseudomembranous Candidiasis (Thrush, Moniliasis)

Predisposing factors: Candida is of low virulence and itself, it is not contagious. It only becomes pathogenic due to some local or systemic changes in the body. The various predisposing factors for oral candidiasis are as follows:
  i. Long-term use of broad-spectrum antibiotics
  ii. Administration of topical or systemic corticosteroids
  iii. Physiologic factors such as infancy, old age and pregnancy

Red and White Lesions of the Oral Mucosa

iv. Immunological deficiency as in leukemia, lymphoma, AIDS, bone marrow transplantation and cancer chemotherapy
v. Radiation to head and neck.
vi. Chronic local irritation from smoking, orthodontic appliances and dentures
vii. Hormonal factors like diabetes mellitus, hyperparathyroidism
viii. Xerostomia
ix. Oral epithelial dysplasia

Clinical features: Acute pseudomembranous candidiasis or thrush is an infection of the superficial layer of the oral mucosa characterized by soft, white, slightly elevated plaques. This plaque is composed of desquamated epithelial cells, inflammatory cells, fibrin and masses of fungal hyphae. The lesions are usually painless and can be removed by rubbing or scraping leaving an area of erythema or shallow ulcers. The lesions may be localized, involving only a smaller area, or generalized, affecting the entire oral mucosa. The other symptoms are bad taste or loss of taste and burning of mouth and throat.

Acute Atrophic Candidiasis

Acute atrophic candidiasis is characterized by red, painful and erythematous patch on oral mucosa that persists for some time with no indication of pseudomembranous white lesion. It is also called antibiotic-sore-mouth as it occurs in patients who have been treated with broad spectrum antibiotics. The patient develops symptoms of bad taste, burning sensation and sore throat. There may be generalized depapillation of tongue.

CHRONIC CANDIDIASIS

Chronic Atrophic Candidiasis

Chronic atrophic candidiasis occurs as three clinical conditions which are denture sore mouth, angular cheilitis and median rhomboid glossitis. The first two conditions are more common and hence are described below.

Denture Sore Mouth

Denture sore mouth is a condition characterized by diffuse inflammation of the denture bearing area. Usually the maxillary denture bearing area is affected. The lesion clinically appears as bright red, velvety area with little keratinization. Pain and burning sensation are present when the disease aggravates but the red erythematous area persists as long as the denture is worn. It may be associated with palatal papillary hyperplasia which appears as granular type involving central hard palate and alveolar ridges.

The denture sore mouth may be caused due to trauma from poorly-fitting denture or due to loosely adapted denture that favours contact of candida with mucosa. The negative pressure under the maxillary denture may exclude salivary antibodies, which favours the growth of candida between denture and mucosa (Fig. 11.12).

Angular Cheilitis

Angular cheilitis is a clinical finding in majority of lesions affecting the lip commissures. Most of the cases of angular cheilitis are associated with candida, and in 80% of such cases, it occurs along with denture sore-mouth. It may also be caused by reduced vertical dimension, which results in overclosure of mouth, and by nutritional deficiency (iron deficiency, vitamin B-complex or folic acid deficiency).

The more severe form of angular cheilitis termed as cheilo-candidiasis affects the full lip and sometimes involves adjacent skin. These lesions are associated with habitual lip-sucking, sunlight and chronic candida infection. (Figs 11.3 and 11.23).

Chronic Hyperplastic Candidiasis

Chronic hyperplastic candidiasis or candida leukoplakia is an extremely chronic form of oral candidiasis. The lesions appear firm, white and leathery and are commonly found on buccal mucosa, lips and tongue. In this condition the candidal mycelia invade deeply into the mucosa and skin. Histopathologic examination exhibits acanthosis,

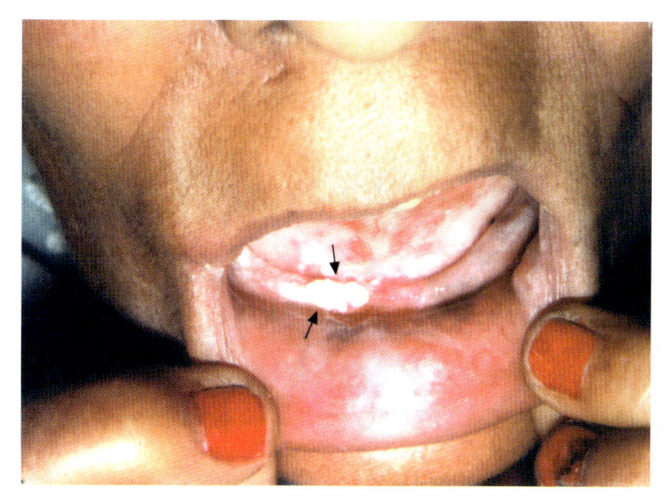

Fig. 11.12: Candidiasis on the mandibular ridge (shown by arrows)

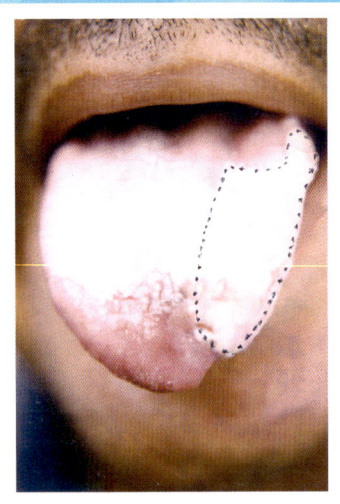

Fig. 11.13: Chronic hyperplastic candidiasis (thrush) is as thick white coating on tongue. Thrush is 0.5 mm above all over the tongue. Thrush dotted area is 0.8 mm raised above the tongue surface (*Courtesy* Dr. Mithilesh Chandra, Noida)

parakeratosis, microabscess formation, pseudoepitheliomatous hyperplasia and chronic inflammatory cell infiltration. Epithelial dysplasia also occurs in candidal leukoplakia.

It may be associated with chronic mucocutaneous candidiasis or immunologic or endocrine abnormalities. The other predisposing factors are smoking, chronic defective denture wearing and chronic candidiasis affecting buccal mucosa, palate, tongue and lip commissures (Fig. 11.13).

Candidiasis Endocrinopathy Syndrome

In this dental hypoplasia and severe caries are commonly observed.

Treatment of Oral Candidiasis

Oral candidiasis of both acute and chronic type can be treated by eating yogurt two to three times a week and improving the oral hygiene and topical and systemic administration of antifungal drugs. The majority of acute oral candidal infections respond to nystatin and amphotericin B and usually do not reoccur if predisposing factors are also eliminated. The more efficient treatment for both acute and chronic candidiasis includes single daily (in very severe cases twice daily) doses of 200 mg ketoconazole or fluconazole or itraconazole oral suspension (100 to 200 mg/d with meals) for 2 weeks. Usually no side effects like abdominal pain, pruritis and increased liver enzymes are seen in two weeks. For treatment of (a) the resistant of lesions of chronic mucocutaneous candidiasis (CMC) and (b) Systemic candidiasis intravenous injections of fluconazole or amphotericin B 50 to 100 mg per day are used. Orally amphotericin B 50 to 100 mg four times a day is also used single oral dose of 150 mg of fluconazole is also effective. Nystatin vaginal tablet may be sucked or it may be crushed and suspended in glycerine and when applied in oral cavity four times a day is effective. Three to four times daily oral rinse with nystatin for 7 to 21 days is also effective. Resistant cases may require a second course of the treatment. Clotrimazole (a derivative of an imidazole) 1% is effective for topical application. Patients with predisposing factors like prolonged use of corticosteroid aerosols, xerostomia and immunodeficiency require repeated treatments to prevent recurrences.

Treatment of angular cheilitis and denture-sore-mouth should involve the elimination of candida from denture surface by applying nystatin suspension or cream, along with systemic antifungal therapy.

NON-KERATOTIC WHITE LESIONS

Burns of Oral Mucosa

The frequent cause of non-keratotic white lesions are burns due to physical, chemical or thermal agents. The lesions of burn are characterized by pseudomembrane consisting of coagulated tissue with an inflammatory exudate. There may be necrosis and scarring of the oral mucosa if the burns are caused by very hot objects or electric current. Common causes for burns of oral mucosa are hot or extremely cold beverages or foodstuffs, chemicals, local application of aspirin tablets, burn due to smoking till end of cigarette and various dental medicaments like silver nitrate, phenol, paraformaldehyde and eugenol (Figs 11.14 and 11.15).

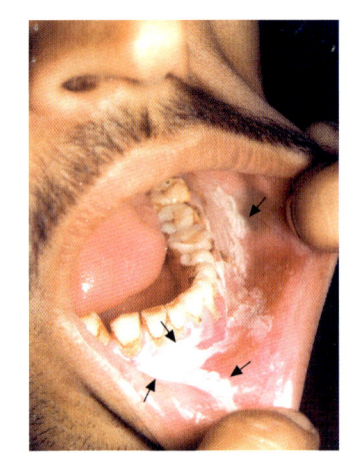

Fig. 11.14: Burn of mandibular labiobuccal gingiva and vestibule due to chemical (shown by arrows)

Red and White Lesions of the Oral Mucosa

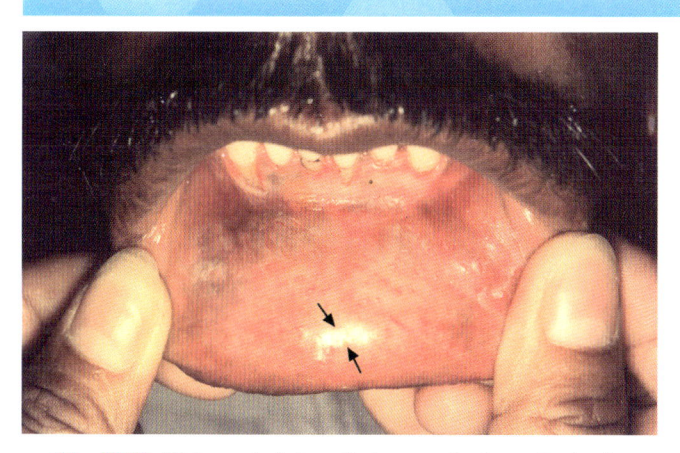

Fig. 11.15: White spot of cigarette burn on the lower lip due to smoking till end of cigarette (shown by arrows)

erythematous base on tongue, lips and buccal mucosa. Such type of white lesions are also caused by infection of oral mucosa by gram-negative bacteria following radiation and immunosuppressive therapy. This condition is referred to as mucositis or bacterial stomatitis.

Treatment of Non-keratotic White Lesions

Non-keratotic white lesions are often painful because of inflammation and erosion. So their treatment includes application of topical analgesic agents. Treatment also includes the elimination of physical, chemical and microbial agents which cause the disease.

KERATOTIC LESIONS WITHOUT PRECANCEROUS POTENTIAL

Traumatic Keratosis

Traumatic keratosis is characterized by thickened whitish patch on the oral mucosa. These lesions occur due to continuous irritation of the oral mucosa by local irritants. The irritants may be sharp edges of dentures and broken teeth, denture clasps and smoking. Majority of these lesions reduce in size or disappear completely after removal of the irritant. Topical antifungal agent can also be used to hasten the healing process. Histologically, lesions show hyperkeratosis, parakeratosis and acanthosis (Figs 11.5 and 11.6).

Focal Epithelial Hyperplasia

Focal epithelial hyperplasia has been discussed in chapter 7.

Intraoral Skin Grafts

Intraoral skin grafts are the pieces of skin grafted in the oral mucosa to cover a defect of extensive oral wound, to repair an oroantral fistula and to cover wide excision of any oral lesion. These skin grafts appear greyish white and wrinkled due to imbibition of water, which are sometimes identified as white lesions and cause suspicion.

Lesions Associated with Dental Restorations

Keratotic white lesions are also seen associated with dental restorations. These lesions are caused due to trauma from rough surface of restorations, adhering dental plaque to restorations and allergy to mercury.

Electrogalvanic current due to large metallic restoration could also be an etiological factor for keratotic white lesion.

Habitual Lip and Cheek Biting

The lesions of habitual lip and cheek biting are characterized by rough, ulcerated and reddened area with partly detached superficial epithelium. These lesions are produced by continuous rubbing, sucking or chewing movements due to which the surface of lip or cheek mucosa gets abraded. Habitual lip and cheek biting occur as an unconscious and unintentional nervous habit. If the habit occurs mostly during the night, a plastic occlusal nightguard and diazepam 5 to 10 mg at bedtime can be used to control the habit.

Uremic Stomatitis

Uremic stomatitis is a rare condition seen in seriously ill patients with renal failure and with blood urea nitrogen level above 50 mg/dl. The lesion is characterized by extensive pseudomembranous white lesion which is caused due to chemical burn resulting from increased ammonia level in saliva. The ammonia is released due to the action of microorganism on salivary urea.

Non-keratotic White Lesion by Infectious Agents like Koplik's Spot

Non-keratotic white lesions are also caused by some specific infectious agents, for example Koplik's spot, syphilitic mucous patch, thrush and bacterial stomatitis. Koplik's spot are caused by measles virus and appear as white lesion on an erythematous and inflamed base on the buccal mucosa.

Syphilitic Mucous Patch

Syphilitic mucous patches are seen in secondary syphilis and appear as greyish white membranous area overeroded

Histologically, they resembles leukoplakia in half of the cases and lichen planus, in the other half.

Psoriasiform Lesions

Psoriasiform lesions include psoriasis, Reiter's syndrome, Benign migratory glossitis and 'ectopic geographic tongue'. In Reiter's syndrome there are painless, red, slightly elevated areas, sometimes granular or even vesicular with a white circinate border on the lips, gingiva and buccal mucosa. 'Munro abscesses' are found in psoriasis. The tetrad of Reiter's syndrome include urethritis, arthritis, conjunctivitis and mucocutaneous lesion. It is observed in males of 20 to 30 years of age. Oral lesion appear in 5 to 50 percent of patients with the disease.

Keratosis Follicularis

It is an autosomal dominant disorder characterized by eruption of keratotic papules. In cytologic smear of keratosis follicularis 'grains' and 'corps ronds' are seen.

RED AND WHITE LESIONS WITH PREMALIGNANT POTENTIAL

Stomatitis Nicotina Palati

Stomatitis nicotina palati is a specific lesion occurring on the palate of those individuals who heavily smoke, smoking rod like cigarettes, cigars or pipe. Lesions are more prominent and well developed on the keratinized hard palate and are restricted to the area exposed to thick jet of tobacco smoke.

Initially the lesion appears red, which gradually becomes pale or greyish white, thick and may be fissured. Openings of the palatal minor salivary glands get thickened and may appear as white nodules with reddish dot at the centre. In rare condition ducts of minor salivary glands may show squamous metaplasia which may lead to obstruction of ducts resulting in the formation of retention cysts. Stomatitis nicotina palati in early stage is a reversible condition, so, it may gradually disappears following cessation of smoking (Fig.11.16).

Erythroplakia (Erythroplasia of Queyrat)

The term erythroplakia is used to describe red, velvety, plaque like lesions of mucous membrane that often represent high frequency of cellular atypia, premalignant and malignant changes.

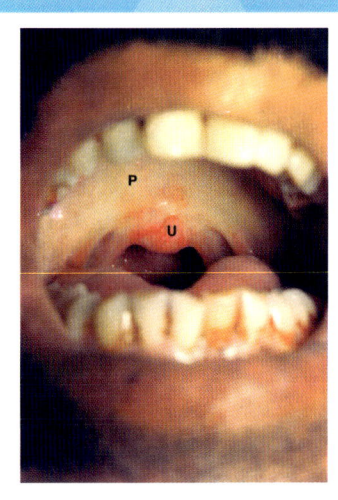

Fig. 11.16: Stomatitis nicotina palati with smoked buccal mucosa with submucous fibrosis of palate (shown by P) tonsillar pillars and buccal mucosa. Uvula is remarkably mobile (shown by U)

Clinical Features

Erythroplakia occurs in four distinct clinical patterns which are as follows:

Homogenous erythroplakia: It appears as bright red, soft and velvety lesion with irregular but well defined margins. It is commonly found on buccal mucosa and sometimes on the soft palate, under the tongue and floor of mouth (Figs 11.17 and 11.18).

Erythroplakia with white raised margins: It is big red colored area like an ulcer with white raised margins usually of triangular shape on buccal mucosa (Fig. 11.19).

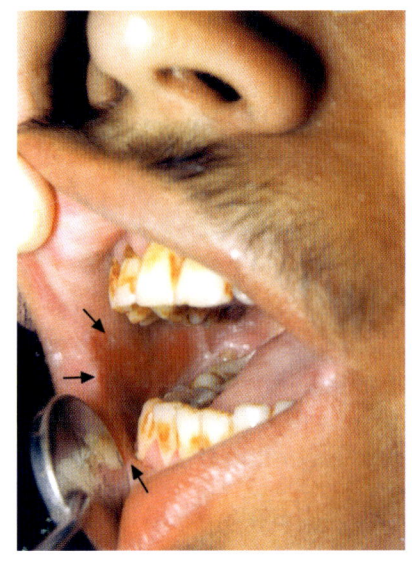

Fig. 11.17: Homogenous erythroplakia of buccal mucosa (shown by arrows)

Red and White Lesions of the Oral Mucosa

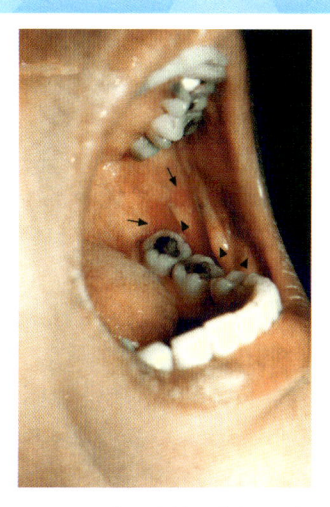

Fig. 11.18: Homogenous erythroplakia of buccal mucosa (shown by arrows) with fibrous bands of SMF. The bands become prominent (shown by arrow heads) on forceful opening of mouth

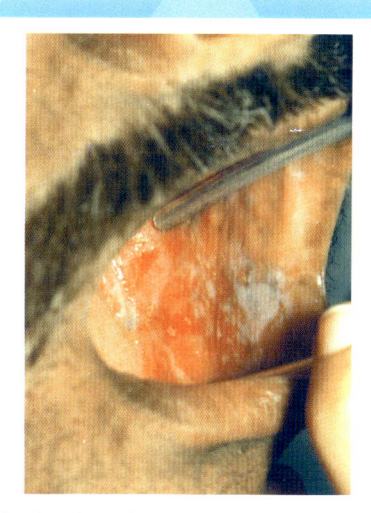

Fig. 11.20: Erythroplakia (red patches) interspersed with patches of leukoplakia (light gray patches) of buccal mucosa

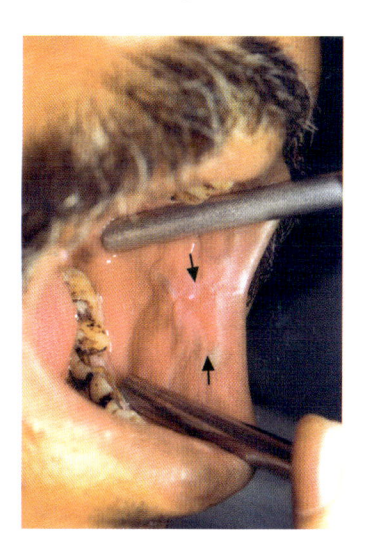

Fig. 11.19: Erythroplakia with white raised margins of buccal mucosa (shown by arrows)

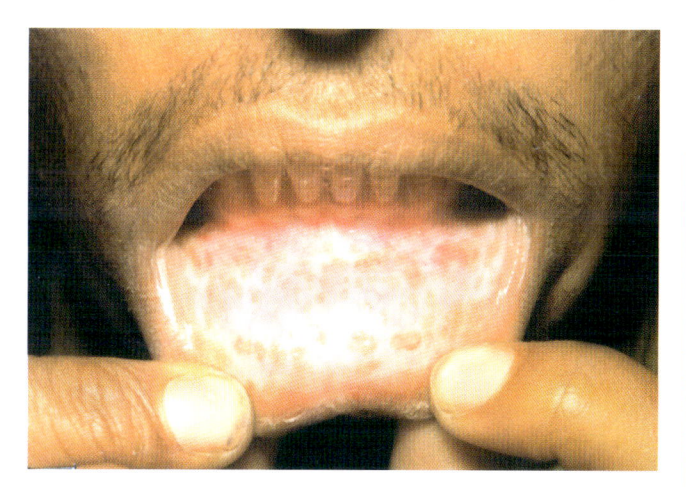

Fig. 11.21: Speckled erythroplakia of the mucosa of the lower lip

Erythroplakia interspersed with patches of leukoplakia: There is presence of irregular erythematous area which is not as bright as homogenous form, along with few white leukoplakic patches. It is most frequently seen on tongue, buccal mucosa and floor of the mouth (Fig. 11.20).

Speckled erythroplakia: Speckled erythroplakia is somewhat identical to speckled leukoplakia. The lesion is granular red, soft, irregular, raised erythematous area of white keratin within or peripheral to the lesion. It may occur any where in the oral cavity.

Malignant transformation of erythroplakia is considerably high. About 80 to 90% of erythroplakia are histopathologically either carcinoma in situ, epithelial dysplasia or invasive carcinoma. Erythroplakia mostly occurs in sixth and seventh decades of life. It is associated with smoking, tobacco and alcohol abuse (Fig. 11.21).

Treatment

Treatment of erythroplakia starts with removal of suspected irritant. If the lesion persists after two weeks of removal of irritant, biopsy is necessary. In case of erythroplakia with severe and extensive epithelial dysplasia, or early carcinoma surgical removal of entire lesion is required. Prompt treatment as per guideline for the malignancy must be done for malignant erythroplakia. Asymptomatic malignant erythroplakic lesions are about 1 to 2 cm in diameter. After treatment long term follow up is a must as there may be recurrence and multifocal involvement.

Leukoplakia

Leukoplakia is a white patch or plaque occurring on the surface of mucous membrane that cannot be removed by rubbing or scraping and cannot be characterized clinically or pathologically as any other disease.

Etiology

The following factors are considered to be of etiological significance.

Local factors: Initiation of condition depends upon a number of extrinsic local factors. Factors most frequently involved are tobacco, alcohol, chronic irritation from sharp margins of teeth and prosthesis, electrogalvanic reactions, candidiasis and sometimes herpes simplex and papilloma viruses. Out of these tobacco is the major factor responsible for the development of leukoplakia.

Tobacco is used in various forms for smoking, chewing and snuffing. In some parts of India tobacco is used in some special and more harmful ways. Among them 'khaini' and 'chutta' are more popular. Khaini (coarse powder of dried tobacco leaves rubbed with slaked lime) is put into the mouth usually, between the lower lip and lower teeth and its juice is sucked very slowly for one to three hours. After this period fresh 'khaini' is placed at the same place depending upon the habit. It is popular in male adults and aged persons in some eastern parts of India. When tobacco is rubbed with lime more strong and harmful products are liberated.

'Chutta' smoking is very popular in adults and aged persons of south eastern parts of India. 'Chutta' is a cigar like tobacco preparation in which burning end is kept inside the oral cavity. Usually it causes pathology of the palate.

Systemic factors: The regional and systemic factors like tertiary syphilis, sideropenic anemia, vitamin B_{12} and folic acid deficiency, and other nutritional deficiencies are all responsible for atrophic changes in the oral mucous membrane which lead to leukoplakia.

Clinical Features

Leukoplakia appears as white patch or plaque which may be either non-palpable or fissured, indurated or papillomatous. It may be either well-localized lesion or diffuse large lesion covering large area of oral mucosa. Leukoplakic patches may be found anywhere in the oral cavity, but frequently involved sites are buccal mucosa, gingivae and vermilion border of lip. Leukoplakia is seen chiefly in older age group and more commonly in males than in females. Clinically, leukoplakia can be categorized into five types.

Homogenous leukoplakia: It is a localized lesion which clinically presents as extensive white patch with wrinkled or corrugated surface (Fig.11.22).

Speckled leukoplakia: In speckled leukoplakia there are many small white specks of leukoplakia very near to each other. Its malignancy rate is very low (Figs 11.23 and 11.24).

Nodular leukoplakia: It refers to mixed red and white lesions with small keratotic nodules scattered over an erythematous base. This clinical type has high rate of malignant transformation (Fig. 11.25).

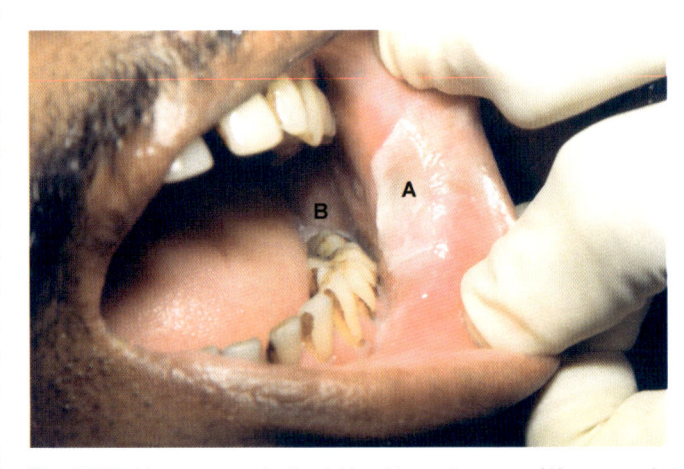

Fig. 11.22: Homogenous leukoplakia of buccal mucosa (A) near angle of mouth white lesion (B) in retromolar area light grey lesion

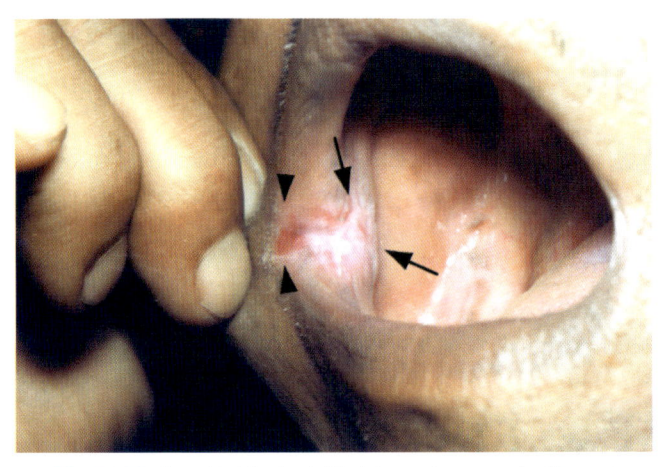

Fig. 11.23: Speckled leukoplakia (shown by arrows) of buccal mucosa with angular cheilitis (shown by arrow heads)

Red and White Lesions of the Oral Mucosa

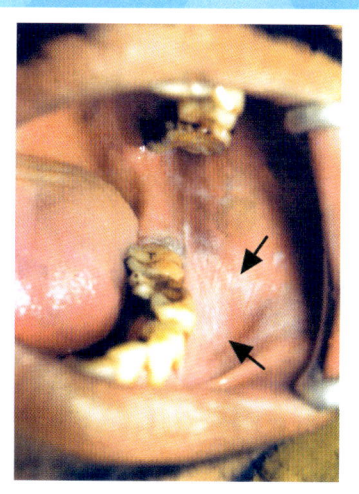

Fig. 11.24: Speckled leukoplakia in vestibule and buccal mucosa (shown by arrows)

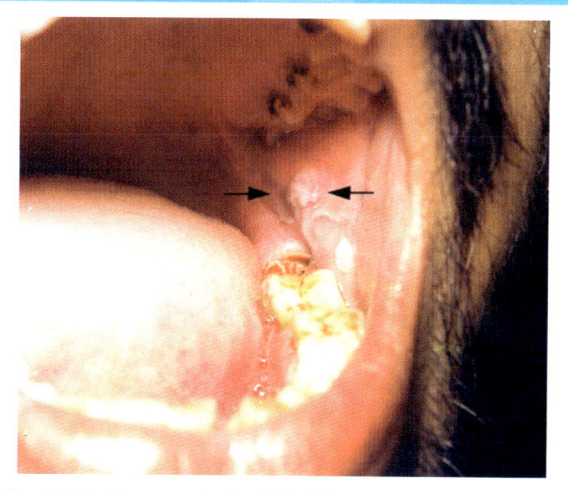

Fig. 11.27: Verrucous leukoplakia (shown by arrows) of buccal mucosa with submucous fibrosis

Verrucous leukoplakia: In verrucous leukoplakia, surface of the lesion breaks into multiple papillary projections, which may be heavily keratinized (Figs 11.26 and 11.27).

Proliferative verrucous leukoplakia (PVL): The lesions of PVL clinically present as extensive papillary or verrucoid white plaques that involve multiple mucosal sites in the oral cavity. This type of leukoplakia has a very high risk for transformation to dysplasia, verrucous carcinoma or squamous cell carcinoma (Fig. 11.28).

Malignant Transformation

Malignant transformation rate of leukoplakia is about 3 to 6 percent. Malignant potentiality of leukoplakia depends

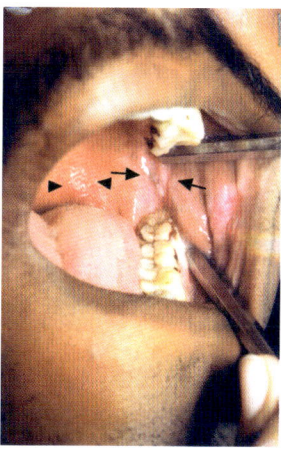

Fig. 11.25: Nodular leukoplakia on buccal mucosa (shown by arrows) and speckled leukoplakia on palate (shown by arrow heads). In buccal mucosa bands of OSMF are visible

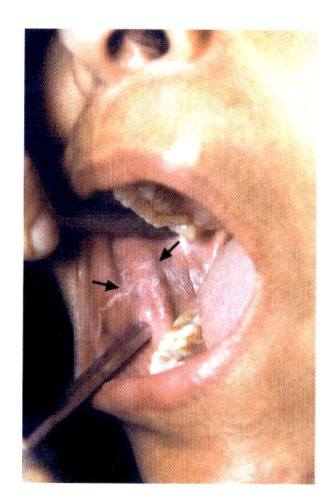

Fig. 11.26: Verrucous leukoplakia of buccal mucosa (shown by arrows)

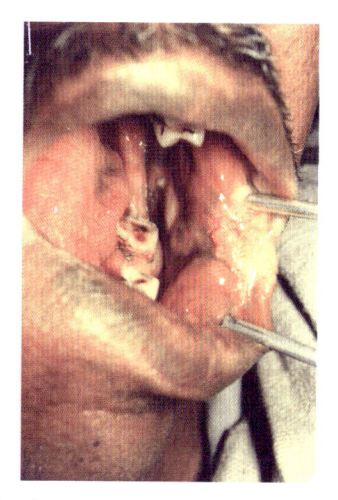

Fig. 11.28: Proliferative verrucous leukoplakia with small raised pointed nodules may be converting into squamous cell carcinoma near the angle of mouth. In buccal mucosa band of OSMF is visible

upon several factors. Following factors increase the chances of malignancy.
  i. Persistence of local irritating factors or continued use of tobacco or presence of irritants.
  ii. Lesion present on floor of mouth, lip and tongue has high risk of malignancy.
  iii. Nodular or speckled type of leukoplakia.
  iv. Female patient of older age.

Classification and Staging of Oral Leukoplakia

Clinical (provisional) diagnosis:

L—Extension of leukoplakia
  L0- No evidence of lesion
  L1- 2 cm or less
  L2- Between 2 to 4 cm
  L3- 4 cm or more
  Lx- Not specified
S—Site of leukoplakia
  S1- All sites excluding floor of oral cavity and tongue
  S2- Floor of oral cavity and/or tongue
  Sx- Not specified
C—Clinical aspect
  C1- Homogenous
  C2- Non homogenous
  Cx- Not specified

Histopathological (definite) diagnosis:
P—Histological features
  P1- No dysplasia
  P2- Mild dysplasia
  P3- Moderate dysplasia
  P4- Severe dysplasia
  Px- Not specified

Staging-4 stages
1. Any L, S1, C1, P1 or P2
2. Any L, S1 or S2, C2, P1 or P2
3. Any L, S2, C2, P1 or P2
4. Any L, any S, any C, P3 or P4

Treatment

Treatment of leukoplakia starts with the elimination of all possible local irritants and systemic predisposing factors along with administration of topical antifungal therapy for one to two weeks. If the lesion does not dissipate significantly within the period of 2 weeks, biopsy is a must to find out degree of dysplasia, if any. The patient should avoid tobacco, alcohol and other irritants. Systemic vitamins A and E are prescribed as an additional treatment for extensive leukoplakia that cannot be removed entirely by surgery.

Vitamins A and E preparation regress the lesions of leukoplakia. Dysplastic form of leukoplakia should be treated by surgical excision, cryosurgery or carbon dioxide or neodymium: yttrium- aluminium- garnet (ND: YAG) laser excision or ablation. Topical application or intralesional injection of cancer chemotherapeutic agents like bleomycin in dimethyl sulfoxide can also be used for treatment of oral lcukoplakia if dysplasia is prcscnt. For pcrsistcnt lcukoplakia careful follow up must be done as they may change to squamous cell carcinoma.

Bleomycin is very effective in dysplastic leukoplakia and squamous cell carcinoma. Adverse effects are mucocutaneous toxicity and pulmonary fibrosis with little mylosuppression. Dose is 30 mg twice daily i.v. or i.m. (total dose 300 to 400 mg). 'BLEOCIN' in 15 mg inj. is used.

Lichen Planus

Lichen planus is a common dermatological disease that occurs on the skin and oral mucous membrane. It is characterized by eruption of flat-topped, violaceous papules on flexor surface of arms, inner aspect of knees and thighs, male genitalia and mucous membrane. Oral lesions are seen in about 50% of patients having lichen planus. In Grinspan's syndrome oral lichen planus, diabetes mellitus and hypertension is present.

Etiology

Though the etiology of lichen planus is not clearly known, there is some role of psychological factors. The lesions are mostly seen during the period of emotional upset, anxiety, over-work and mental strain. The other major etiological factor associated with lichen planus is an immunologic and cell-mediated degeneration of basal cell layer of the epithelium.

Lichen planus is also caused due to drug-induced lichenoid reactions. These toxic reactions are caused by various drugs like antihypertensives, antimicrobials, NSAIDS and dental restorative materials.

Clinical Features

The lesions of the oral lichen planus are of following types:
Reticular form: The typical lesion of lichen planus is reticular form which consists of 'Wickham's striae which are slightly elevated white lines that produce either a lacy

Red and White Lesions of the Oral Mucosa

or annular lesion. This is the most common form of lichen planus and most often seen on the cheek and tongue (Fig.11.29).

Papular form: This type of lichen planus consists of 0.5 to 1 mm elevated white lesion, or papules, usually seen on keratinized area of oral mucosa (Fig. 11.30).

Plaque form: The plaque type lichen planus appears as an elevated smooth or irregular pearly white or greyish plaque on the oral mucosa. It commonly occurs on cheek, tongue and gingivae. It resembles leukoplakia (Fig. 11.31).

Atrophic form: Atrophic lichen planus appears as smooth, poorly defined, inflamed area of the oral mucosa covered by thinned red epithelium. The lesion commonly involves buccal vestibule and gingiva (Fig.11.32).

Bullous and Erosive Lichen Planus: It has already been described in chapter 10.

The lesions of the lichen planus are usually painless and remain asymptomatic in many patients before they are recognized during a routine dental examination or by the patient himself, noticing that the mucosa is rougher than normal. Lichen planus most frequently affects the mucosa of cheek and tongue. Reticular and papular lesions are generally asymptomatic, whereas atrophic, erosive and bullous forms are associated with pain (Figs 11.33 and 11.34).

Treatment

The asymptomatic lesions of lichen planus such as of reticular type do not require any treatment and heal spontaneously. The plaque like and erosive form of lichen planus is managed by vitamin B-complex supplements, high potency topical and intralesional corticosteroids. Oral and

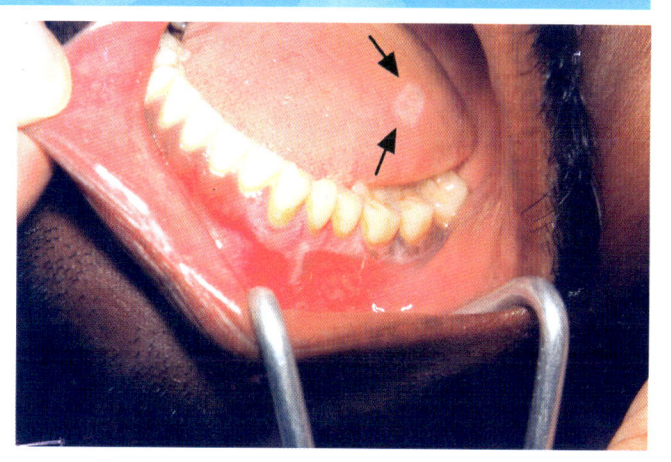

Fig. 11.30: Papular form of lichen planus of tongue (shown by arrows)

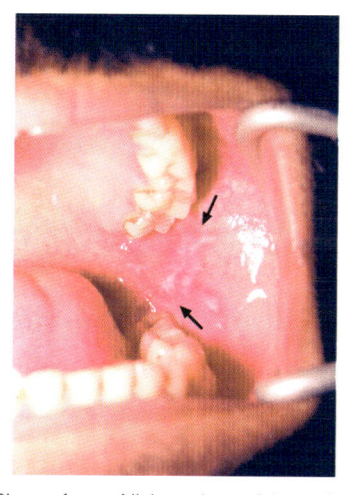

Fig. 11.31: Plaque form of lichen planus (shown by arrows) and patches of leukoplakia on buccal macosa

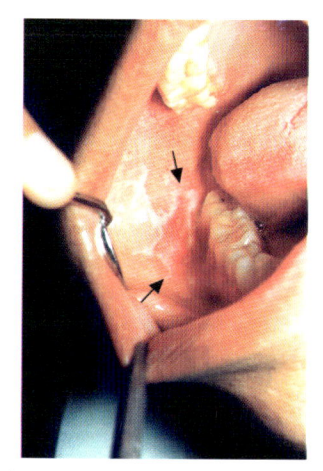

Fig. 11.29: Lichen planus of buccal mucosa (shown by arrows)

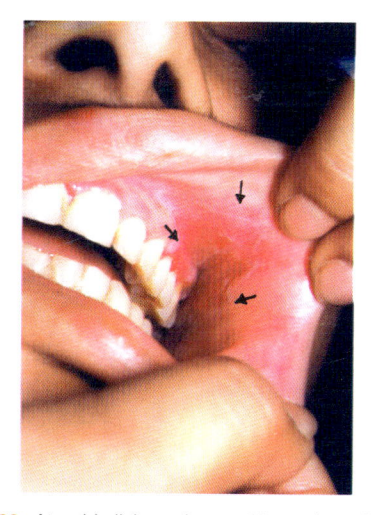

Fig. 11.32: Atrophic lichen planus of buccal vestibule and gingiva (shown by arrows)

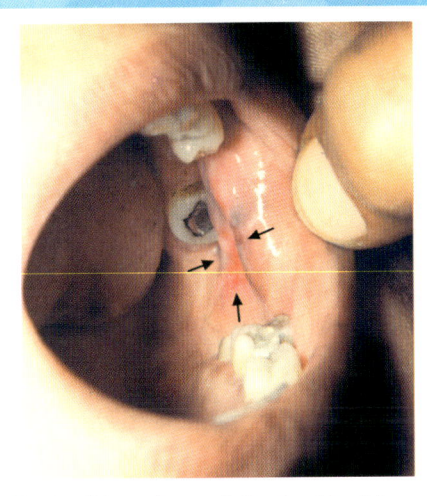

Fig. 11.33: Erosive lichen planus of alveolar ridge (shown by arrows)

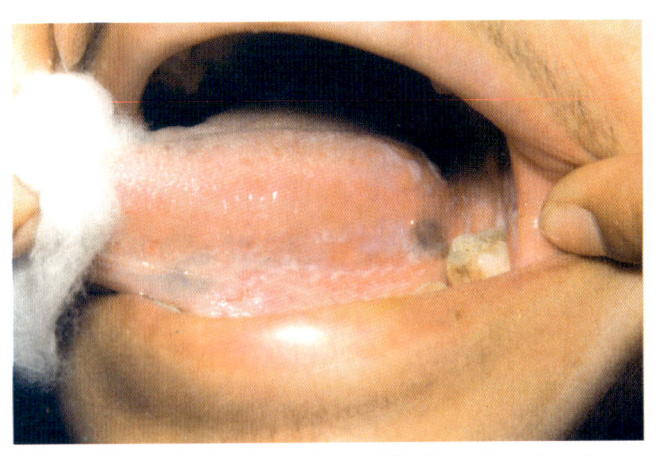

Fig. 11.34: Erosive lichen planus of the floor of mouth and base of the tongue

systemic administration of corticosteroids like Betamethasone and dexamethasone oral 0.5 mg to 5 mg per day or injection 4 to 20 mg i.m., or i.v. inj. of betnesol, betacortril, and dexona may be indicated. Oral tablet 0.5 mg. each and inj. 4 mg/ml (as sod. phosphate), 0.5 mg/ml oral drops 0.1% topical are also available. The lesions of the oral lichen planus are usually too diffuse for surgical removal. Cauterization and cryosurgery can be done for such lesions. Symptomatic treatment can be provided by topical analgesics and topical corticosteroids. Topical corticosteroids also promote the healing of erosive areas. The non-responsive and extensively eroded areas of mucosa can be treated by intralesional injection of steroid in a 50% mixture with lidocaine.

Malignant Potential

About 1.5 to 2 percent of oral lichen planus gets transformed into squamous cell carcinoma. Malignant transformation is seen especially in erosive type of lichen planus which may be due to exposure of deeper layers of the epithelium to the environmental carcinogens. Most of the carcinoma developing in the areas of lichen planus is found on the tongue. Lichen planus exhibiting dysplastic changes is found on the cheek.

Lichenoid reactions: Rarely administration of some drugs etc. produce lichen planus type lesions. Histologically these lesions are similar to lichen planus.

On the following basis lichenoid reactions are clinically differentiated from lichen planus.
a. The lichenoid reactions are associated with the use of a drug, systemic disease, materials used in dentistry or food flavors and edible colors etc.
b. The lichenoid reactions gradually disappear by themselves by discontinuation of the etiological factor. Leukoplakia does not exhibit Lichenoid tissue reaction.

Lichenoid reactions induced by drugs: With lichenoid reactions there will be a history of use of new drug, dental material, food flavour and edible color etc. The reactions can be of oral mucosa and skin. Any drug can produce these reactions but NSAIDs and antihypertensive drugs are more commonly produce these reactions.

Graft-versus-host-disease (GVHD): GVHD is a complex multisystem immunologic phenomenon. It is recognized by interaction of immuno-competent cells from one person (donor) to another person (recipient) who is immuno-deficient and also possesses transplantation isoantigens which are foreign to the graft and may stimulate it. Among all the reactions the epidermal (skin and mucous membrane) reactions are always present in all GVHD. Histologically GVHD resemble oral lichen planus.

Clinical features: There may be mild rash to diffuse severe sloughing and toxic epidermal necrolysis (Lyell's disease). Lyell's disease is a type of erythema multiforme. In this large flaccid bullae develop with detachment of the epidermis in large sheets resulting into the appearance of the scalded skin.

Oral mucous membrane is also affected. Both skin and oral mucosa are affected in chronic GVHD cases. Burning sensation in oral mucosa may be present. Rarely lichenoid lesions may be extensive involving cheeks, tongue, lips, and gingivae. Oral cavity is the mirror showing early oral changes due to transplantation related complications. Most of these infections are opportunistic candida infections.

Red and White Lesions of the Oral Mucosa

Treatment: Strict matching of histocompatibility and careful use of immunosuppressive drugs are essential to present GVHD lesions. Topical corticosteroid and palliative medication heal ulcerations. In resistant lesions ultraviolet A irradiation with oral psoralen is effective. Topical azathioprine suspension is used as oral rinse. After about two minutes of rinsing the solution is swallowed as it is also effective systemically.

Oral Submucous Fibrosis (OSMF)

Oral submucous fibrosis is a chronic disease in which fibrous bands are formed in the oral cavity resulting in restriction of the mouth opening and movement of tongue. It is characterized by juxta-epithelial inflammatory reaction followed by fibroelastic change of the lamina propria with subsequent epithelial atrophy.

Etiology

The exact etiology of the condition is not clearly known. In most of the cases of OSMF, excessive consumption of red chillies or areca nut (betel nut) chewing has been found to be an important etiological factor. Therefore, it is predominantly seen in India, where spices and betel nut are excessively consumed. Other possible etiological factors may be deficiency of vitamin B complex and iron, and immunological disorders.

Clinical Features

The disease is common between 30 to 50 years of age. The patient complains of reduced mouth opening and redness followed by whiteness, ulceration and burning sensation in the mouth. Fibrotic changes are seen in buccal mucosa, retromolar area, soft palate, tongue, pharynx and esophagus. In advanced stage, mucosa loses its resiliency and becomes blanched leading to trismus, difficulty in mastication, speech and swallowing. Leukoplakia and epithelial dysplasia often develop as secondary changes in areas of affected epithelium (Figs 11.16 and 11.35 to 11.37).

Management of OSMF

Patient should stop chewing betel nuts, betels and smoking, and consuming chillies, alcohol and spicy food. The definitive treatment of oral submucous fibrosis includes intralesional injection of hydrocortisone and collagenase to cause fibrinolysis. Systemic corticosteroid therapy can also be administered. If restriction of mouth opening is

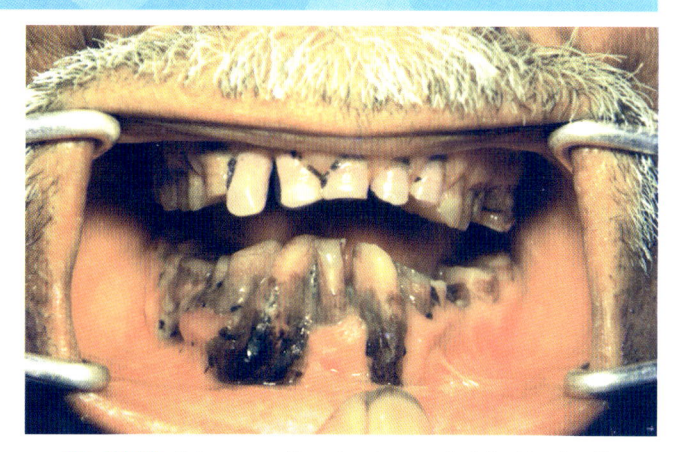

Fig. 11.35: Submucous fibrosis, sharp and attrited teeth with black tartar on the exposed roots

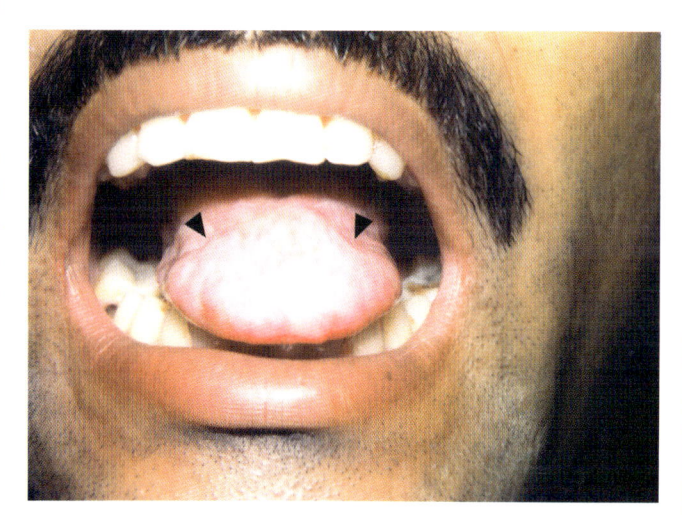

Fig. 11.36: Submucous fibrosis of tongue with restricted protrusion and mouth opening. Keratinization of dorsal surface of anterior one third is seen (shown by arrowheads)

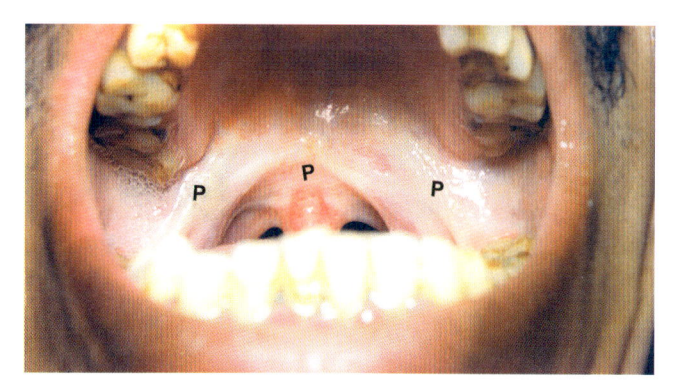

Fig. 11.37: Stomatitis nicotina palati (shown as black palate) and submucous fibrosis of soft palate, tonsillars pillars, (shown as P) retromolar areas and buccal mucosa with restricted mouth opening in a 'chutta' smoker, who keeps the burning end inside the mouth.

present even after the therapeutic treatment, surgical excision of fibrotic bands is carried out. About 7.6 percent of cases of oral submucous fibrosis may undergo malignant transformation hence its early management is very essential.

Prevention of OSMF: For prevention and interception following precautions should be observed.
A. Stoping chewing betelnut and betels.
B. Avoid spicy, chilly and very hot food
C. Elimination of local irritants
D. Use of internal supplements (for interception only) like
   a. Vitamin A 10,000 to 20,000 I.U. daily
   b. Antioxidants
E. Periodical check-up

Therapeutic management: Intralesional injection of the following.
a. Corticosteroid (dexamethasone) and hyaluronidase (hylase) and their combinations.
b. Placental extract
c. Collagenase—Collagenase is an enzyme that catalyzes the degradation of collagen.
d. Chymotrypsin—It is a proteolytic enzyme.

Corticosteroid: Corticosteroid prevent and suppress inflammatory reaction and prevent fibrosis by lowering fibroblastic proliferation and deposition of collagen.

Dosage: Long acting corticosteroid betamethasone (betnesol, betacortril) or dexamethasone [decadron, dexona 4 mg (1 ml)] is injected intralesionally and submucosally at 2 to 4 days intervals for one to four months, as per requirement.

Hyaluronidase: Hyaluronidase (hylase or hynidase) is an enzyme which acts by depolymerizing hyaluronic acid which is an essential component in intercellular ground substance, which detects the permeability of tissues by breaking down hyaluronic acid. It lowers collagen formation and also lowers viscosity of intercellular substance. 1500 IU in 1 ml of 2% lignocaine hydrochloride is injected intralesionally.

Combination: A combination of 4 mg (1 ml) betnesol, 1500 IU (i.v.) hyaluronidase and 1 ml of lignocaine hydrochloride can be injected intralesionally submucously in the fibrous bands at 4 to 8 days interval for one to four months.

Collagenase: Two mg of collagenase in one ml of distilled water is injected in the area of fibrosis at weekly or biweekly intervals. With this a more mouth opening is achieved and burning sensation is also reduced to appreciable extent.

Placental extract (placentre*): Placental extract (placentrex) is an aqueous extract of human placenta. It contains nucleotides such as DNA, RNA, enzymes, alkaline phosphatase etc. vitamins such as B_2, B_6, B_{12}, E, folic acid pentothanic acid etc. It also contain amino acids, steroids, ketosteroids, fatty acids and trace elements. The placental extracts acts as a biogenic stimulator;
It has the following actions.
a. It accelerates cellular metabolism
b. Aids in absorption of exudate
c. Stimulates regenerating process
d. Increases physiological formation of organ or organs.

ORAL MANAGEMENT

Oral iron preparations and topical vitamin A and steroids have also been used with variable results.

Orally following may be given daily or on alternate days for few weeks.
A. Vitamin A 10,000 IU
B. Vitamin B_1, B_6, B_{12}
C. Capsule Antioxidant
D. Capsule vitamin B-complex with zinc and selenium
E. Capsule vitamin E and C

LOCAL APPLICATION

Combination of the following ointments (approximately 200 mg of each) may be applied locally four times a day.
1. Hydrocortisone
2. Metrogyl
3. Chlorhexidine Gluconate
4. Local antibiotics

Surgical management: Surgery is the treatment of choice in patients with very limited mouth opening and in cases where biopsy has shown dysplastic or neoplastic changes. In this same fibrous bands are cut at two places about one cm. apart and middle portion of about one cm long is removed.

Grafting techniques: Split skin graft technique which now a days is usually done has given good results.

Irreversible stomatitis nicotina palati: In the long term in chain smokers and tobacco chewers the palatal mucosa become grey or black. It is called stomatitis nicotina palati. It becomes irreversible and sometimes a premalignant lesion. The chances are more in chronic habitual tobacco chewers and chain smokers of long standing specially of reverse smoking. In reverse smoking the burning end of the smoking rod like cigar, bidi, cigarette, 'chutta' is kept inside the mouth. This habit is popular in the areas where the winds are very fast and/or misty due to which the burning end if kept outside the mouth stops burning. To keep the burning end glowing, the smoker keep it inside the mouth and the other end outside the mouth. Reverse smoking is seen in south American and Asian populations. In this more tar is deposited in the mucosa of the oral cavity specially on palate (Figs 11.37 and 11.38).

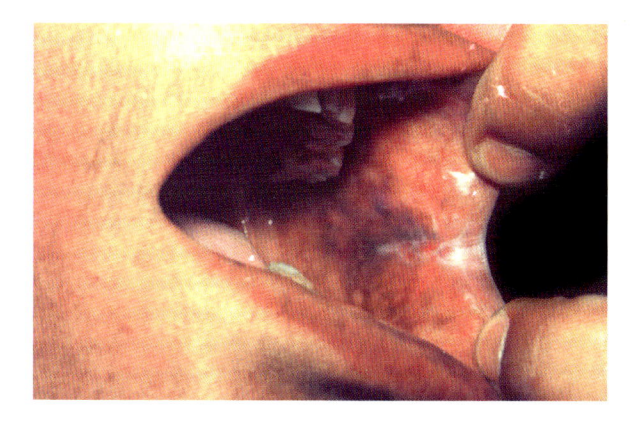

Fig. 11.38: Buccal mucosa of a heavy reverse smoker. Leukoplakia is present at the angle of the mouth. Black stains on buccal mucosa, palate and lower lip are due to smoking

Erythroleukoplakic and premalignant changes take place in the oral mucosa. Histologically, there is hyperkeratosis and acanthosis with squamous metaplasia and hyperplasia of salivary duct opening. These openings clinically appear as slightly elevated papules with punctate red centers which represent inflamed and metaplastically changed minor salivary gland ducts. Rarely atypical or dysplastic changes are seen which show malignant changes.

The abnormal discoloration or elevation in the palate if do not disappear within one month after totally leaving the tobacco chewing or smoking habit, then histological examination should be carried out. Usually all discolorations and elevations must disappear within one month.

No specific treatment is required except antioxidants, multivitamin capsules, warm saline gargle and total discontinuation of the habit.

Lesions Associated with Smokeless Tobacco and Alcohol Use

Cigarettes, cigars and pipes have been the traditional method of tobacco use, but with increased awareness against the hazard of tobacco smoking; use of smokeless tobacco has been increased. Smokeless tobacco like chewing tobacco mixed with betel nut and lime, practice of holding tobacco in the oral vestibule and snuff inhaling are common in India and southeast Asian countries. About 60 to 70% of the oral mucosal white lesions are associated with the use of tobacco.

Tobacco used in the form of snuff, chewing tobacco and placing tobacco rubbed with lime (*Khaini*) in the vestibule is responsible for high rate of oral and pharyngeal cancer. Cigarette smoking combined with chronic snuff inhaling results in localized leukoplakia of vestibule and gingiva which ultimately increases the risk of cancer. Similar mucosal lesions are produced by taking tobacco in the form of 'or along with Paan', '*Khaini*', paste, powder and viscous liquid forms and '*gutkha*' which are popular in India and other countries of the subcontinent.

'*PAAN*' contains a special green leaf, on which paste of slaked lime and catechu made with water are applied. Over these pastes on the pan leaf few small pieces of arecanut, cardamom and tobacco are placed and then paan leaf is wrapped in a small packet form. Paan can also be used without tobacco. This paan packet is kept in the buccal vestibule of one side in the oral cavity and slowly chewed and its juice is sucked.

'Khaini' has been described earlier. 'Gutkha' is a mixture of lime, catechu, cardamom, tobacco, menthol, thymol and other spices in the ground powder form. 'Gutkha' powder is placed in the vestibule of one side of the oral cavity and its juice is slowly sucked for about an hour. Then depending upon the habit fresh 'Gutkha' is placed in the oral cavity. Tobacco mixed with spices in paste, viscous liquid and powder forms is also consumed. Tobacco in fine powder form mixed with or without chemicals and spices is also used in 'snuff' form.

'Gutkha' and tobacco in various forms are consumed several times in a day specially after meals, depending upon the habit of the person.

These various forms of tobacco chewing are associated with verrucous carcinoma of the site where the tobacco quid, '*paan*' or '*gutkha*' is habitually held. Alcohol is considered as oral co-carcinogen particularly in tobacco users.

Oral Lesions Associated with Reverse Smoking

Reverse smoking is the practice of holding burning end of the smoking rod like 'chutta', 'cigarette' or 'bidi' in the mouth, which allows smoking in occupations or localities which are exposed to water spray or/and high winds. Various palatal changes are associated with reverse smoking, possibly caused by high intraoral temperature and combustion products. Ulcerations result from intense heat from the lighted end of smoking rod. Smoke and combustion products result in hyperpigmentation of oral mucosa. Leukoplakia and stomatitis nicotina are also seen associated with reverse smoking which may result into carcinoma of palate (Figs 11.16, 11.37 and 11.38).

Lupus Erythematosus (Systemic and Discoid)

Systemic lupus erythematosus (SLE) causes multiorgan damage. The oral lesions of systemic lupus are similar to discoid lupus. They are usually observed on buccal mucosa. The lesion consists of erythema, ulceration, keratotic plaques and white striae or papules. On taking hot and spicy foods lesions become more painful. Discoid lupus erythematosus (DLE) is present in both localized and disseminated forms. DLE is present on the oral mucosa and skin and has better prognosis than SLE.

Discoid Lupus Erythematosus (DLE)

Discoid lupus erythematosus is an autoimmune disease characterized by keratotic or mixed red and white lesions of the oral mucosa. The oral lesions of discoid lupus erythematosus are slightly elevated, circumscribed white patches surrounded by telangiectatic ring or hale. The early lesions appear as irregular red patches without keratosis. The characteristic appearance of the lesions is alternating red (atrophic), white (keratotic) and red (telangiectatic) zones. The disease may be associated with lichen planus and candida. The majority of lesions occur on the cheeks, labial mucosa, gingival tissue and vermilion border of the lip. Lesions may produce burning sensation during taking hot and spicy food.

Topical and systemic corticosteroid therapy is the treatment of choice.

The skin lesions appear on sun-exposed areas of the face and are red scaly patches. Rarely oral lesions may appear without skin lesion. The oral lesions of DLE are like erosive lichen planus and appear on buccal mucosa, tongue, palate and vermilion border of the lips. Oral lesions of DLE resemble leukoplakia. Hence for confirmation of diagnosis the following must be considered:
a. Clinical appearance of the lesions
b. Co-existence of cutaneous lesions
c. Histological examination
d. Direct immunofluorescence testing

Histopathologic Characteristics

Histological features of oral lesions in discoid form and systemic form are almost similar. In oral lupus there are following changes:

a. Hyperorthokeratosis with keratotic plugs
b. Atrophy of the rete ridges
c. Liquefactive degeneration of the basal cell layer
d. Edema of the superficial lamina propria.
e. Direct immunofluorescence testing of lesional tissue in lupus shows the deposition of various immunoglobulins and C3 in a granular band of basement membrane zone. This is called 'positive lupus band' test. This is absent in discoid lesions.

Malignancy Potential

Rarely squamous cell carcinoma and very rarely basal cell carcinoma may develop in healing scars of discoid lupus erythematous, usually in the presence of other contributory factors. Oral ulcers are mostly present in lupus erythematous. Oral ulcers are observed in SLE patients who have higher level of disease activity.

Developmental White Lesions: Ectopic Lymphoid Tissue

Oral lymphoepithelial cyst which is a cystic ectopic lymphoid issue is rarely observed in the form of small nodules or cysts in several locations. Usually it is observed in the floor of the mouth, ventral surface and lateral border of the tongue, the posterior soft palate, oropharynx and facial tonsillar area. Due to allergy or other inflammatory conditions they become hyperplastic nodules and are diagnosed by clinical features alone. If they become large and cause discomfort biopsy should be taken and removed surgically.

Dyskeratosis Congenita

Dyskeratosis congenita is a well recognized but rare genokeratosis. In this three typical signs are present which are oral leukoplakia, dystrophy of the nails and pigmentation of the skin. And there is high incidence of oral cancer in the young age of about 10 years. Mostly males are affected. It is a rare X-linked disorder.

Treatment

There is no specific treatment for the disease. Careful periodic examinations of patient for malignant transformation of oral lesion must be done.

BIBLIOGRAPHY

1. Bud FZ, Jorgensen E, Mojon P, et al. Effect of an oral health program on the occurrence of oral candidiasis in a long-term care facility. Community Dent Oral Epidemiol 2000;28(2): 141-9.

2. Daley T, Birek C, Wysocki GP, Oral bowenoid lesions. Differential diagnosis and pathogenetic insights. Oral Surg Oral Med Oral Pathol Oral Radiol Enodod 2000;90 (4): 466-73.
3. Guggenheimer J, Moore PA, Rossie, K, et al. Insulin-dependent diabetes mellitus and oral soft tissue pathologies: II Prevalence and characteristics of Candida and candidal lesions. Oral Surg Oral Med Oral Pathol 2000;89(5): 570-6.
4. Horn KA, Gao X, Dino GA, Kamal-Bhal S. Determinants of youth tobacco use in West Virginia: A comparison of smoking and smokeless tobacco use. Am J Drug Alcohol Abuse 2000;26 (1): 125-38.
5. Hashibe M, Mathew B, Kuruvilla B, et al. L Chewing tobacco, alcohol, and the risk of erythroplakia. Cancer Epidemiol Biomarkers Prev 9(7): 639-45, 2000.
6. Khanna JN, Andrade NN. Oral Submucous fibrosis. A new concept in surgical management. Report of 100 cases. Int J Oral Maxillofac Surg 1995;24(6):433-9.
7. Koch P, Bahmer FA. Oral lesions and symptoms related to metals used in dental restorations. A clinical, allergological, and histologic study. J Am Acad Dermatol 1999;41(3pt 1):422-30.
8. Mirbod SM, Ahing SI. Tobacco-associated lesions of the oral cavity. Part I. Nonmalignant lesions. J Can Dent Assoc 2000;66(5):252-6.
9. Rigotti NA, Lee JE, Wechsler H. US college students use of tobacco products. Results of a national survey. JAMA 2000;284(6):699-705.
10. Sciubba JJ. Improving detection of precancerous and cancerous oral lesions. Computer-assisted analysis of the oral brush biopsy. J Am Dent Assoc 1999;130:1445-57.
11. Satish Chandra. Incidence of oral leukoplakia and pan chewing in Varanasi Dental outdoor patients, JIDA 1966;38(6).

12

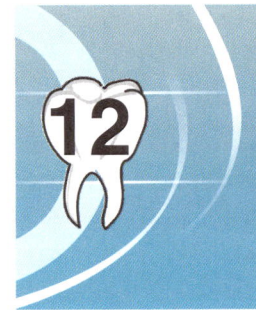

Pigmented Lesions of the Oral Tissues

INTRODUCTION

During the course of disease, the oral mucosal tissues undergoes different types of discolorations. Disease process results into the formation of pseudomembranes, increased keratinization (white lesion), or increased vascularization (red lesion). The various pigmented lesions of the oral mucosa are due to blue, brown and black discolorations of the oral mucosa. These color changes are due to either exogenous or endogenous pigmentations. Endogenous pigmentation of oral mucous membrane is mainly due to melanin, hemoglobin and hemosiderin. Exogenous pigments may be deposited systemically or directly into the submucosa. The sources are silver amalgam, heavy metals and chromogenic bacteria. According to color, configuration and distribution, oral pigmentations can be clinically classified into the following:
1. Brown melanotic lesions
2. Brown heme-associated lesions
3. Blue/purple vascular lesions
4. Gray/black pigmentations.

BROWN MELANOTIC LESIONS

The melanin pigment is derived from tyrosine. Melanin is synthesized in melanocytes. Melanin granules are transferred into adjacent basal cells. When melanocytes over-synthesized or over populate increase in melanin pigment occurs.

Oral Melanotic Macule (Ephelis, Focal Melanosis, Solitary Labial Lentigo)

Oral melanotic macule is the oral counterpart of ephelis or freckle. Ephelis is caused due to increase in melanin pigment synthesis by basal layer melanocytes. The lesion is macular and can be seen on vermilion border of the lower lip. The melanotic macules on the oral mucosa are oval or irregular in shape. They may be brown or black in color and mostly occur on the gingiva, palate and buccal mucosa.

Microscopically, a normal epithelial layer and basal cells containing numerous melanin pigment granules are seen, without proliferation of melanocytes. The oral melanotic macule is harmless and does not predispose to melanoma (Fig. 12.1).

Drug-induced Melanosis

A number of drugs induce oral mucosal pigmentations. These pigmentations may be localized, usually on the hard palate or diffuse, throughout the mouth. The major drugs associated with melanosis are anti malarials like quinoline, hydroxyquinoline, and amodiaquine. Such pigmentation can also be seen in minocycline, drug used in the treatment of acne. Oral contraceptives and pregnancy can occasionally induce hyperpigmentation of facial skin, specially in the perioral region. This condition is referred to as melasma or chloasma.

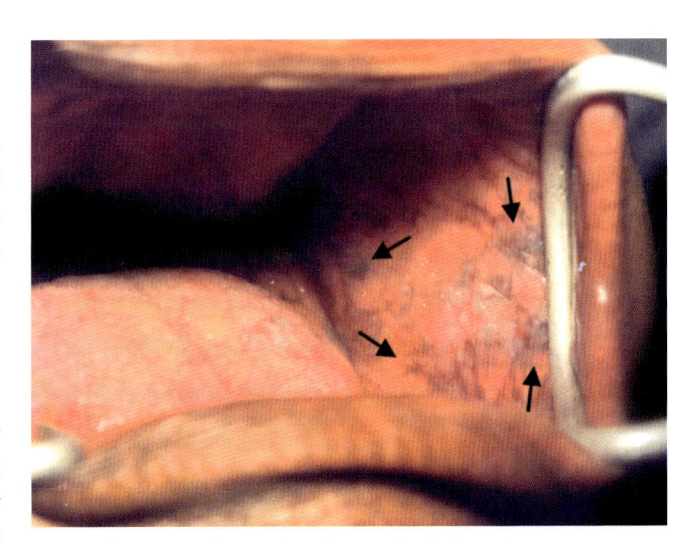

Fig. 12.1: Oral melanotic maculae in buccal mucosa (shown by arrows)

Pigmented Lesions of the Oral Tissues

Malignant Melanoma

Malignant melanomas of oral mucous membrane are very rare. They mostly occur on the anterior labial gingiva and anterior aspect of the hard palate. In the early stage, oral melanomas appear as brown macule and black plaques with an irregular outline. They may be focal or diffuse during early stages, which gradually become more nodular and diffuse.

Excision with wide margins is the treatment of choice. If lesion has metastasized, CT scan and MRI (magnetic resonance imaging) should be done to investigate regional metastasis to the submandibular and cervical lymph nodes. Chemotherapy and immunotherapy can be employed in such condition (Figs 12.2 and 12.3).

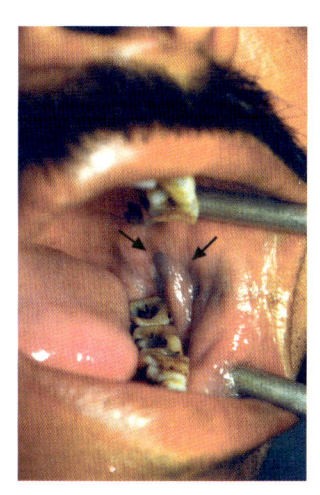

Fig. 12.2: Initial stage of oral melanoma of buccal mucosa (shown by arrows)

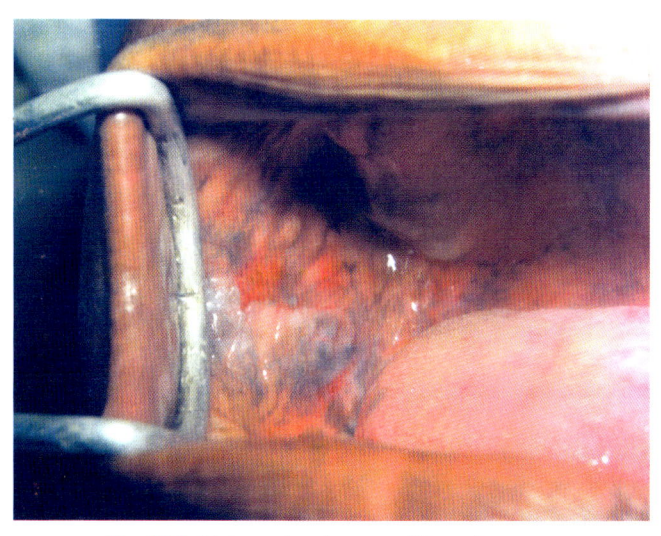

Fig. 12.3: Malignant melanoma of buccal mucosa

Normal Racial or Physiological Pigmentation

Physiological pigmentation occurs as a common characteristic of darker races like negros. There may be diffuse melanosis of the facial gingiva. Tongue and lingual gingiva may exhibit multiple, diffuse and reticulated brown macules. Racial pigmentation usually takes place in childhood (Fig. 12.4).

Smoker's Melanosis

Oral mucosa of smoking rod like cigarette, cigar, bidi smokers and tobacco chewers may show pigmentation due to tobacco products. These pigmentation appear as diffuse macular melanosis of the lips, palate, floor of the mouth, lateral margins of tongue and buccal mucosa, which are referred as "Smoker's melanosis". The lesions are brown, flat and irregular. In dark individuals, who exhibit physiologic pigmentation, tobacco stimulates an increase in oral pigmentation. These lesions have no premalignant potential (Figs 12.5 to 12.7).

Nevocellular and Blue Nevi

Nevi are the benign proliferations of the melanocytes. The two major types of Nevi are nevocellular nevi and blue nevi. Nevocellular nevi arise from basal layer melanocytes, whereas cells of blue nevi are derived neuroectodermally. Nevocellular and blue nevi appear brown in the oral mucosa and may be nodular or macular. They can appear at any age and are most frequently found on palate and gingiva and sometimes on the buccal mucosa and lips. Once they reach a given size, their growth stops and the lesion remains static.

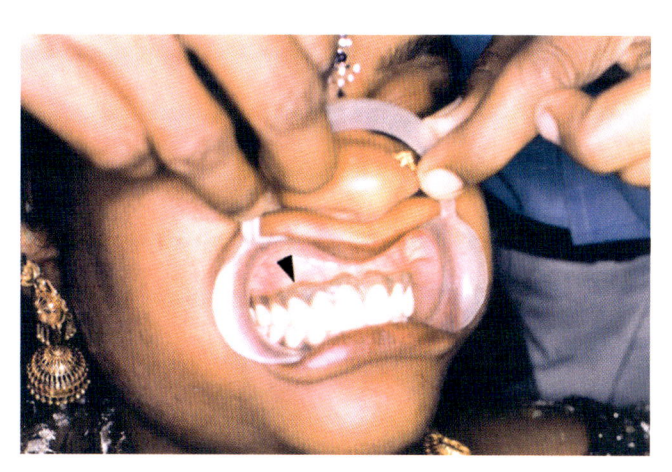

Fig. 12.4: Normal racial or physiological pigmentation (shown by arrowhead)

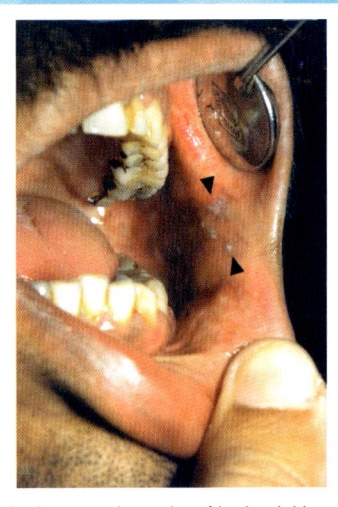

Fig. 12.5: Greyish pigmented specks of leukoplakia on buccal mucosa in the mouth of a chain reverse smoker (shown by arrowheads)

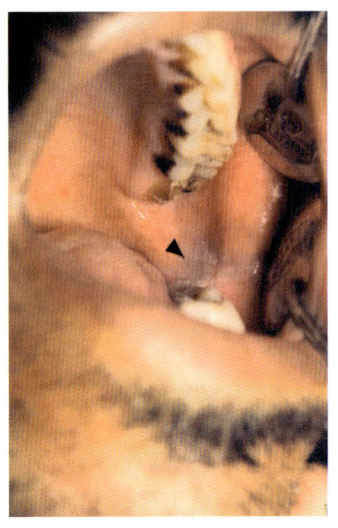

Fig. 12.6: Greyish pigmented leukoplakia of retromolar area in chain smoker (shown by arrowhead)

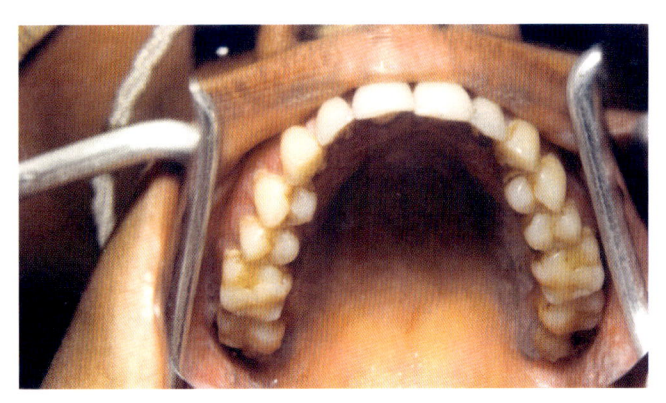

Fig. 12.7: Burnt hard palate of reverse smoker

The treatment of choice is simple excision by surgery or laser.

Endocrinopathic Pigmentation

Pigmentation due to disorder in the function of an endocrine gland is seen in Addison's disease and Cushing's syndrome. The cause of hyperpigmentation in both of these endocrine disorders is the oversecretion of adrenocorticotropic hormone (ACTH), which has melanocytic stimulating properties. The clinical sign of Addison's disease and Cushing's syndrome is patchy melanosis of the oral mucosa. The skin may appear tanned and the gingiva, palate and buccal mucosa may be blotchy. By treatment of endocrine problem pigmentation disappears.

Neurofibromatosis

Neurofibromatosis is an autosomal dominant inherited disease characterized clinically by patches of hyperpigmentation and cutaneous and subcutaneous tumors. The hyperpigmented areas may be present anywhere on the body surface and rarely on oral mucosa, and are called 'café-au-lait' spots. These hyperpigmented areas have the color of coffee with cream and vary from small macule to broad diffuse lesion. Microscopically, café-au-lait spots exhibit basilar melanosis without melanocyte proliferation. Surgical removal is done for cosmatic reasons. Rarely it undergoes malignant changes and require early management.

Peutz-Jeghers Syndrome

In Peutz-Jeghers syndrome, oral pigmentation is a characteristic symptom. The pigmentation is usually seen on the lips, and appears as multiple, focal melanotic brown macules. Such lesions may also occur on the anterior part of tongue, buccal mucosa and mucosal surface of the lips. The macules appear as ephelides or freckles of less than 0.5 cm in diameter. Microscopically, lesions show basilar melanogenesis without melanocytic proliferation. Surgical removal is done for cosmatic reasons. Rarely it undergoes malignant changes and require early management.

HIV-Oral Melanosis

HIV- positive patients may show hyperpigmentation of the skin, nails and mucous membranes. The lesion may appear as diffuse, multifocal and brown macules. The most frequently affected site is buccal mucosa, but palate, tongue and gingiva may also be involved. HIV associated pigmentation is characterized by basilar melanin pigment.

Albright's Syndrome or Café-au-lait Pigmentation

Albright's syndrome is due to endocrine disturbances. Albright's syndrome is associated with polyostotic fibrous dysplasia, bony deformities, precocious puberty and café-au-lait spots on skin. Café-au-lait spots are brown patches of cutaneous pigmentation usually less than six in number, which may be quite large with irregular border. Lips are the common site of pigmentation.

Pigmented Lichen Planus

Lichen planus is a disease which generally presents as a white lesion on the oral mucosa. Sometimes, erosive lichen planus can be associated with diffuse melanosis. The lesion appears as reticulated white patch overlied by brown macular foci. This increase in melanogenesis is stimulated by the infiltrate into the basal layer of T-lymphocytes that contributes to basal cell degeneration.

BROWN HEME-ASSOCIATED LESIONS

Petechiae

Petechiae are the very minute purplish red hemorrhagic spots of pinpoint to pinhead size, which are not blanched by pressure. They are less than 2 mm in diameter. These capillary hemorrhages appear purplish red initially but turn brown in few days due to lysis of extravasated red cells and its degradation into hemosiderin. Disorders of platelet aggregation, idiopathic thrombocytopenic purpura, aspirin toxicity, myelophthistic lesions and myelosuppressive chemotherapy lead to purpura which ultimately leads to petechiae. Most of the oral petechial hemorrhage are seen on soft palate and are caused due to suction. Excessive suction of the soft palate against the posterior tongue is seen in patients of viral or allergic pharyngitis. If petechiae are caused due to suction or trauma, the patient should be instructed to stop the activity which is responsible for causing the lesion. Usally within 2 weeks the lesions disappear.If they fail to disappear, it may be due to hemorrhagic diathesis which should be ruled out by platelet count and platelet aggregation studies.

Ecchymosis

Ecchymosis is a brown irregularly formed patch larger than 3 mm in diameter, caused by extravasation of blood into skin or mucous membrane. The common cause of ecchymosis is trauma and is mostly seen on the lips and face, but occasionally on oral mucosa. Immediately after the trauma, red corpuscles extravasate into the submucosa, which then appears as bright red or blue red macule or swelling if hematoma forms. After few days lesion assumes brown color due to degradation of hemoglobin to hemosiderin. Patients taking anticoagulant drugs may show ecchymosis on cheek or tongue, which usually gets traumatized during mastication (Fig. 12.8).

Hemochromatosis

In hemochromatosis there is deposition of hemosiderin pigment in tissues, organs and skin. It is multifocal pigmentation of oral tissue. It is a disorder of iron metabolism, characterized by excessive absorption of ingested iron and saturation of iron binding protein. It may occur in primary heritable disease or may be secondary to various diseases and conditions like cirrhosis of liver, chronic anemia, porphyria and excess intake of iron either by oral route, by injection or in the form of blood transfusion therapy.

The lesion of hemochromatosis in oral mucosa appears as brown to gray macules and mostly occur on palate and gingiva. As the condition can be the consequence of systemic diseases the physician should be consulted. Treatment include phlebotomy (i.e. removal of blood from the patient) done at regular intervals until the hematocrit returns to normal. If phlebotomy is not possible the iron chelators like deferoxomine are administered parenterally.

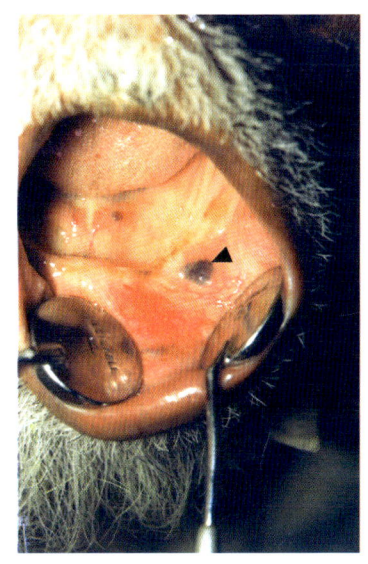

Fig. 12.8: Ecchymosis due to impingement of the denture border (shown by arrowhead)

BLUE/PURPLE VASCULAR LESIONS

Kaposi's Sarcoma

Kaposi's sarcoma is a multifocal malignant neoplasm of putative vascular origin occurring in two different clinical forms (a) in elderly men, in the oral mucosa and on the skin of lower extremities, (b) and in the lymph nodes of children. It is an inactive and painless tumour with slow progressive growth. Kaposi's sarcoma is the most common oral neoplasm to accompany HIV infection. The oral lesions in Kaposi's sarcoma usually appear in hard palate and begin as flat red, blue or purple macules of variable size and irregular configuration. The typical lesions are multifocal with numerous isolated and coalescing plaques. The lesions gradually increase in size to become nodular growth and may cover the entire palate. These oral tumors may be red, blue or purple in color. Hard palate and facial gingiva are the most favored oral site (Fig.12.9).

Microscopically, Kaposi sarcoma lesions show extravasation of red corpuscles and hemosiderin granules. If more hemosiderin is present, tumor will appear more brown.

Treatment of Kaposi's sarcoma depends upon the stage of tumor. The early macular or plaque stage is painless and does not require treatment. Large nodular lesions protruding below the plane of occlusion may interfere in mastication and need electrocauterization or surgical or laser excision followed by coagulative hemostasis. Intralesional injection of 1% sodium tetradecyl sulfate may be given for necrosis of the swelling. This injection is very painful and patient should be on analgesic before injection. One percent vinblastine sulfate intralesional injection is beneficial and cause very less pain as it is not a sclerosing agent. Multiple biweekly intralesional injections of 1% vinblastine sulfate can be given to eradicate the tumor. The dose of Vinblastine is 0.1 to 0.15 mg per. kg. body weight IV injection, weekly 3 doses.

Hemangioma

Hemangioma is a tumor of dilated blood vessels. Hemangioma may be a congenital anomaly, in which proliferation of blood vessels leads to a mass that resembles a neoplasm. They arise in childhood and are found on the skin, in the scalp and within the connective tissue of mucous membrane. They may also occur within muscles, so-called intramuscular hemangiomas. Most of the hemangiomas are raised and nodular, some may be flat, macular and diffuse. The color of hemangioma depends upon the depth of vascular proliferation within the oral submucosa, the lesion close to the overlying epithelium appear reddish blue, or if it is present deeper in the connective tissue, it will be a deep blue.

Most oral hemangiomas are located on tongue and may extend deeply between its intrinsic muscle. Tongue hemangiomas are multinodular and bluish red in color. The other common sites for hemangioma in children are lip and buccal mucosa, where it appears blue, raised and localized. Most hemangiomas get blanched under pressure, but if intraluminal clots are formed within the lesion, they become palpable and will usually not blanch. Most of the congenital hemangiomas undergo spontaneous regression at a relatively early age. Cases which do not show such remission may be treated by surgery, either conventional or laser or cryosurgery. Intramuscular and large-sized hemangiomas may be treated by administration of intralesional injection of sclerosing agents such as 1% sodium tetradecyl sulfate. These agents cause post injection pain, which should be controlled with a moderate level of analgesic such as aspirin with codeine. Subcutaneous tattooing or organ laser is used to treat cutaneous port-wine stains (Fig. 12.10).

Sturge-Weber Syndrome (Disease) (Encephalotrigeminal Angiomatosis)

Sturge-Weber syndrome is a rare congenital vascular condition. In this there are seizures. Sometimes angiomatous lesions also involve the gingiva and buccal mucosa along

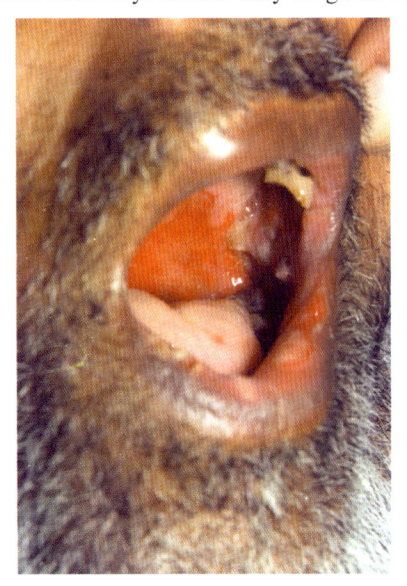

Fig. 12.9: Kaposi's sarcoma with pemphigus vulgaris having reddish purple irregular macule on the palatal mucosa and erosion on the lips in a HIV seropositive patient

Pigmented Lesions of the Oral Tissues

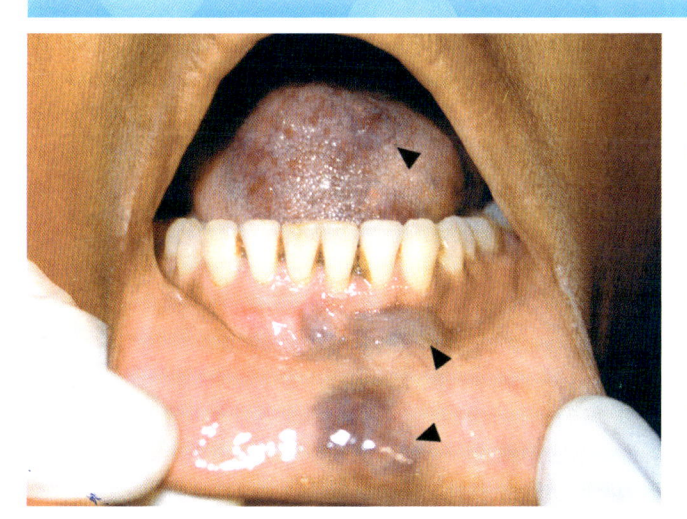

Fig. 12.10: Hemangioma of tongue, lip and gum (shown by arrowheads)

with facial lesions. Treatment is neurosurgical and anticonvulsant drugs.

Varices

Varices or varicosities refer to a condition characterized by pathologic dilation of veins or venules. Varicosities tend to occur in adults and aged persons. In the oral tissues, chief site of involvement is ventral portion of the tongue. They appear as tortuous blue, red and purple elevation over the ventrolateral surface of the tongue. They are usually painless and do not rupture and bleed.

A focal dilation of vein is known as varix. They are mostly located on the lower lip. They appear as focal raised pigmentation of blue, red or purple color with lobulated or nodular surface mucosa. Varix arises in older individuals and once formed, does not usually regress. Varix may result from trauma, such as lip and cheek biting.

Though varices are painless and of no clinical consequence, they may sometimes interfere with mastication and require excision either by conventional surgery, electrosurgery, cryosurgery and laser. One percent sodium tetradecyl sulfate injected with a tuberculin syringe intralesionally into the lumen is effective but more painful than simple excision. Hence strong analysis should be done before injection.

Hereditary Hemorrhagic Telangiectasia

Hereditary hemorrhagic telangiectasia is a genetically transmitted disease, inherited as an autosomal dominant trait. The onset of the disease is usually after puberty but may also be seen during infancy. The lesion appears as round or oval purple papule measuring less that 0.5 cm in diameter. Hundreds of such purple papules may be present on tongue, buccal mucosa and vermilion and mucosal surfaces of the lips. The facial skin, neck and nasal mucosa may also be involved.

There is no treatment. For cosmetic reasons telangiectatic areas may be removed under LA by electrocautery or laser.

Angiosarcoma

Angiosarcoma is vascular neoplasm not associated with HIV, hence it is different from Kaposi's sarcoma. It can arise anywhere in the body from blood or lymph vessel but rarely in oral cavity. It appears red, blue or purple colored nodular tumors. Treatment is radical excision and prognosis is poor.

GREY/BLACK PIGMENTATIONS

Heavy Metal Ingestion

A number of metallic compounds like lead, mercury and bismuth were used medicinally many years ago. These heavy metals or metal salts are used in industries, which leads to occupational hazards. Heavy metals may also result in oral pigmentation as they get deposited in oral tissues if ingested either in sufficient quantities or for a long period of time.

Lead

Exposure to lead results in a condition called "plumbism" or "saturnism". Exposure may be through paints, medicaments, cooking vessels or industries. Oral manifestations are metallic taste, excessive salivation and a grey-black line along the gingival margin. Lead ingestion is also associated with systemic symptoms of toxicity like lead encephalopathy, peripheral neuritis and gastrointestinal disturbances.

Mercury

Mercury poisoning or mercurialism is caused by ingestion or inhalation of mercury or mercury compounds due to occupational exposure or use of drugs containing mercury. Mercury poisoning is associated with increased salivation, metallic taste, ulceration of the mouth and loosening of teeth. The pigmentation is usually found along the free marginal gingiva due to deposition of the dark sulfide compound.

Bismuth

Bismuth was once used for the treatment of syphilis, but it has been replaced by antibiotics. The metal is still used in treating dermatologic disorders. The oral manifestation is characterized by bismuth pigmentation of the oral mucosa, particularly of gingival and buccal mucosa. The pigmentation appears as narrow blue-black line along the gingival margin. Pigmentation may also be seen on buccal mucosa, lips and ventral surface of the tongue.

Silver

Chronic exposure to silver compound may lead to condition called argyria. It results in permanent pigmentation of skin and mucous membrane due to silver compounds. The pigmentation of oral mucous membrane is dispersed throughout the oral cavity and appears bluish gray.

Amalgam Tattoo

Amalgam tattoo is the most common source of focal pigmentation in the oral mucosa. The pigmentation appears as bluish gray or black macules on buccal mucosa, gingiva or palate. It is relatively common finding in dental practice and generally occurs due to iatrogenic consequences. The amalgam particles may get deposited into mucosa lacerated by dentist's bur during removal of old amalgam restorations. It may also get deposited in oral tissue from amalgam particles introduced into a socket or beneath periosteum during tooth extraction and entering a surgical wound during root canal treatment with retrograde amalgam filling. Silver amalgam tattoos are harmless, so their removal is not required.

Graphite Tattoo

Graphite tattoo is commonly seen on the palate of school going children. It is caused due to traumatic implantation of lead from pencil. The lesion appears as focal gray or black macules.

Hairy Tongue

Hairy tongue is an unusual condition of unknown etiology characterized by hypertrophy of the filiform papillae. The lesion usually involves the middle and posterior one-third of the dorsum of the tongue. The hyperplastic papillae get pigmented by colonization of chromogenic bacteria that gives various colors ranging from green to brown to black. The papillae often show staining from coffee, tea and tobacco.

Hairy tongue is a benign condition. Food debris may collect deep between the papillae and produce irritation of the tongue. Treatment consists of brushing the tongue to promote desquamation and debris removal. Use of tea, coffee and tobacco should be avoided (Figs 12.11 and 12.12).

MISCELLANEOUS CONDITIONS

Carotenemia

Carotenemia is a rare condition characterized by generalized yellowish discoloration of skin and oral mucous membrane. It is due to increased quantities of carotene in the blood, due to high intake of food containing carotene pigments,

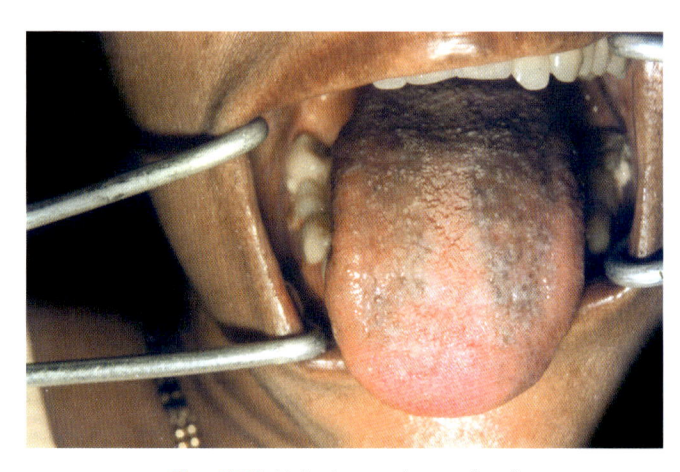

Fig. 12.11: Hairy tongue (generalized)

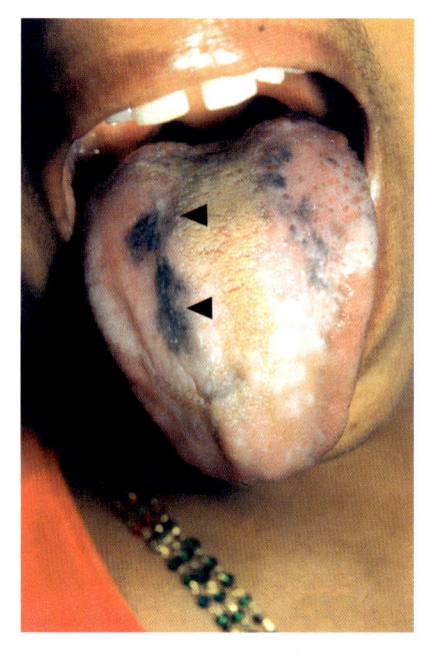

Fig.12.12: Hairy tongue (localized patches) (shown by arrowheads)

such as carrots. Other conditions that may cause yellowish discoloration are hyperlipemia, nephritis, diabetes mellitus, hypothyroidism and conditions associated with impaired conversion of carotene to vitamin A.

Bilirubin Pigmentation

Jaundice is yellow discoloration of the skin and mucous membrane with bile pigments. It results when the serum bilirubin level exceeds 2 to 3 mg/dl. The yellow discoloration in the oral cavity is more pronounced on the buccal mucosa and palate.

BIBLIOGRAPHY

1. Doval DC, Rao CR, Saitha KS, et al. Malignant melanoma of the oral cavity. Report of 14 cases from a regional cancer centre. Eur J Surg Oncol 1996;22:245-9.
2. Eisen D, Hakim MD. Minocycline-induced pigmentation. Incidence. Prevention and management. Drug Saf 1998;18:413-40.
3. Kleinegger CL, Hammond HL, Finkelstein MW. Oral Mucosal hyperpigmentation secondary to antimalarial drug therapy Oral Surg Oral Med Oral Pathol Oral Radiol Endod 2000;90:189-94.
4. Nandapalan V, Roland NJ, Helliwell TR, et al. Mucosal melanoma of the head and neck. Clin Otolaryngol 1998;23:107-16.
5. Peters E, Gardner DF. A method of distinguishing between amalgam and graphite in tissue. Oral Surg Oral Med Oral Pathol 1986;62:73.

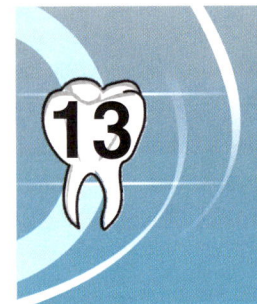

Benign Oral Tumors

INTRODUCTION

Stedman's medical dictionary describes benign tumor as the "tumor that does not metastasize and does not invade and destroy adjacent normal tissue". According to Mosby's dental dictionary "benign tumor is a neoplasm unable to metastasize". However, benign tumor is a non-malignant swelling or enlargement that does not transfer from one organ or part of the body to another.

NORMAL STRUCTURAL VARIATIONS

Structural variations of jaw bones and oral soft tissues are sometimes mistaken as tumors. Ectopic lymphoid nodules and tori are the examples of such structural variants.

Tori

Tori are the localized nodular enlargement that occur frequently on the cortical bone of the palate (torus palatinus) and jaws (torus mandibularis). Histologically they consist of layers of dense cortical bone covered by a thin epithelium with less rete pegs development. Tori may cause problem in the construction of dentures. Due to their prominent position and thin epithelial covering they are frequently traumatized and resulting ulcers are slow to heal. Sometimes tori on the palate or lingual mandibular ridge may become very large to interfere with eating and speaking (Fig. 7.17).

Ectopic Lymphoid Nodules

Ectopic lymphoid nodules or "Oral tonsils" are small, slightly reddish nodular elevations of a localized area of the oral mucosa.

INFLAMMATORY (REACTIVE) HYPERPLASIAS

Inflammatory hyperplasia is a commonly occurring nodular growth of the oral mucosa histologically resembling inflammatory granulation tissue. The major etiological factor for the lesions is chronic trauma which may be produced by calculus, fractured teeth, ill fitting dentures and overhanging dental restorations. Most of the inflammatory hyperplasia are subjected to continuous masticatory trauma and usually get ulcerated and hemorrhagic.

These inflammatory hyperplasia may appear swollen, distended and red to purple due to dilated blood vessels, acute and chronic inflammatory exudates and localized abscesses.

Fibrous Inflammatory Hyperplasia

Fibrous inflammatory hyperplasias may appear on any surface of the oral mucous membrane. They are identified as follows.

Oral Squamous Papilloma

Squamous papillomas are inflammatory hyperplasia which are either sessile or pedunculated and keratinized. Recently it has been proved as a virus induced benign growth, hence described under as the same heading (Fig. 13.1).

Fibroma

Fibroma are the inflammatory hyperplasias which are sessile, firm and covered by thin squamous epithelium. On gingiva the similar lesion is called epulis. Most of the epulis remain smaller than 1 cm in diameter except the epulis fissuratum. Rarely epulis is large and pedunculated (Fig. 13.2).

Treatment and prognosis: Fibroma or fibrous inflammatory hyperplasias are benign and do not have any malignant potential. Their etiology is a chronic irritation. Surgical or laser excision is successful if etiological chronic irritation

Benign Oral Tumors

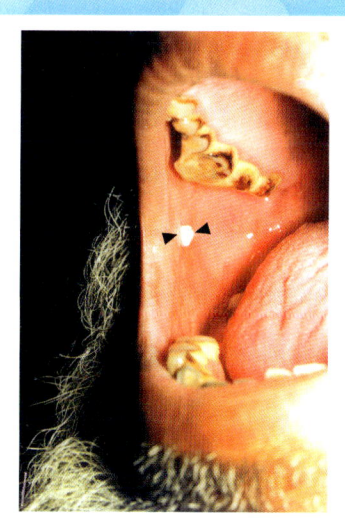

Fig. 13.1: Papilloma of buccal mucosa (shown by arrowheads)

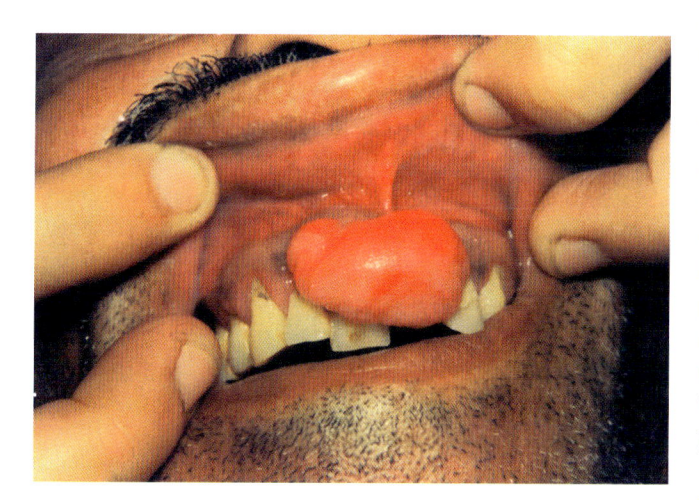

Fig. 13.2: Very large pedunculated midline epulis or fibroma

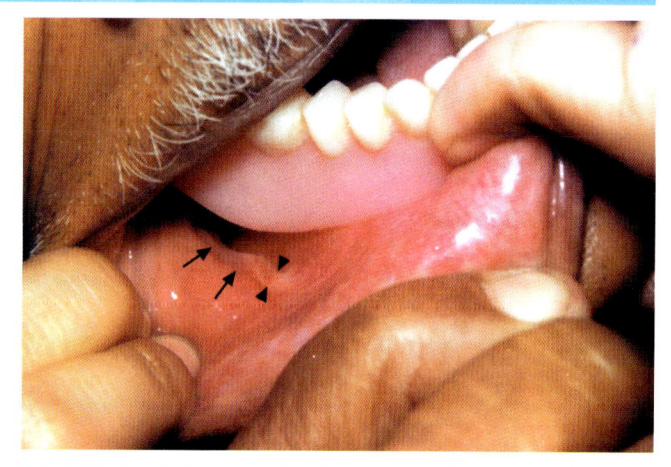

Fig. 13.3: Epulis fissuratum is a fibrous hyperplasia due to impinging denture border (shown by arrow). An ulcer is also present (shown by arrowheads)

is also removed. Microscopic examination of the excised tissue must be carried out to confirm the benign nature of the lesion. Very rarely there are reports of squamous cell carcinoma due to chronic irritation by denture but as a precautionary step all excised tissues must be histologically examined.

Epulis Fissuratum

Epulis fissuratum occurs in the tissues at the periphery of ill-fitting dentures in which the overgrowth of tissue is split by edge of denture. Approximately half part of the lesion lies under the denture and other part between the lips or cheek and outer denture surface (Fig. 13.3).

Treatment: Treatment is removal of the chronic irritation and surgical or laser excision of the overgrowth of the tissues.

Pulp Polyp

Pulp polyp (chronic hyperplastic pulpitis) is a hyperplastic granulation tissue growing out of the exposed pulp chamber of grossly decayed teeth which fills the cavity in the tooth. Fibrous inflammatory hyperplasias have no malignant potential. They mostly do not recur after excision unless the source of chronic irritation is not eliminated. All the fibrous inflammatory hyperplasias of the oral cavity should be treated by local excision. The excised tissue must be histologically examined to confirm the benign nature.

Pyogenic Granuloma

Pyogenic granuloma is an elevated, pedunculated or sessile mass of highly vascularised granulation tissue with a smooth, lobulated or warty surface, which frequently gets ulcerated and shows tendency for hemorrhage. It occurs most frequently on gingiva and has a strong tendency to recur after excision.

As they are located close to gingival margin, calculus and overhanging margins of dental restoration are thought to be an important etiological irritant. They must be eliminated when the lesion is excised. Pyogenic granuloma may get mature and become more collagenous and less vascular, gradually converting into a fibrous epulis. The treatment of pyogenic granuloma includes elimination of sublingual irritants and gingival pockets throughout the mouth, as well as excision of the gingival growth (Fig.13.4).

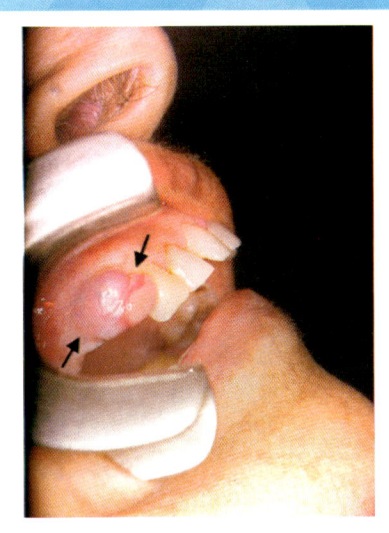

Fig. 13.4: Pyogenic granuloma partially covering maxillary right lateral incisor and fully covering canine and first and second premolar teeth (shown by arrows)

Treatment: Surgical or laser excision.

Pseudoepitheliomatous Hyperplasia

It is a common benign proliferation of the oral epithelium, in which there is marked increase and downgrowth of epidermal cell. The rete pegs are extended in an irregular manner deep into the underlying connective tissue. Pseudoepitheliomatous hyperplasia is treated by local excision along with elimination of chronic initiating irritant.

Peripheral and Central Giant Cell Granuloma

Giant cell granuloma is the non-neoplastic lesion characterized by the proliferation of granulation tissue containing numerous multinucleated giant cells. It occurs either as peripheral exophytic lesion on the gingiva and alveolar mucosa or as a centrally located lesion within the jaw, skull or facial bones. These lesions are highly vascularized and present as soft, red-blue hemorrhagic nodular swelling.

Central giant cell granuloma occurs predominantly anterior to the first molar in the mandible. Peripheral are five times more common than central giant cell granulomas. Increased level of parathormone in primary and secondary hyperthyroidism stimulates the occurrence of these lesions.

Treatment of giant cell granuloma includes conservative surgical treatment (curettage). Recurrent giant cell lesion should be treated by repeat curettage or curettage with cryosurgery of the walls of bony cavity. In 12 to 37 % recurrence cases repeat curettage is required which usually prevents further recurrence. Rarely some lesions behave aggressively in which segmental jaw resection with a margin of normal tissue is required.

Palatal Papillomatosis (Palatal Papillary Hyperplasia)

Palatal papillomatosis is a common lesion occurring on the hard palate due to chronic denture irritation caused by 'relief areas' or 'suction chambers'. The lesion appears as numerous, closely arranged, red, edematous papillary projection involving nearly all the hard palate. It is usually associated with denture-sore mouth (stomatitis) due to chronic candidal infection. In candidal infection, the lesions of palatal papillary hyperplasia appear as red, swollen, tightly packed projections. Such lesions are friable, often bleed with minimal trauma and may be having thin whitish exudate.

It occurs in 3 to 4% of denture wearers. Discontinuing the use of the ill-fitting dentures or construction of new dentures without surgical removal of the excess tissue generally results in regression of the edema and inflammation, but the papillary hyperplasia persists. Electrocauterization, cryosurgery or laser surgery prior to new denture construction return the mouth to normal state.

When florid papillomatous of the palate is observed and persists in nondenture users, the differential diagnosis should also include several granulomatous diseases which appear in this fashion. This must be done when papillary lesions are white in color and extend over the alveolar mucosa. These diseases include infectious granulomas, Cowden's syndrome and verrucous carcinoma.

Benign Lymphoid Hyperplasia

As a result benign (reactive) processes and lymphoid neoplasms, uncapsulated lymphoid tissues which are normally present in the oral cavity become enlarged. This lymphoid tissue is normally present on the soft palate, foliate papillae on the posterolateral aspects of the tongue dorsum.

Uncapsulated lymphoid aggregates which are normally present on the soft palate, the foliate papillae on the posterolateral aspects of the dorsum of the tongue and the anterior tonsillar pillar in the oral cavity increase in size due to benign processes and form benign lymphoid neoplasms.

HAMARTOMAS

(Hamartion = a bodily defect,+ oma = tumor). Hamartoma means a tumor like bodily defect. Hamartoma is a tumor

Benign Oral Tumors

like growth. It is benign self limiting new growth of normal tissues. Hamartoma is a focal malformation resembling a neoplasm, but results from faulty development in an organ. Hamartomas are hereditary malformations. Oral hamartomas usually occur along with other developmental abnormalities.

It is characterized by the presence of particular histologic tissues in improper proportions or distribution with prominent excess of one type of tissue. Hamartomas are usually congenital and once they achieve their full size, they do not extend to involve more tissue. Neoplastic and malignant transformation and compression on the adjacent tissues like tumor are unusual in hamartomas.

Hemangioma

Hemangioma is a common benign tumor characterized by proliferation of blood vessels. It may be present at all sites in the oral cavity and face and may involve deeper structures like salivary glands, muscles, facial bones and jaw, temporomandibular joint, mucous membrane and skin. They appear as red patches or birthmarks and may occur as isolated lesions in the oral cavity or multiple lesions affecting different parts of body. Two main histological types commonly described are capillary hemangioma and cavernous hemangioma. Capillary hemangioma consists of small proliferating blood capillaries whereas cavernous hemangioma consists of large, dilated blood pools. In both the types, the vessels are lined by single layer of endothelial cells with little connective tissue stroma. Hemangioma of oral mucosa and skin usually consists with similar lesions of CNS and meninges.

Most of the hemangiomas are present from birth which gradually increase in size with body growth. On palpation, large lesions are warm and pulsatile. Such lesions may bleed profusely on trauma or during damage to epithelium.

Centrally located hemangioma occurs in either maxilla or mandible and care should be taken during taking of biopsy or excising such lesion because of their tendency of excessive bleeding and also due to difficulty of knowing their extent into bone. CT scan, conventional and doppler ultrasound, microangiography should be used to know the extent of lesion (Fig. 13.5).

Hemangioma can be treated in the following ways:
A. Conventional surgery
B. Cryosurgery and laser surgery
C. Injection of sclerosing solution
D. Intravascular embolization with plastic spheres
E. Intralesional corticosteroid therapy

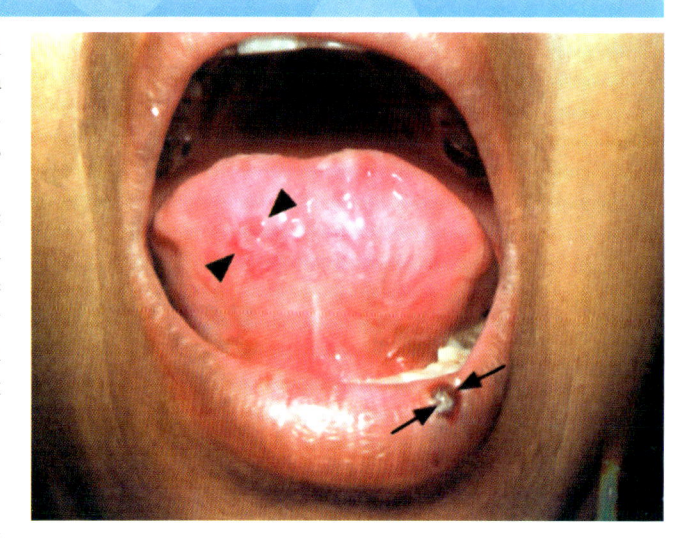

Fig. 13.5: Small hemangioma on lower lip (shown by arrows), macroglossia and ulcer on tongue tip (shown by arrowheads)

Lymphangioma

Lymphangioma is a benign tumor of lymphatic vessels. It is like hemangioma but the abnormal vessels are filled with a clear, protein rich fluid containing lymph rather than blood. Lymphangioma may occur alone or in association with hemangioma or other anomalous blood vessels with which the lymphangiomatous vessels are anastomosed. Oral lymphangioma clinically appear as a racemose surface.

The intraoral lymphangioma most commonly occurs on the tongue but is also seen on palate, buccal mucosa, gingiva and lips. An unusual form of lymphangioma termed alveolar lymphangioma occurs on the alveolar mucosa of the neonates, which disappears spontaneously with chewing and tooth eruption. Large sized lymphangioma spreading into the neck is referred to as cystic hygroma. The management of lymphangioma is like that of hemangioma.

Granular Cell Tumor

Granular cell tumor is an important oral hamartomatous lesion, as it frequently occurs as a nodule on the dorsum of the tongue and on the gingiva in its variant form or other mucosal site. These lesions are composed of large eosinophilic, granular cells interspersed with a collagenous stroma.

Most of the granular cell tumors occur on the tongue but may occasionally occur on the palate, floor of mouth, buccal mucosa and lips. Treatment of these lesions both on tongue and other extralingual sites is by simple excision.

Neurofibroma

Neurofibroma is the most common benign tumor of nerve tissue, arising from the perineural fibroblasts. It may occur as solitary lesion or multiple lesions associated with neurofibromatosis. Solitary neurofibroma is an innocuous lesion but multiple neurofibromas have tendency to develop sarcoma. It occurs as small, asymptomatic nodule mostly on tongue, floor of mouth and buccal mucosa. Histologically neurofibroma is composed of a proliferation of delicate spindle cells with thin, wavy nuclei intermingled with neuritis in an irregular pattern as well as delicate, intertwining connective tissue fibrils. Neurofibromas are treated by surgical excision or laser and usually do not recur.

Neurilemmoma (Schwannomas; Neuro-Lemmoma; Perineural Fibroblastoma; Neurinoma; Lemmoma)

Neurilemmoma are the benign neoplasm arising from the Schwann cells of the nerve sheath. The lesion is usually single, circumscribed, painless nodule of varying size. The common site of occurrence are the tongue, palate, floor of mouth, buccal mucosa, gingiva and lips.

Histologically neurilemmoma is same as neurofibroma, but it also exhibits palisading of nuclei and organoid nuclei which are absent in neurofibroma. The treatment of neurilemmoma is surgical excision.

Melanoameloblastoma

Melanoameloblastoma or melanotic neuroectodermal tumor of infancy is a rare tumor of neuro-ectodermal origin, usually occurring in children under six months of age. It occurs in both intraoral and extraoral sites but most often involves the anterior maxilla of infants. Melanoameloblastoma presents clinically as rapidly growing blue-black lesion which may protrude into the mouth causing elevation of upper lip and thus prevents suckling.

Histologically, it shows cuboidal or slit like spaces lined by melanin containing epithelial cells. It is treated by conservative surgical excision.

Dermoid/Epidermoid/Sebaceous Cyst

Dermoid cyst a type of cystic teratoma arising mainly from embryonic germinal epithelium. Rarely it also contain structures of other germ layers. These cysts are derived from epithelial remnants in the midline during closure of the mandibular and hyoid branchial branches. When it contain fat and arise from sebaceous gland it is also called as sebaceous cyst.

Dermoid cyst is an inclusion cyst found in face, neck, floor of mouth and in submaxillary and sublingual areas. These cysts are derived due to cystic degeneration of epithelium trapped in these tissues during closure of mandibular and hyoid branchial arches. These cysts contain keratin and sebaceous material in cyst cavity and epidermal tissues, hair follicle, sweat and sebaceous glands in the cyst wall. These lesions are not neoplastic.

Clinical Features

The epidermoid cyst mainly occurs in young adulthood in both sexes, because of increased glandular secretory activity of the trapped epithelium. Usually dermoid cyst produce a bulge in the floor of the mouth resulting difficulty in eating and talking. It may also arise below the mylohyoid muscle. It feels like a 'dough' on palpation. Its size is usually several centimeter in diameter. Rarely these cysts become infected they may develop a sinus. Very rarely they become malignant.

The following lesions resemble with dermoid cyst. (a) ranula (b) branchial cleft cyst (c) blockage of Whartson's duct of submandibular salivary gland (d) cystic hygroma (e) acute infection of the floor of the mouth (f) thyroglossal tract cyst (g) tumors of the floor of the mouth (h) infection of submandibular and sublingual salivary gland (Figs 13.6 and 13.7).

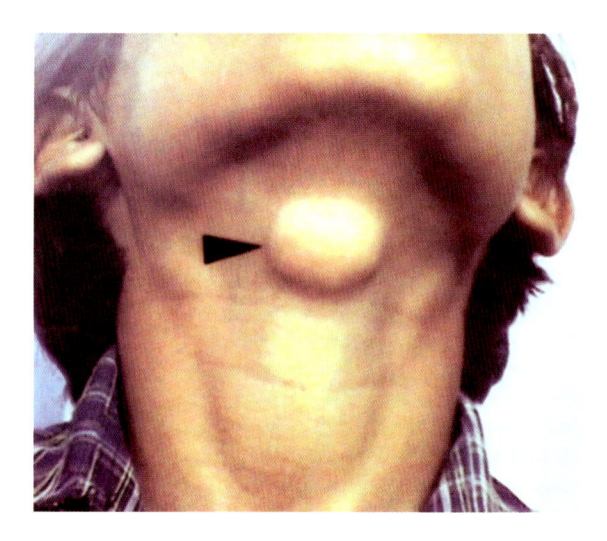

Fig. 13.6: Dermoid cyst of midline (shown by arrowhead) (*Courtesy* Dr. Rohit Chandra, Noida)

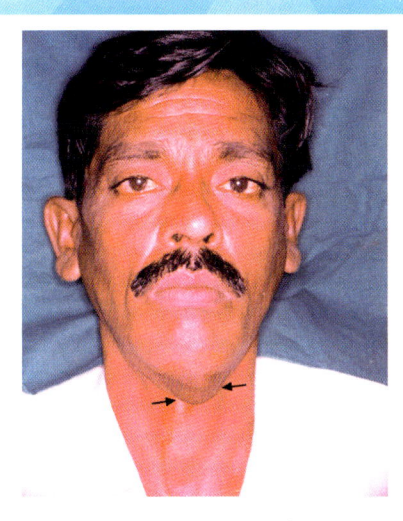

Fig. 13.7: Implantational sebaceous (dermoid) cyst in submental region, front view (shown by arrows) (*Courtesy* Dr. Rohit Chandra, Noida)

Treatment and Prognosis

Dermoid cysts are removed surgically. Recurrence is very rare. Rarely transformation to squamous cell carcinoma may take place. Dermoid cysts which are above the geniohyoid muscle can be removed intraorally and those below the geniohyoid muscle require an extraoral approach.

Fibrous Dysplasia of Bone

Fibrous dysplasia of bone is one of the most complicated diseases of osseous tissue. It results from disturbances in the development of bone forming mesenchyme, due to which bone undergoes physiologic lysis and is replaced by fibrous tissue. The bones of face and jaws are frequently involved. The lesion often acquires large size, resulting in asymmetric distortion and expansion of bone. It occurs more in maxilla and less in mandible.

It may be confined to a single bone (monostotic fibrous dysplasia) or may have many bones affected (polyostotic fibrous dysplasia). The former type is more common than latter. Technetium Tc-99 m bone scans and computed tomography provide great help in diagnosing the extent of lesions of fibrous dysplasia.

Surface contouring of the affected bone, curettage of bony cavity and packing with bone chips are the mode of treatment.

Ossifying Fibroma

Ossifying fibroma occur more often in mandible than maxilla. Histologically it is like fibrous dysplasia, both are slow growing and occur in young age. Fibrous dysplasia grow endosteally following general structure of affected bone, mostly producing irregular thickening of the bone. Ossifying fibroma grows by destroying surrounding bone and fills cavities like nasal cavity and accessory sinuses.

Ossifying fibromas are treated by surgical enucleation. Juvenile aggressive types are treated by enbloc resection.

ANEURYSMAL BONE CYST, TRAUMATIC BONE CYST AND STATIC BONE CYST

These cysts rarely occur in jaws, more in mandible than in maxilla in younger age groups (upto 30 years of age). These cysts involve both the sexes equally. For treatment of all these cysts a through curettage of the lesion with its walls and then packing with the bone chips result in the healing of the defect.

Teratomas and Dermoid Cysts

Teratomas are neoplasms which are composed of a combination of tissues and more than one of these tissues show neoplastic proliferation. They are congenitally acquired. Mainly they are found in ovary. Rarely they are found in oral cavity or protruding into the oral cavity from the base of the skull in children. In new born infants in which teratomas arise from base of the skull and extend into cranial cavity and oral cavity rarely survive. Dermoid cysts are mostly found in the floor of the mouth. Surgical or laser excision is the treatment of choice.

Cherubism

Cherubism is a rare fibroosseous disease of the jaws of children. It is of genetic nature. It is characterized by swollen jaws, missing or displaced teeth and raised eyes. Radiographically lesions show multiple well defined multilocular radiolucencies in the mandible and maxilla. Cherubism progresses rapidly in childhood but become static and may even show regression in puberty.

There is no active treatment except extraction of teeth in the involved areas and in post puberty age surgical correction for cosmetic purpose may be done. Surgical contouring of expanded jaw bones and complete curettage may be done.

BENIGN ODONTOGENIC TUMORS

Odontogenic tumors are the rare tumors of the oral cavity and account for 9% of all tumors in the oral region. Odontogenic tumors arise from dental lamina or any of its derivative. It can be classified as follows:

1. Tumors of ectodermal origin
   A. Ameloblastoma
   B. Adenomatoid odontogenic tumor
   C. Calcifying odontogenic cyst
   D. Calcifying epithelial odontogenic tumor
   E. Squamous odontogenic tumor
2. Tumors of mesodermal origin
   A. Cementoma
      a. Cementifying fibroma
      b. Cementoblastoma
      c. Periapical cemental dysplasia
   B. Central odontogenic fibroma
   C. Odontogenic myxoma
3. Tumors of mixed origin
   A. Ameloblastic fibroma
   B. Ameloblastic fibro-odontoma
   C. Odontoma
      a. Complex odontoma
      b. Compound odontoma
   D. Ameloblastic odontoma
   E. Ameloblastic fibrosarcoma.

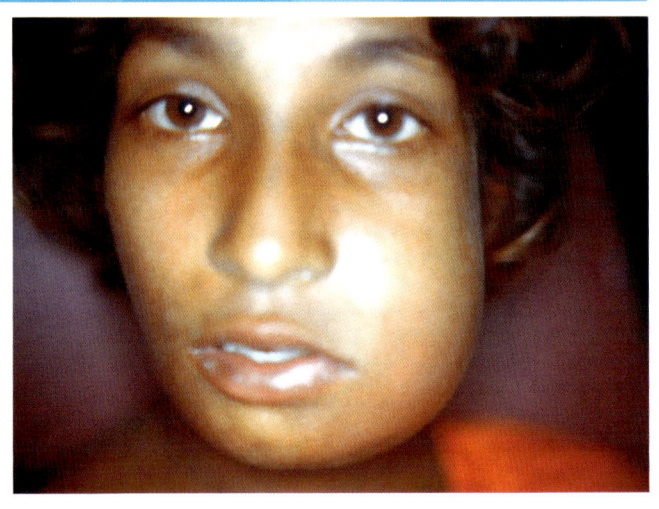

Fig. 13.8: Ameloblastoma of left angle of the mandible

Tumors of Ectodermal Origin

Ameloblastoma

It is most prevalent odontogenic tumor. Ameloblastoma is a benign odontogenic epithelial neoplasm. It is slowly growing expansile radiolucent tumor. Ameloblastoma is prevalent in individuals of 20 to 40 years of age, and occurs most commonly in posterior region of the mandible. Rarely it occurs in maxilla. Occasionally malignant ameloblastoma may be observed.

It clinically presents as slow, enlarging, painless, bony hard swelling of jaw. Lesions of ameloblastoma may cause expansion and thinning of cortical plates which results in loosening of teeth. Curettage is least desirable treatment as it is associated with high incidence of recurrence. Block excision and complete removal of the lesion with good margin of unaffected bone is the treatment of choice. Hemimandibulectomy is indicated for large-sized lesions (Fig.13.8). Prognosis is good as it is essentially a local problem and metastases is very rare.

Adenomatoid Odontogenic Tumor (AOT)

It is benign epithelial odontogenic tumor that usually arises from the cells of the outer enamel epithelium, during the stage of follicle formation, and is characterized by the formation of duct like structures. The site of occurrence is greater in anterior part of the maxilla. The lesion is asymptomatic in nature and mostly develops anterior to the cuspids. It is well-encapsulated lesion that rarely recurs after conservative surgical excision.

Calcifying Odontogenic Cyst (Gorlin Cyst, Keratinizing and or Calcifying Epithelial Odontogenic Cyst; Cystic Keratinizing Tumor)

Calcifying odontogenic cyst is a benign odontogenic tumor with the features of both a cyst and solid tumor. They are found to be associated with ameloblastomas or other odontogenic tumors. It may occur at any age in life and may be either intraosseous or extraosseous lesion. It is treated by total surgical enucleation.

Calcifying Epithelial Odontogenic Tumor (Pindborg Tumor)

It is benign epithelial odontogenic neoplasm resembling an ameloblastoma and is identified as unilocular or multilocular swelling. It is slow-growing, painless lesion mostly occurring in molar-ramus area. Treatment is by enucleation or local block excision.

Squamous Odontogenic Tumor

It is a rare epithelial odontogenic tumor, thought to be arising from epithelial cell rests of Malassez. The lesion equally involves maxilla and mandible. The presenting manifestations are pain, tenderness and mobility of involved teeth. It is treated by enucleation.

Benign Oral Tumors

Tumors of Mesodermal Origin

Cementoma

Cementoma is a benign cementum-producing tumor. Its three types are recognized which are as follows:

Cementifying fibroma: Cementifying fibroma occurs in mandible of older individuals. It is a slow-growing tumor and may produce swelling and mild deformity. It should be treated by enucleation.

Cementoblastoma: Cementoblastoma usually occurs around the root of mandibular premolar or molar. The lesion may cause expansion of cortical plates.

Periapical cemental dysplasia: The lesion mostly occurs near the periodontal ligament around the apex of a tooth, usually a mandibular incisor. The lesions are asymptomatic and are usually small and multiple in number. No specific treatment is required.

Odontogenic Myxoma

The odontogenic myxoma is a tumor of the jaws arising from mesenchymal portion of the tooth germ. It is a slow growing invasive tumor that may gain quite large size which expands the bone and may cause destruction of the cortex. Invasion of antrum in lesions of maxilla and displacement of teeth by tumor mass is a common finding. The treatment of odontogenic myxoma is surgical excision.

Central Odontogenic Fibroma

It is very uncommon tumor of the jaw. The odontogenic fibroma occurs more frequently in children and young adults. It is painless, slow-growing and non-aggressive lesion. It is generally asymptomatic except for swelling of jaw. It is treated by surgical excision.

Tumors of Mixed Origin

Ameloblastic Fibroma

Ameloblastic fibroma is an odontogenic tumor of mixed epithelial and mesenchymal origin. It arises most commonly in the mandibular molar region. It presents clinically as a slow growing, painless lesion which may cause mild swelling of the jaw. Ameloblastic fibroma usually occurs among children and young adults. It may be treated by local excision or curettage.

Ameloblastic Fibro-odontoma

Ameloblastic fibro-odontoma is made up of both mesenchymal and epithelial tissue along with calcified dental tissue. It usually occurs in children and most often in the mandible.

There is swelling and failure of tooth eruption. The ameloblastic fibro-odontoma is treated by curettage.

Odontomas

Odontoma is a hamartomatous odontogenic tumour composed of enamel, cementum, dentin or pulp tissue. They are small, non-aggressive lesions. Odontomas are of two types:

Complex odontoma: In complex odontoma, odontogenic tissues are poorly differentiated and are organized in a haphazard arrangement not resembling a tooth. They usually involve the posterior part of jaw.

Compound odontoma: In compound odontoma, odontogenic tissues are organized and resemble a tooth. It is found mainly in anterior part of the jaw.

CYSTS OF THE JAWS

Cyst is an abnormal sac lined by epithelium which contains fluid, gas or semi-solid material. Cysts may be present in jaw bone and soft tissues of the face, floor of the mouth and neck. It may cause intraoral or extraoral swelling that may resemble a benign tumor. The WHO classification of jaw cysts is as follows.

Developmental Cysts

A. Odontogenic cysts
   a. Odontogenic keratocyst (primordial cyst)
   b. Follicular cyst
   c. Eruption cyst
   d. Alveolar cyst of infants
   e. Gingival cyst of adults
   f. Developmental lateral periodontal cyst
   g. Dentigerous cyst
B. Non-odontogenic cysts
   a. Nasolabial cyst
   b. Midpalatal cyst of infants
   c. Nasopalatine duct cyst.

Inflammatory Cysts

A. Radicular cyst
B. Inflammatory lateral periodontal cyst
C. Inflammatory follicular cyst

Out of these cysts, radicular cyst and nasopalatine cyst, follicular cyst, odontogenic keratocyst constitute 95% of all epithelial jaw cysts. Their salient features are as follows:

Radicular cyst: Radicular cyst is an inflammatory cyst, associated with the apex of a non-vital tooth. It is most frequently caused from infection through the pulp chamber and root canal of carious tooth (Fig.13.9).

Nasopalatine cyst: Nasopalatine or incisive canal cyst is found near the incisive canal and is derived from epithelial remnants of vestigial oronasal duct tissue. Clinically, it appears as small, painful swelling on the anterior part of the hard palate near the midline.

Follicular cyst: Follicular or dentigerous cyst arises from reduced enamel epithelium. It surrounds the crown of impacted, embedded or unerupted teeth. The most common sites of the cyst are mandibular and maxillary third molar area and maxillary canine area. It clinically presents as slow enlarging swelling that may cause expansion of cortical plates and displacement of teeth with subsequent facial asymmetry.

Odontogenic keratocyst: Odontogenic keratocyst or primordial cyst is found in place of a tooth due to cystic degeneration of the enamel organ. It is mainly located in third molar region. It may cause expansion of the bone and displacement of the teeth.

Dentigerous cyst: Dentigerous cyst is an epithelium lined sac filled with fluid or semifluid material which surrounds or includes the tooth or its part usually crown of an unerupted tooth or odontoma (Fig. 13.10).

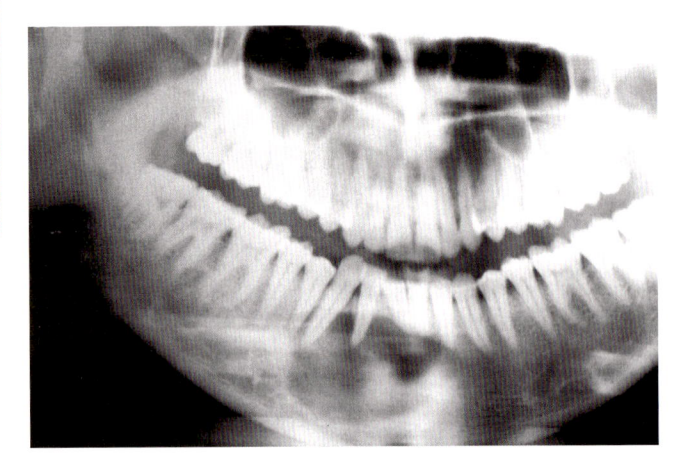

Fig.13.9: Radicular cysts in the mandible (shown by arrows), and alveolar abscess in the maxilla (shown by arrowhead) and attrited incisors as seen in orthopentograph

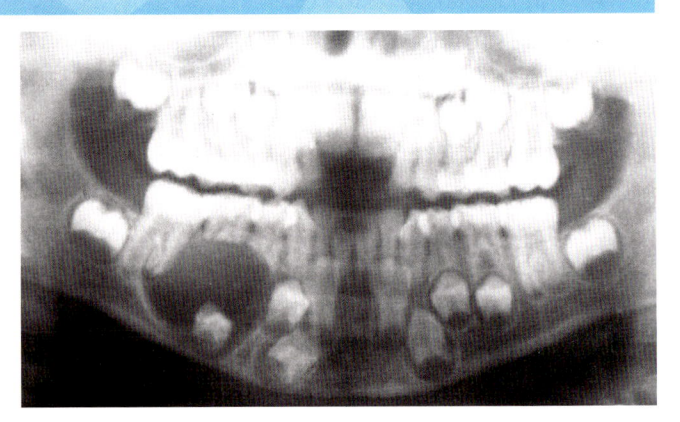

Fig. 13.10: Dentigerous cyst in relation of second premolar in the mandible as seen in orthopentograph

Treatment of cyst: Local excision with complete removal of cystic lining is the treatment of choice for a cyst. Enucleation and marsupialization can be done in case of larger cysts.

"VIRUS INDUCED" BENIGN TUMORS

Oral Squamous Papilloma

It is a benign tumor of epithelial tissue origin and is caused by human papilloma virus (Types HPV 6 and 11). Squamous papilloma usually occurs in third to fifth decades of life. These small epithelial tumors are most commonly found on tongue, buccal mucosa, lips, palate and alveolar gingiva.

It usually appears as pedunculated, cauliflower-like mass. Their surface appear as surface of a cauliflower with small finger like projections. These may be white and keratotic or normal in color. After reaching a certain size their growth is essentially arrested. Recently molecular biological studies have revealed that the viral DNA may be found in a number of oral mucosal lesions. Sometimes the normal oral mucosa harbour few strains of virus specially human papilloma virus (HPV) subtype 16. There are eighty strains of papilloma virus herpes, simplex virus and Epstein-Barr virus.

Usually the papillomas and warts remain benign. Very rarely they convert in malignancy specially in immunosuppressed patients for long periods. Therefore all precautions should be taken when immunosuppressive medicaments (like corticosteroids, cyclosporine and azathioprine) are used for prolonged periods.

Oral papillomas and warts (verrucae vulgaris) are similar in many respects. Both of them are proliferative epithelial lesions caused by HPV with subtype 6 and 11. Squamous papillomas usually occur between thirty to fifty years of age. When on keratinized surface they are well keratinized and wart-like. On unkeratinized mucosal surface they may appear soft and redder. Virus-induced tumor characterized by soft, flat, sessile papules is found in Heck's disease (Focal Epithelial Hyperplasia).

Treatment

The following treatments are usually successful and reoccurrence is very rare if completely removed:
A. Local surgical excision.
B. Electrocoagulation is done on the lips and face where the lesions cause a cosmetic problem.
C. Carbon dioxide laser removal is also successful.

Molluscum Contagiosum

Molluscum contagiosum is a dermatologic infection caused by virus of pox group. The infection is common in children and young adults and manifests as clusters of tiny firm nodules of 5 mm in diameter. The oral lesions occur frequently on tongue, lips and buccal mucosa. They are usually treated by curettage, followed by cryotherapy or topical application of caustics, podophyllin and cantharidin.

Condyloma Acuminatum (Verruca Acuminata; Venereal Wart)

Condyloma acuminatum is caused by a virus which belongs to group of Human papilloma virus. The lesions appear as small, multiple keratotic warts involving hard palate, tongue, lips, cheeks, gingiva and floor of mouth.

Surgical excision, CO_2 laser therapy, cryotherapy and topical podophylline are the various methods of treatment.

Keratoacanthoma (Self Healing Carcinoma, Molluscum Sebaceum; Verrucoma; Molluscum Pseudocarcinomatosum)

It is a rapidly growing tumor that usually occurs on sun-exposed area of the skin. Majority of cases occur between 50 to 70 years of age. The lesion appears fixed to the surrounding tissue covered by thick keratin layers. The lesion may sometimes get matured, exfoliates and heals by itself. The lesion that does not regress by itself is treated by block excision by surgery or laser.

GRANULOMATOUS LESIONS OF THE ORAL CAVITY

Cervicofacial Actinomycosis

Actinomycosis is a granulomatous disease caused by anaerobic, gram-positive, rod-shaped bacteria, Actinomyces israelii. Cervicofacial actinomycosis is the most common form and accounts for 60% of all actinomycosis infection. The most frequent site of involvement is submandibular region. The infection spreads from the periapical region into the soft tissues, salivary glands and rarely the skull. This soft tissue swelling develops into abscess which tend to discharge pus.

The skin surrounding the fistula appears purplish. Treatment involves administration of penicillin and tetracyclines. Four million units of penicillin daily intramuscularly or tetracycline 500 mg every 6 hours is the recommended dose. Nowadays penicillin and tetracycline have been replaced by newer antibiotics.

ANTIFUNGAL DRUGS

Systemic

Amphotericin: B: 0.3-0.78 mg/kg IV over 6-8 hrs. daily 50-100 mg QID oral (for GIT action), 3% topical;
Griseofulvin: 0.5-1.0 g/day in divided doses with meals.
Flucytosine: 100-150 mg/kg/day in 4 divided doses, oral.
Ketoconazole: 200 mg OD-BD oral
Miconazole: 3-15 mg/kg.
Itraconazole: 100-200 mg OD/BD,
Fluconazole: 50-100 mg. OD, 150 mg. weekly oral.

Topical

Miconazole: 1-2% topical;
Clotrimazole: 100 mg vaginal, 1% topical;
Econazole: 150 mg vaginal, 1% topical;
Tolnaflate: 1% cream/solution
Benzoic acid: 3-5% ointment
Quiniodochlor: 3% ointment
Sod. thiosulfate: 20% solution.

Leprosy (Hansen's Disease)

Leprosy is a chronic granulomatous infection caused by Mycobacterium leprae. The oral lesions in leprosy appear as reddish yellow or brown, sessile or pedunculated mucosal nodules. These nodules have a tendency to break down and ulcerate and are found on hard palate, lips, pharynx and tongue. Syndrome is a group of signs and symptoms usually on different parts of the body which occur together and characterize a disease.

Syndromes Associated with Benign Oral Tumors

Gardner's Syndrome

This syndrome is characterized by multiple osteomas of cranial and facial skeleton, hypercementosis, compound odontomes and epidermoid cysts.

Nevoid Basal Cell Carcinoma Syndrome

This syndrome consists of multiple jaw cysts, facial abnormalities and dilaceration of teeth adjacent to cyst.

Multiple Mucosal Neuroma Syndrome (Multiple Endocrine Neoplasia Type III)

It is characterized by multiple neuromas of lips, tongue and buccal and pharyngeal mucosa.

Acanthosis Nigricans

It is associated with perioral and oral mucosal papillomatosis with greyish-brown pigmentation.

Tuberculous Sclerosis

This disorder is characterized by the fine wart like lesions (adenoma sebaceum) on buccal mucosa, pitted enamel hypoplasia, gingival fibromas and cranial defects.

Xanthomas

Xanthomas are deposits of lipoprotein occurring on the face and intraorally. They appear as pale-yellow nodules and are commonly found on lips and cheeks.

Cowden's Syndrome

It is characterized by appearance of multiple papules on the lips and gingiva and papillomatosis of buccal, palatal and oropharyngeal mucosa. The tongue appears fissured or scrotal.

Langerhan's Cell Granulomatosis

It is characterized by radiolucent jaw bone lesions, root resorption; floating teeth and gingival swelling.

Amyloidosis

Amyloid deposits frequently occur in oral cavity. They appear as waxy deposits on lips, gingiva and tongue and lead to macroglossia and gross enlargement of oral tissues.

Von Recklinghausen's Neurofibromatosis

This syndrome is characterised by intraoral neurofibroma especially of tongue which leads to macroglossia.

Peutz-Jeghers Syndrome

Frecking and pigmentation of lips and oral mucosa is seen. The similar lesions are also seen on fingers and toes.

Albright's Syndrome

The presence of solitary and multiple foci of fibrous dysplasia of jaw bones. Rarely coffee with cream colored oral pigmentation is also present. Pigmentation spots are present on the skin.

Paget's Disease of Bone (Osteitis Deformans)

In this there are localized or generalized bony jaw growth and hypercementosis. There are large head, curved back and bowed legs. There is raised serum alkaline phosphatase, usually with normal calcium and phosphorus levels.

BIBLIOGRAPHY

1. Blanas N, Freund B, Schwartz M, Furst IM. Systematic review of the treatment and prognosis of the odontogenic keratocyst. Oral Surg Oral Med Oral Pathol Oral Radiol Endod; 2000;90(5):553-8.
2. Flaitz CM. Peripheral giant cell granuloma: A potentially aggressive lesion in children. Pediatr Dent 2000;22:232-3.
3. Li TJ, Wu, YT, Yu SF, Yu GY. Unicystic ameloblastoma: A clinicopathologic study of 33 Chinese patients. Am J Surg Pathol 2000;24(10):1385-92.
4. Motamedi MH, Behnia H, Motamedi MR. Surgical technique for the treatment of high-flow arteriovenous malformations of the mandible. J Maxillofac Surg 2000;28(4):238-42.
5. Nileema RK, Tinky BC, Amita B. Oral manifestations in HIV infection JIAOMR 2006;18:01.
6. Philipsen HP, Reichart PA. Calcifying epithelial odontogenic tumor. Biological profile based on 181 cases from the literature. Oral Oncol 2000;36(1):17-26.
7. Sunitha M, Shanmugan S. Intraoral Non-Hodgkin's lymphoma in a HIV patient JIAOMR 2006;18:01.
8. Vuillemin-Bodaghi V, Parlier-Cuau C, Cywiner-Golenzer C, et al. Multifocal osteogenic sarcoma in Paget's disease. Skeletal Radiol 2000;29:349-53.

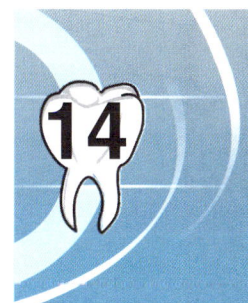

Malignant Oral Tumors

INTRODUCTION AND EPIDEMIOLOGY

Oral cancer is one of the most prevalent cancers all over the world. It is one of the top 10 most common causes of death. In south east Asia oral cancer is the most prevalent cancer and accounts for five percent of all malignant tumors affecting the body. About eighty percent of oral/oropharyngeal malignancies worldwide are squamous cell carcinomas arising in the mucous membrane. Other malignant neoplasms of head and neck region occur in salivary glands, lymph nodes, thyroid gland, soft tissues and bone, but these are less common. This chapter focuses on squamous cell carcinoma of oral cavity.

Oral cancer is a disease of old age. About 95% of cases occur in people older than 40 years. The majority of oral carcinomas involve the oropharynx, tongue and floor of mouth. The least common sites are lips, palate and gingiva.

ETIOLOGY AND RISK FACTORS OF ORAL CANCER

Various predisposing factors are suggested in etiology of oral cancer. Tobacco and alcohol use, physical irritants, environmental factors like exposure to actinic radiation, natural carcinogenic agents, industrial pollutants, chemical irritants, viral infections, hormonal effects, malnutrition, cellular aging, immunologic surveillance and hereditary and immune factors increase the risk of development of cancer.

The persons who have history of cancer are at high risk of developing a second oropharyngeal cancer. Immunosuppression increases the risk of the development of squammous cell carcinoma (SCC). Tobacco contains strong carcinogens which include nicotine, polycyclic aromatic hydrocarbons, nitrosodicthanolamine, nitrosoproline and polonium. Nicotine is a strong addicting chemical. Tobacco smoke contain nicotine, carbon monoxide, hydrogen cyanide, and thiocyanate.

Tobacco and alcohol use are the most serious contributing risk factors in development of oral cancer. Tobacco and tobacco smoke contain potent carcinogens and the smokeless tobacco (*Paan*, *khaini*, *gutka*, etc.) lead to benign hyperkeratosis and epithelial dysplasia, which is associated with increased incidence of malignant lesions. Alcohol along with tobacco use leads to synergistic effect on the development of oral cancer. The mechanism of synergism is as follows.

Alcohol causes dehydration of mucosa which cause a increase in mucosal permeability and the effect of carcinogens present in alcohol and tobacco. Liver dysfunction and malnutrition also increase chances of oral cancer.

CLINICAL FEATURES

Oral squamous cell carcinoma in the initial stages is mostly asymptomatic. The patient knows about the disease only after the appearance of symptoms with progression of disease. The most common symptom which is present at the time of diagnosis and for which patient seeks help is discomfort. Patient also complains of a mass in mouth or neck. Dysphagia, otalgia, oral bleeding and limited movement may also occur.

The high risk areas like buccal mucosa, tongue, floor of mouth and hard and soft palate should be carefully examined for tissue changes like red, white or mixed red and white lesion, smooth, granular or rough lesion or the presence of mass or ulceration. The initial lesion is flat or raised and ulcerated or non-ulcerated, and may be palpable or indurated. Lesions present on tongue can affect normal functioning like speech, mastication and deglutition.

Normally, oral carcinoma is painless unless it gets traumatized or secondarily infected. Involvement of lymph nodes depends upon the stage of the tumor, so cervical and submandibular lymph nodes should be examined carefully.

Lymph nodes associated with carcinoma become enlarged, hard in consistency and fixed to adjacent tissues Figs (14.1 to 14.25).

SQUAMOUS CELL CARCINOMA (SCC) OF LOWER RIGHT SIDE OF LIP, INCLUDING ANGLE OF MOUTH

Sixty-five years old male patient with history of smoking and drinking since 40 years. Exophytic proliferative growth of lower lip and buccal mucosa of right side with pigmented exophytic growth having squamous cell carcinoma of lower right side of lip including angle of mouth (Figs 14.23 and 14.24).

VERRUCOUS CARCINOMA OF UPPER LIP

Verrucous carcinoma is a type of slow-growing, low grade squamous cell carcinoma of oral cavity. Verrucous carcinoma usually occurs in persons who smoke or use snuff or chewing tobacco. This lesion was first defined as a separate entity by Ackerman in 1948.

Clinical appearance is that of a large, broad lesion with minimal to moderate extension and elevation above the surface mucosa. Generally the lesions appear initially as a broad base, warty and fungating mass. The surface is rough, pebbly with cauliflower like growth.

Verrucous carcinoma is frequently associated with leukoplakia at its periphery.

Fifty-five years old male patient with history of smoking since 30 years having verrucous carcinoma of the upper lip, which is a type of squamous cell carcinoma (Fig. 14.25).

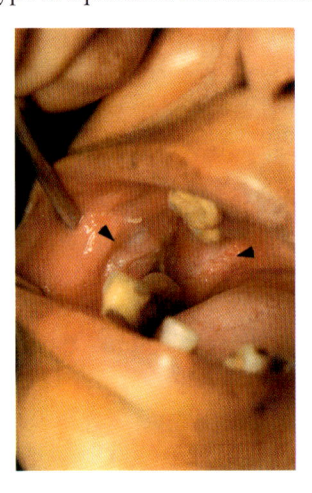

Fig. 14.1: Squamous cell carcinoma (SCC) of cheek and retromolar area in initial stage (shown by arrowheads)

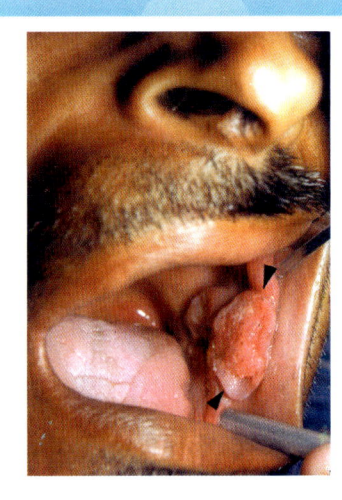

Fig. 14.2: Squamous cell carcinoma (SCC) of cheek in advanced stage (shown by arrowheads)

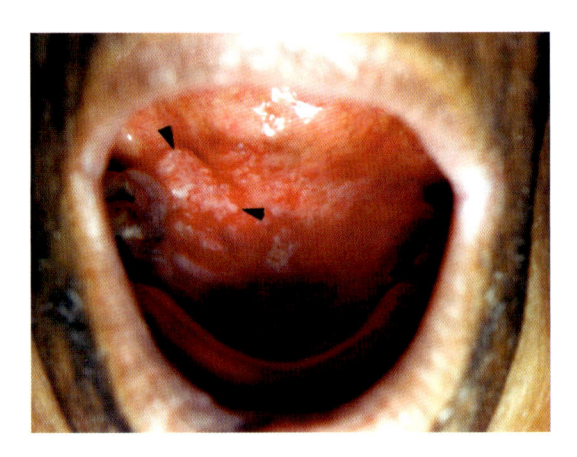

Fig. 14.3: Squamous cell carcinoma of gingiva and palate in initial stage (shown by arrowheads)

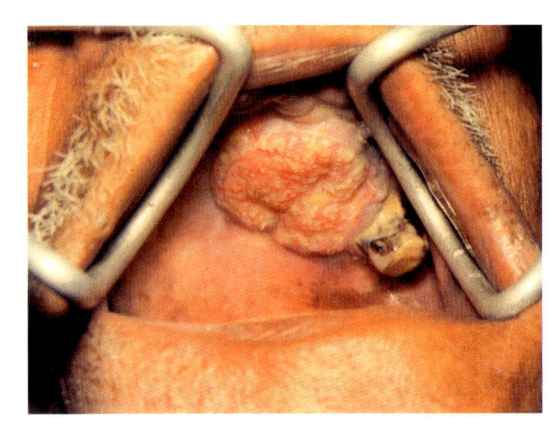

Fig. 14.4: Squamous cell carcinoma of palate in advanced stage

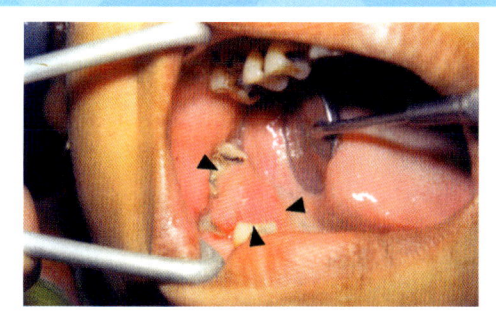

Fig. 14.5: Carcinoma of alveolar mucosa of mandibular molar region in initial stage (shown by arrowheads)

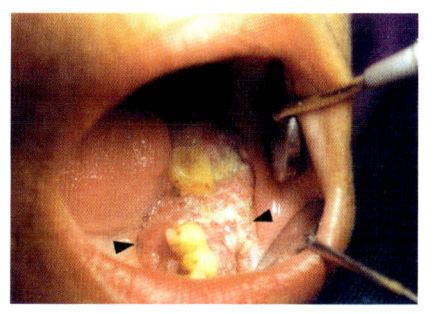

Fig. 14.6: Carcinoma of alveolar mucosa of mandibular molar region in advanced stage (shown by arrowheads)

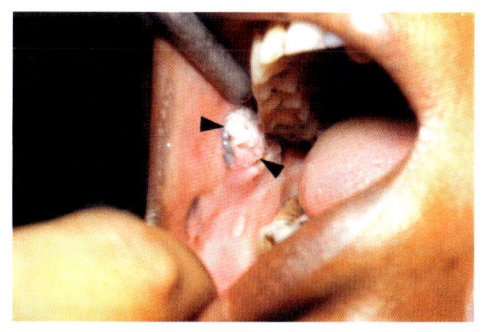

Fig. 14.7: Squamous cell carcinoma of cheek probably due to sharp edges of teeth (shown by arrowheads)

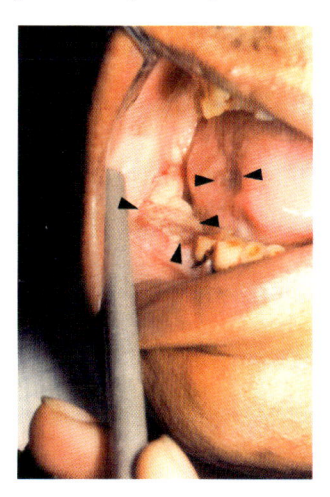

Fig. 14.8: Squamous cell carcinoma of alveolus of mandibular molar region and margin of tongue (shown by arrowheads)

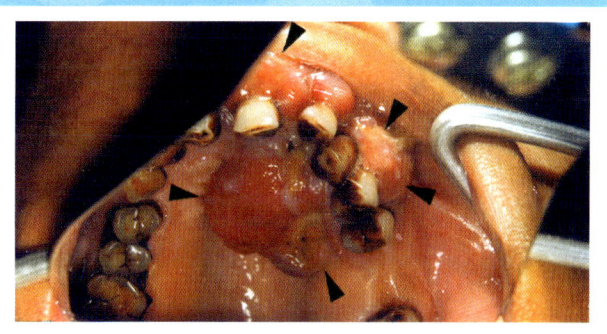

Fig. 14.9: Carcinoma of alveolar mucosa of maxillary anterior and premolar region and palate (shown by arrowheads)

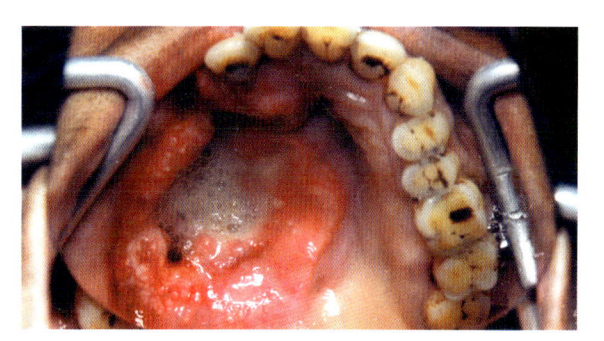

Fig. 14.10: Kaposi's sarcoma perforating palate in HIV positive patient

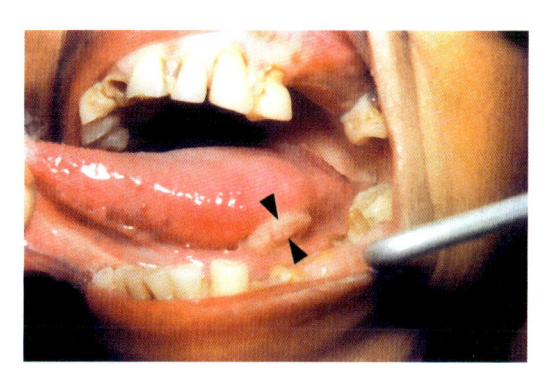

Fig. 14.11: Squamous cell carcinoma of lateral border of base of tongue, whitish oval structure (shown by arrowheads)

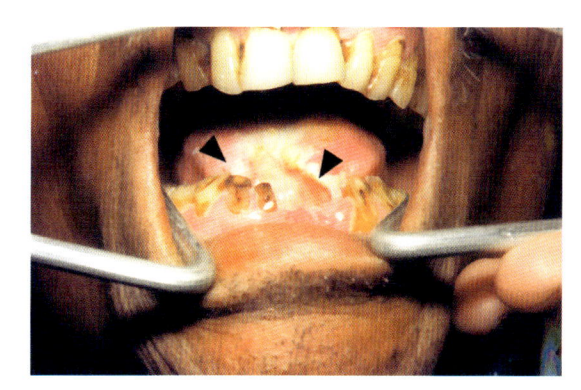

Fig. 14.12: Squamous cell carcinoma of anterior part of tongue due to attrited sharp teeth. There is also restricted mobility of tongue

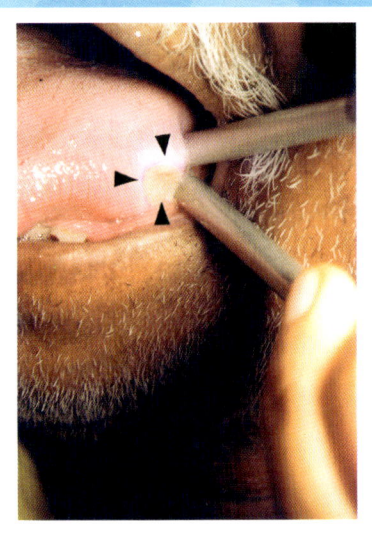

Fig. 14.13: Squamous cell carcinoma of lateral border of tongue (shown by arrowheads)

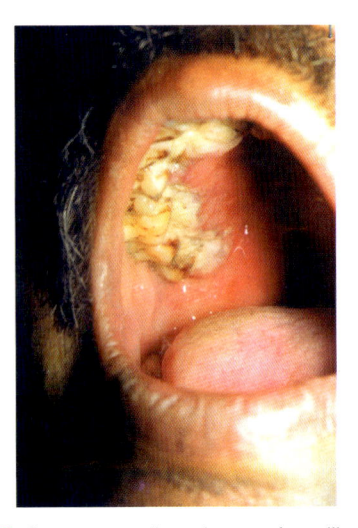

Fig. 14.14: Squamous cell carcinoma of maxillary palatal gingiva in initial stage

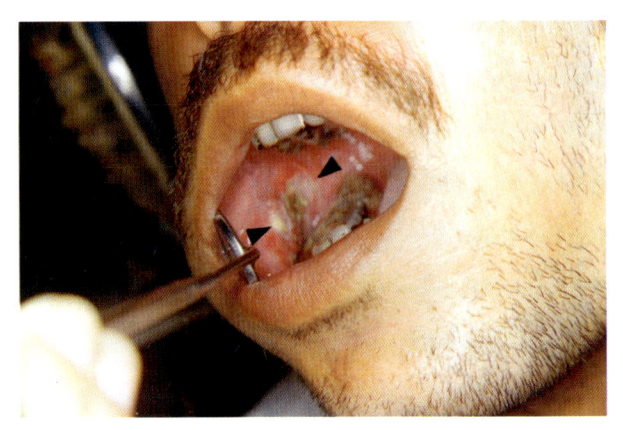

Fig. 14.15: Squamous cell carcinoma of buccal mucosa in initial stage (shown by arrowheads)

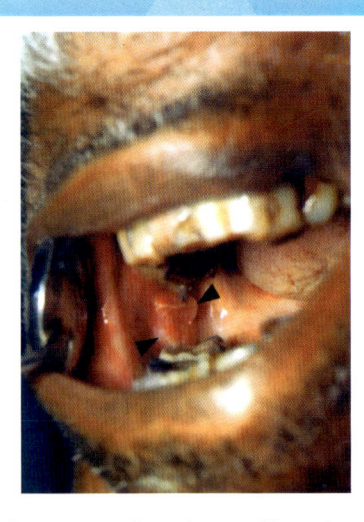

Fig. 14.16: Squamous cell carcinoma of buccal mucosa due to chronic cheek biting in initial stage (shown by arrowheads)

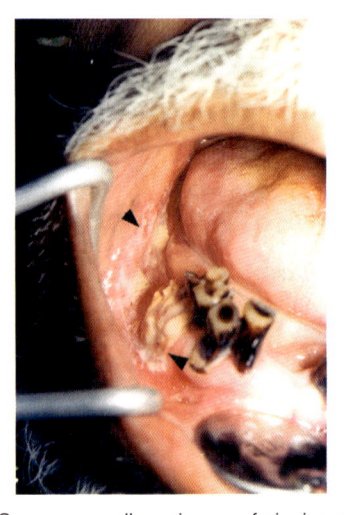

Fig. 14.17: Squamous cell carcinoma of gingiva and cheek in advanced stage (shown by arrowheads)

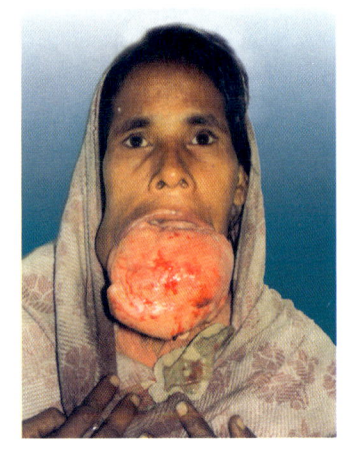

Fig. 14.18: Squamous cell carcinoma of lower lip in advanced stage

Malignant Oral Tumors

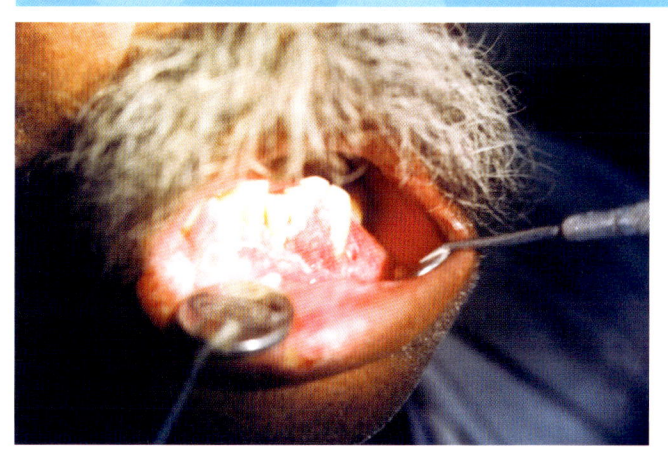

Fig. 14.19: Squamous cell carcinoma of labial gingiva of mandibular anterior teeth in advanced stage

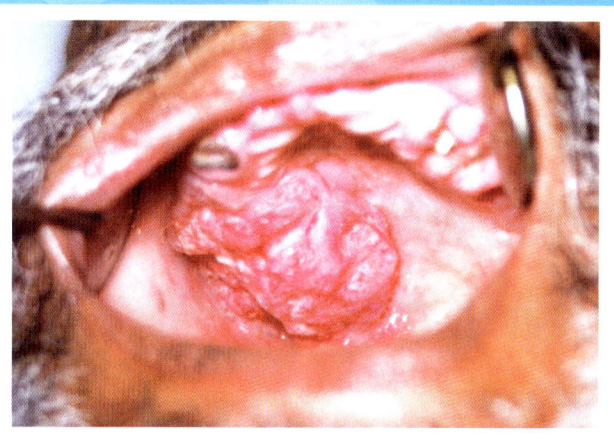

Fig. 14.22: Squamous cell carcinoma of alveolus and hard palate (advanced stage)

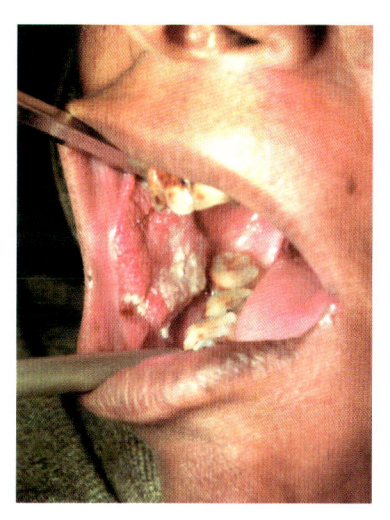

Fig. 14.20: Advanced stage of carcinoma of cheek

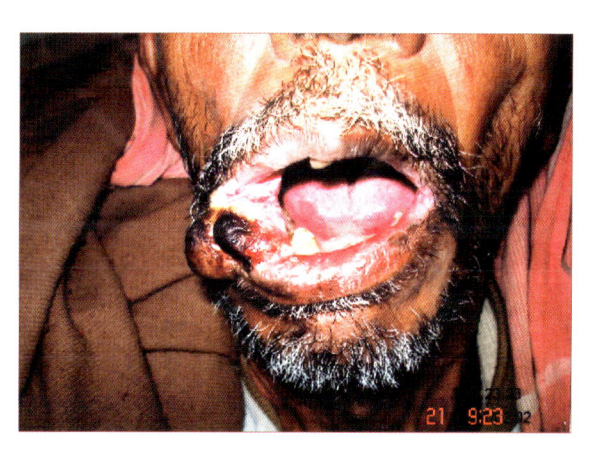

Fig. 14.23: Squamous cell carcinoma of right angle of mouth and right cheek —extra oral view. It is exophytic and beginning to show central pigmentation. It showed fairly deep invasion into the lip and cheek

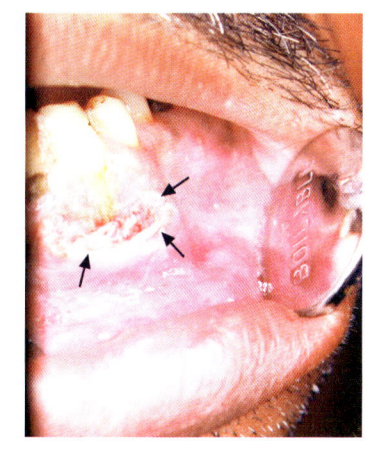

Fig. 14.21: Initial stage of squamous cell carcinoma of the labial vestibule of mandibular anterior teeth in a 'KHAINI' chewer (shown by arrows). 'Khaini' chewers keep it at this place. Khaini is freshly prepared by rubbing tobacco leaves powder with the slaked lime for about 15 minutes

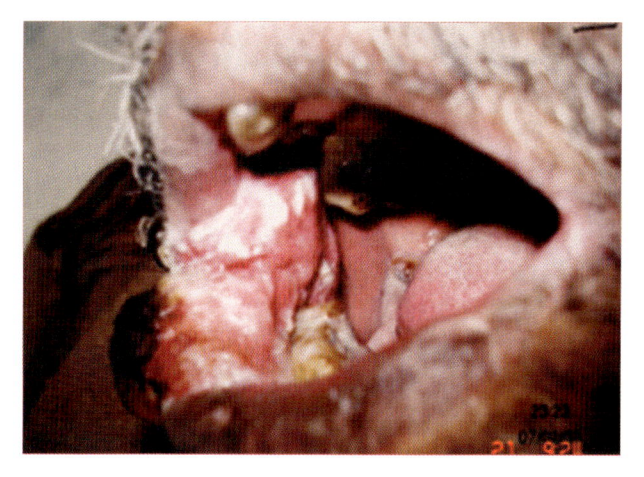

Fig. 14.24: Squamous cell carcinoma (ulcerative) of right angle of mouth and right cheek —Intra oral view of SCC shown in Fig. 14.23.

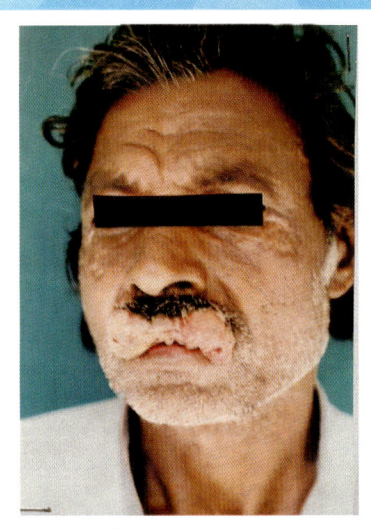

Fig. 14.25: Verrucous carcinoma (a type of squamous cell carcinoma) of upper lip. It is remarkably exophytic in its growth. Although this lesion is extensive but there was relatively little deep invasion

PATHOGENESIS

Oral squamous cell carcinoma (OSCC) is caused by multi-stage process. Normal → dysplastic lesion (premalignant lesion) → OSCC. WHO has defined premalignant lesion as 'a morphologically altered tissue in which cancer is more likely to occur'. It includes oral leukoplakia, oral erythroplakia and oral lichen planus.

On the basis of histomorphology dysplastic lesions are classified as follows:

Mild Dysplasia

In mild dysplasia dysplastic cells are limited to the basal layer of the epithelium.

Moderate Dysplasia

In moderate dysplasia there are moderate changes in cellular morphology and moderate increase in thickness of epithelium.

Severe Dysplasia

In severe dysplasia there are severe increasing changes in cellular morphology and excessive increase in the thickness of epithelium.

INVESTIGATIONS

Imaging

Imaging techniques like radiographic films, ultrasound, magnetic resonance imaging (MRI), computed tomography and nuclear scintiscanning provide extent of soft tissue lesion and bone involvement. Evaluation of bone involvement is important in staging, treatment planning and determining the prognosis.

MRI is helpful in showing distortion of bony trabeculae, and nuclear scintiscanning provide evidence of bone involvement by tumor and necrosis of bone due to radiation therapy. Soft tissue involvement and status of cervical lymph nodes can be determined by CT scan and MRI.

Cytologic Examination

Toluidine blue is used to identify the site to be biopsied and indicates site at risk for malignancy. It also helps in determining the margins of the lesion for treatment planning. The dye toluidine blue is applied over the suspected area for one to two minutes. Thereafter the area is wiped with the cotton swab dipped in absolute alcohol. The area which retains the dye is the area having dysplasia.

The tissue is acquired for histopathology by standard biopsy techniques and fine needle aspiration cytology.

DIFFERENTIAL DIAGNOSIS

- Verrucous carcinoma
- Papillary squamous cell carcinoma
- Basal cell carcinoma
- Verruciform xanthoma
- Keratoacanthoma

Most lip carcinomas are well differentiated lesions, often classified as grade I carcinoma.

DIAGNOSIS OF ORAL CANCER

Investigations for early detection of oral cancer are as follows:

Types of Diagnostic Tools

    A. Non-invasive
    B. Invasive

Non-Invasive
    i. Exfoliative cytology
    ii. Toluidine blue staining

Invasive
    i. Biopsy
    ii. Chemiluminescence and LED
    iii. Immunohistochemical techniques
    iv. Lasers

Malignant Oral Tumors

EXFOLIATIVE CYTOLOGY

Exfoliative cytology is the diagnosis from cells scraped from the surfaces of the lesions. The indications are as follows
1. Adjunct to clinical diagnosis
2. Suspicious chronic lesions
3. Detecting field change in oral cancer

Advantages are as follows:
1. Non-invasive
2. Simple for general clinician

Disadvantages are as follows:
A. Requires a trained cytopathologist
B. Moderate to high index of suspicion for malignancy, definitive biopsy specimen is indicated not exfoliative cytology
C. False negatives are reportedly as high as 37 percent

TOLUIDINE BLUE STAINING

1. Ninety-five percent toluidine blue [vital staining]
2. Adjunct to clinical impression before biopsy of a lesion.
3. Basic metachromatism nuclear stain to survey the oral mucosa or evidence of multiple primary tumors.
4. As a post therapeutic surveilance list aiding in the early diagnosis of tumor recurrence
5. Sensitivity 93.5 to 97.8 percent.
6. Specificity 73.3 to 92.9 percent

For a persistent lesion, definitive diagnosis is established by a tissue biopsy. Adjunctive methods such as vital staining with toluidine blue (toloniun chloride) are helpful in accelerating the biopsy and or selecting the most appropriate spot at which to perform the biopsy

The stain uses a one percent aqua solution of the dye that is decolorized with 1 percent acetic acid. The dye binds to dysplastic and malignant epithelial cells with a high degree of accuracy.

It gives excellent results with false negative (under diagnosis) and false positive (over diagnosis) rates of well below 10 percent.

PROCEDURE

1. Rinse mouth with tap water twice for 30 seconds each time, to remove food particles and debris. Rinse mouth with 1% acetic acid for 30 seconds followed by toluidine blue spot application or toluidine blue rinse.
2. Rinse mouth with 4 to 5 ounces of 1% acetic acid for 1 minute to remove excess stain.
3. Rinse mouth with tap water
4. Wipe with a cotton swab dipped in absolute alcohol.
5. Examine for purplish blue colored spots which show dysplastic and malignant epithelial cells.

Advantages
1. Simple
2. Inexpensive
3. No mutagenic effect is reported till date.

Disadvantage
Rarely may give false negative and false positive results.

BIOPSY

Following are the types of biopsy:
1. Excisional biopsy
2. Incisional biopsy
3. Fine needle aspiration
4. Brush biopsy
5. Punch biopsy.

EXCISIONAL BIOPSY INDICATIONS

A. Whenever a lesion is small enough that complete removal is possible without significant morbidity.
B. Both a therapeutic as well as a diagnostic procedure.
C. Generally for lesions of 1 cm or less than 1 cm in diameter.
D. Additional advantage is that–it does not transect the tumor.

BRUSH BIOPSY

Advantages are as follows:
A. It is simple
B. It is reliable
C. It is non- invasive
D. It is less time consuming

ORAL CDX BRUSH BIOPSY PROCEDURE

1. Moisten the brush with water/saliva
2. Apply pressure on the surface of the lesion with the brush.
3. Rotate until pin point bleeding appears, 5 to 10 times or more depending on the thickness of the lesion.
4. Remove the cells with brush
5. Transfer to glass slides
6. Fixation is done
7. Air drying and staining is done
8. Examine under microscope

INTERPRETATION

1. No epithelial abnormality
2. Atypical abnormal epithelial cells, uncertain diagnostic significances.
3. Positive or negative

CHEMILUMINESCENCE AND LED

The early detection of primary oral cancer, or recurrent cancer is important for improving the survival rates. Advancements in cancer research have led to the innovation of contemporary diagnostic tools for early oral cancer detection. Vizilite and glucosides based on the principle of 'chemiluminescence' and light emitting diodes (LED) are the reliable tools available for this purpose

Advantages

Advantages are as follows:
a. Reliable and advanced diagnostic tool
b. Early diagnosis is possible
c. Chemical energy released as light
d. LED is inexpensive
e. It is safe and non-invasive
f. Findings can be documented.

Principles

Principles are as follows:
A. Density of the nuclear content and mitochondrial matrix of abnormal cells is greater than normal cells.
B. Increased molecular density may reveal increased proliferative rate and mitotic activity of precancerous cells
   i. It enhances the examiners ability to see the differences in the nuclear/cytoplasmic ratio of dysplastic cells (Fig. 14.26).
   ii. After rinsing with one percent acetic acid solution the dense nucleus of the abnormal squamous epithelium appears white when viewed under diffused low-energy wavelength light.
   iii. Normal epithelium will absorb light and appear dark.

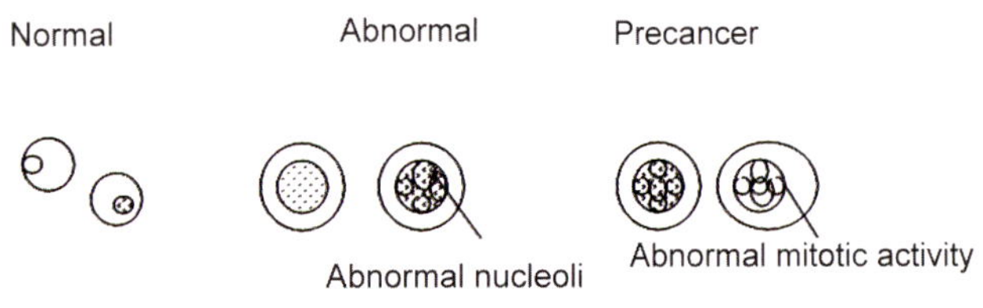

Procedure

Procedure is as follows:
1. Rinse the mouth with one percent acetic acid
2. Activate the device and insert into the holder.
3. Dim ambient room lights preferred.
4. Examine the oral cavity using the device.
5. Effected mucosa appears as an opaque (acetowhite)

This method shows a sensitivity of 100 percent indicating no false negative findings. There are a fewer false positive findings with the glucosides and LEDs and therefore their specificity is rationally greater than for vizilite. Although all 3 tools seem to be equally effective in the identification of early dysplastic changes. Differences exist in terms of cost effectiveness, duration of use and usage on multiple patients.

IMMUNOHISTOCHEMICAL TECHNIQUES

1. Detection of antigens is a routine diagnostic procedure.
2. Technique sensitive
3. Antigen needs to be preserved (Table 14.1)
4. Sample is snap frozen in liquid nitrogen and preserved.
5. Used for definitive diagnosis
6. Enzymes are of diagnostic significance if present in large quantities. Enzyme are visualized by immunocytochemistry
7. Basis is the immunogenic properties of enzymatic protein.

Immunohistochemical techniques also can be used for detection of oral cancer.

LASERS

1. Lasers are promising tool for the early detection of precancerous and cancerous conditions.
2. Cancerous changes in the mouth not visible clinically can be detected by lasers.
3. Cancerous tissues are subjected to laser light fluoresce.

Histological Diagnosis of Carcinoma

Carcinoma in Situ

In this abnormal cells involve the entire thickness of epithelium without invading the basement membrane.

Fig. 14.26: Altered cytoplasm nuclear ratio

Table 14.1: Tumor associated antigens which are useful in immunohistochemical diagnosis

Neoplasm	Antigens
• Carcinomas	Keratins
• Adenocarcinomas	Keratins
• Salivary gland tumors	S-100 protein, actins, calponin
• Rhabdomyosarcoma	Desmin, myoglobin, actin, myogenin, muscle specific actin
• Leiomyosarcoma	Smooth muscle actin
• Neurosarcoma	Neurofilaments, S-100
• Angiosarcoma and Kaposi's related antigen	CD 31, CD 34, factor VIII
• Melanoma	HMB45, S100 protein
• Langerhans cell disease	CD la
• Lymphomas	CD 45, CD 45, RB is form
• B-cell lymphomas	CD 20, CD 791, CD 45 RA
• T-cell lymphomas	CD 3, CD 43, CD 45 RO isoform
• Anaplastic large cell (Ki I)	CD 30 (Ber H2 clone), ALK-1
• Hodgkin's disease (RS cells)	CD 15, CD 30
• Plasma cell myeloma	k/l light chains
• Leukemic infiltrates	TdT, myeloperoxidase
• Paraganglioma and neuroendocrine Carcinoma	Synaptophysin, chromogranin, neurofilament
• Olfactory neuroblastoma	Synaptophysin, chromogranin neurofilament
• Ewing's sarcoma and PNET's	CD 99
• Solitary fibrous tumor	CD 34, CD 99 Bcl-2

Bowen's Disease

Bowen's disease is a localized intraepithelial squamous cell carcinoma. It occurs on genital mucosa and rarely on oral mucosa. Particularly in patients who have ingested arsenic.

Treatment

Excision, irradiation, cauterization and exposure to solid carbon dioxide. If left untreated, carcinomatous invasion may occur.

Carcinoma

The carcinoma is diagnosed when the basement membrane is disrupted and the connective tissue is invaded.

Most of the leukoplakia gradually disappear after removal of irritant and totally stopping the oral habit. They do not progress to malignancy. The severity of dysplasia is a scale to measure the malignant risk of premalignant lesion. The presence of candida colonies increases the risk of malignancy.

Prediction of Malignancy—Molecular Changes in Premalignancy and Oral Malignancy

The progression to malignancy is a genetic process. This process leads to change in cellular behavior and morphology. The important genes taking part in squamous cell carcinoma (HNSCC) are proto-oncogenes and tumor suppressor genes (TSGs).

Prediction of malignancy potential can be done more accurately by molecular staging then by clinicopathological features. Molecular staging provides the fundamental biologic characteristic of each tumor. Therefore molecular markers are very important clinical markers in diagnosis, staging and treatment planning. TSGs negatively regulate cell growth and differentiation. In carcinogenesis process there is functional loss of TSGs.

Loss of heterozygosity (LOH) predict the malignancy risk of low grade dysplastic oral epithelial lesions. This is very important because majority of oral precancerous lesion do not become cancerous. Malignancy prone and non-malignancy prone lesions do not differ histomorphologically but they definitely differ genetically.

PROGNOSIS

TNM Staging of Tumor of Oral Cavity

Tumor, node and metasis (TNM) system of cancer classification has been developed by the American Joint Committee on Cancer (AJCC). In this classification T is the size of primary tumor, N is the presence of tumor in lymph nodes and M is distant metastasis. The spread of oral SCC is very common and has big influence on treatment planning. T, N and M have been combined to classify stages 1 to 4. Cervical node metastases is common. Distant metastases below the clavicle are unusual. Posterior lesions are diagnosed in advanced stages after becoming symptomatic, hence prognosis is usually poorer (Table 14.2).

In oral cancer the diagnosis and treatment in initial stage is very important as the second chance of treatment is very rarely available. Head and neck cancer become fatal due to erosion of cranial base, major vessels, secondary infection of respiratory tract, weakness, loss of weight and atrophy. Oral cancer treatment team must include oral and maxillofacial surgeon, head and neck surgeon, genetic experts, radiation oncologists, oral pathologists, medical oncologists, plastic surgeon and auxiliary health care workers.

Table 14.2: TNM classification of oral cavity tumor for staging of oral cancer

Stage	Size of Primary Tumor (T)	Metastasis of Regional Lymph Node (N)	Distant Metastasis (M)
0	Tis Carcinoma *in situ*	N0- No lymphnode metastasis	M0- No distant metastasis
I	T1 smaller than 2 cms	N0	M0
II	T2 Larger than 2 cms but smaller than 4 cms	N0	M0
III	T1	N1 single ipsilateral node smaller than 3 cms	M0
	T2	N0 or N1	M0
	T3 Larger than 4 cms	N0 or N1	M0
IV	T4 Tumor invade adjacent structure	N0 or N1	M0
	Any T	N2a- single ipsilateral node larger than 3 cms and smaller than 6 cms or N2b- Multiple ipsilateral node smaller than 6 cms or N2c- Bilateral or contralateral node smaller than 6 cms or N3 node more than 6 cms	M0
	Any T	Any N	M1 Distant metastasis

Adapted from the report of American Joint Committee on Cancer.

Virus in Oral Cancer

About one half of oral squamous cell carcinomas contain HPV type 16 or 18 (HPV-16 or18).

Tumor Biology

In oral carcinoma oncogene amplification has been observed. There is no definite conclusion on genetic risk and cocarcinogenesis. In oral squamous cell carcinoma there may be role of cytokines. In patients with oral cancer carcinoembryonic antigens are elevated. Depending on the degree of cellular dysplasia intercellular enzymes are also lost or altered.

Immunosuppressed patients are more prone to malignant disease which indicate the importance of an intact immune response. In patients with head and neck malignancy total number of T cells are decreased and there is reduced inflammatory response like migration of microphages.

Spread

Squamous cell carcinoma mainly spreads by direct local extension and occasionally by submucosal spread. The regional extension is by the lymphatics, due to invasion break down of laminin and collagen takes place in the basement membrane.

Nutritional Prevention of Oral Cancer

Vitamin A and carotenoid play a role in prevention of oral cancer. Heavy dose of Vitamin A (10,000 to 30,000 IU daily) for few weeks may regress the premalignant leukoplakia, oral submucous fibrosis and other premalignant oral lesions.

Signs and Symptoms

In initial stages oral cancer is asymptomatic and is identified during routine examination or when the symptoms appear. The symptoms is presence of growth in oral cavity. Less frequent symptoms are dysphagia, otalgia, odynophagia, restricted movement of tongue or cheek, restricted mouth opening and oral bleeding. The lesion may be palpable, indurated, flat, elevated, ulcerated or non ulcerated.

Lymph nodes of malignancy become enlarged and firm to hard in texture usually nontender. Lymphatic drainage of oral cancer is mostly in submandibular and diagastric nodes, than cervical nodes.

TREATMENT OF ORAL CANCER

The main aim is to cure the patient of cancer. The treatment of choice for oral cancer depends upon the following factors:
 i. Site, size and location of primary lesion
 ii. Cell type and degree of differentiation
 iii. Status of lymph node involvement

Malignant Oral Tumors

iv. Extent of bone involvement
v. Achievement of adequate surgical margins
vi. Ability to preserve speech and swallowing
vii. Physical and mental status of patient
viii. Age of the patient
ix. Assessment of complications of each therapy
x. Capability and experience of surgeon and radiotherapist
xi. Cooperation and preferences of the patient

Surgery and radiotherapy are the treatment of choice for oral cancer and they are used with intention of curing the disease. Chemotherapy is used as a supplemental therapy. In T1 and T2 lesions either radiotherapy or surgery may be used; both the modalities in combination are usually needed for advanced stages.

Surgery

Surgery is indicated in the treatment of the following:
A. Tumor in primary stage and involved lymph nodes
B. Tumor involving the bone where side effects of surgery are less significant than radiation therapy.
C. Tumor that is not responding to radiotherapy.
D. Recurrent tumor that has already received maximum dose of radiotherapy
E. Tumor involving the bone where radiotherapy alone is not sufficient to give successful results.

Surgery is the treatment of choice for tumors with lymph node involvement. Surgery may also be used to reduce the bulk of tumor and to facilitate drainage from a blocked cavity. Surgery may sometimes get failed due to inadequate margins of resection, incomplete excision and lymphatic or hematogenous spread.

Tumors involving lymph nodes should be treated aggressively due to poor prognosis. Radical neck dissection with involved lymph nodes is carried out for 'en bloc' resection of tumor. It can be combined with radiation therapy and chemotherapy.

Laser Surgery

Surgical excision of dysplastic and malignant lesion can be carried by laser excision/ablation using carbon dioxide laser and neodymium-aluminium-garnet (Nd:YAG) laser. Advantages of laser surgery are as follows:
1. It is well tolerated and improves healing.
2. It reduces bleeding.
3. It reduces hospitalization period.

Disadvantage: Laser limits the evaluation of the margins for histopathological confirmation. However some surgeons prefer to control malignancy of the cells by chemotherapy before surgery.

Radiation Therapy

Radiation therapy may be given alone, or as a part of combined surgical and radiation therapy, with intention of curing the tumor, or reducing the severity of symptoms. In palliative care, radiation provides symptomatic relief from pain, ulceration, bleeding and oropharyngeal obstruction. Radiation therapy uses high energy electromagnetic radiation or high energy particulate matter to destroy tumor cells. Radiation kills malignant cells by disrupting DNA configuration and by chromosomal damage. The radiated cells may die or become incapable of division.

Radiation therapy is the treatment of choice for the following.
a. T1 and T2 tumors
b. Early lesions of squamous cell carcinoma
c. Exophytic and well oxygenated tumors
d. Squamous cell carcinoma limited to mucosa

The radiation treatment planning depends upon size and site of the tumor, total volume to be irradiated, total days of treatment and tolerance of patient. Radiation can be delivered by various methods which are as follows:

I. *Teletherapy*
   i. External beam therapy—External beam therapy is the treatment of choice for tumors of posterior part of tongue, oropharynx and tonsillar pillar.
   ii. Intraoral cone therapy
   iii. Electron beam therapy

II. *Brachytherapy*—Interstitial therapy or intracavitary radiation.

Radiation Sources

A. *For superficial tumors of skin, lip, parotid gland and cervical nodes*: Electron beam therapy provides superficial radiation and better control over the depth of penetration then low kilovolt radiation (50 to 300 kV).
B. *For deep seated tumors*: Heavy particle radiation like neutron beam radiation. Megavoltage radiation using cobalt 60 and use of linear accelerator of ≥ 4 MeV is safe for skin and bone. Variable penetration is provided by linear accelerator due to its ability to vary the energy of the photons.

Treatment Planning

Treatment planning is determined by the following.
a. Tumor size
b. Tumor site
c. Total volume to be radiated
d. No. of treatment of fractions
e. Tolerance of the patients
f. Total no. of days of treatment
g. Sparing of uninvolved tissues and organs

Radiation Dose

For most oral epithelial malignancies radiation delivered in 1.8 to 2 Gy per fraction for 5 weeks to a total dose of 6000 to 6500 c Gy.

Chemotherapy

Chemotherapy is employed for the treatment of advanced tumors or recurrent tumors where surgery and radiation have failed to achieve a cure. Various chemotherapeutic agents used in the treatment of oral cancer in combination or alone are methotrexate, cisplatin, bleomycin, taxol 5- fluorouracil and platinum derivatives.

Chemotherapy may result in temporary reduction in tumor size, but does not help in controlling the primary tumor or incidence of metastasis. The side effects of chemotherapy include nausea, vomiting, mucositis and bone marrow suppression.

Anti Cancer Drugs

The anticancer drugs either kill cancer cells or modify their growth. However, selectivity of majority of drugs is limited and they are one of the most toxic drugs used.

Acting directly on cells (Cytotoxic Drugs)

A. *Alkylating Agents*
 i. *Nitrogen mustards*
 Mechlorethamine 0.4mg/kg i.v in 1-4 days; courses may be repeated at suitable intervals,
 MUSTINE HCl 10 mg dry powder in vial.
 Cyclophosphamide: Chloramphenicol retards the metabolism of cyclophosphamide.
 Dose: 2- 3 mg/kg/day oral 10-15 mg/ kg i.v. every 7 to 10 days, i.m. use also possible ;
 ENDOXAN, CYCLOXAN 50 mg tab; 200, 500, 1000 mg inj.

Chlorambucil:
Dose: 4-10 mg (0.1-0.2mg/kg) daily for 3 to 6 weeks, then 2 mg daily for maintenance; LEUKERAN 2, 5 mg tab.
Melphalan:
Dose: 10 mg daily for 7 days or 6 mg /day for 2 to 3 weeks -4 weeks gap 2 to 4 mg daily for maintenance orally. Also used for regional perfusion in malignant melanoma.
ALKERAN 2, 5 mg tab, 50 mg per vial for inj.

 ii. *Others*
 Thio-TEPA: It has high toxicity: rarely used now.
 Dose: 0.3 to 0.4 mg/kg i.v. at 1 to 4 week intervals; THIOTEPA 15 mg per vial inj.
 Busulfan: 2-6mg/day/ (0.06mg/kg/day) orally; MYLERAN, BUSUPHAN 2 mg tab
 Carmustine: 50-200 mg/m^2 BSA (Body surface area) by i.v. infusion over 1hr, repeat after 6 weeks.
 Lomustine: 100-130mg/m^2 BSA single oral dose every 6 weeks; LOMUSTINE 40, 100 mg cap.
 Dacarbazine: 3.5mg/kg/day i.v for10 days, repeat after 4 weeks.
 Semustine (methyl CCNU): 100 to 200 mg/m^2 BSA single oral dose, repeat after 6 weeks.

B. *Antimetabolites*
 i. *Folic acid antagonist*
 Methotrexate: 15 to 30 mg daily for 5 days oral or 20-40 mg/m^2 BSA IM/IV twice weekly; NEOTREXATE 2.5 mg tab, 50 mg/2 ml inj; BIOTREXATE 2.5 mg tab, 5, 15, 50 mg/vial inj.
 Carcinoma of the lips (Figs 14.23 to 14.25 have been treated by surgical excision, radiotherapy and chemotherapy.

 ii. *Purine antagonists*
 Mercaptopurine (6-*MP*) *and thioguanine (6-TG) are highly effective antineoplastic drugs.*
 6-Mercaptopurine (MP): 2.5 mg/kg/day oral, half dose for maintenance;
 PURINETHOL 50 mg tab.
 6-Thioguanine (TG): 2mg/kg/day, oral.
 Azathioprine: 3-5mg/kg/day, oral, maintenance 1 to 2 mg/kg/day;
 IMURAN, TRANSIMUNE 50 mg tab.

 iii. *Pyrimidine antagonists*
 5-fluorouracil (FU): 1g, alternate day, oral, (6 doses) then 1g weekly or 12 mg/kg/day i.v. for 4 days -6 mg /kg i.v. on alternate days;

FLURACIL, FIVE FLURO 250 mg cap, 250 mg / 5 ml for i.v. inj, also 1% topical solution.
Cytarabine: 1.5-3 mg/kg i.v. BD for 5-10 days; (also by continuous i.v. infusion):
CYTARABIN 100 mg/5 ml, 500 mg /25 ml and 1000 may /20 ml inj.

C. *Vinca Alkaloids*
Vincristine (Oncovin): 1.5 mg/m² BSA IV weekly;
VINCRISTIN 1 mg, 5 mg vial,
NEOCRISTIN, RICRISTIN 1 mg/vial inj.
Vinblastine: 0.1-0.15 mg/kg i.v. weekly × 3 doses;
VINBLASTIN 10 mg/vial inj.

D. *Antibiotics*
Actinomycin-D (Dactinomycin) : 15 micro g/kg i.v. daily for 5 days;
Doxorubicin (Rubidomycin), Doxorubicin°: 60-75mg/m² BSA slow i.v. injection every 3 weeks
ADRIAMYCIN 10 mg/vial inj.
Daunorubicin: 30-60mg/m² BSA i.v. daily for 3 days, repeat weekly
Bleomycins: 30mg twice weekly: i.v. / i.m. (total dose 300 to 400 mg);
BLEOCIN 15 mg inj.
Mitomycin-C:2 –10mg/m² BSA, repeated according to blood count;
MITOMYCIN-C2, 10 mg/injection.
Mithramycin (plicamycin): 25 micro g/kg by slow i.v. infusion daily or on alternate days (total 8 to 10 doses)

E. *Radioactive Isotopes:* ^{131}I, ^{32}P, ^{198}Au.

F. *Miscellaneous Cytotoxic Drugs*
These drugs (except L-asparaginase) have been developed by random synthesis and testing for antitumor activity.
Hydroxyurea: interferes with DNA synthesis. Its primary therapeutic value is in chronic myeloid leukemia, polycythemia vera and in some solid tumors. Myelosuppression is the major toxicity. 20-30mg/kg/daily or 80 mg /kg twice weekly;
HYDREA 500 mg cap.
Procarbazine: 100-300 mg oral daily; maintenance dose 1 to 2 mg/kg /day
L-Asparaginase: 50-200 KU/kg i.v. infusion daily for 2 to 4 weeks; LEUNASE 10,000 KU per vial inj.
Carboplatin: It is better tolerated and has a toxicity profile different from cisplatin. Nephrotoxicity, ototoxicity and neurotoxicity are low. Nausea and vomiting is milder and is delayed: only infrequently limits the dose. The dose limiting toxicity is thrombocytopenia and less often leukopenia. It is rapidly eliminated by the kidney (4 to 6 hr.). It is primarily indicated in ovarian carcinoma of epithelial origin, and has shown promise in squamous carcinoma of head and neck, small cell lung cancer and seminoma.
ONCOCARBIN 150 mg inj.
KEMOCARB 150, 450 mg/vial inj. 400 mg/m² as an i.v. infusion over 15 to 60 min, to be repeated only after 4 weeks

HORMONES

Act by Altering Hormonal Milieu

1. Glucocorticoids
2. Estrogens
3. Antiestrogens
4. Progestins
5. Androgens

They are not cytotoxic, but modify the growth of hormone dependent tumors. All hormones are only palliative.

GENERAL PRINCIPLES IN CHEMOTHERAPY OF CANCER

1. In cancer chemotherapy, analogy is drawn with bacterial chemotherapy; the malignant cell being viewed as an invader.
2. A single clonogenic malignant cell is capable of producing progeny that can kill the host. To affect cure, all malignant cells must be killed or removed.
3. In any cancer, subpopulations of cells differ in their rate of proliferation and susceptibility to cytotoxic drug.
4. Drug regimens which can effectively palliate large tumor burdens may be curative when applied to minute residual tumor cell population after surgery and /or irradiation.
5. Whenever possible, complete remission should be the goal of cancer chemotherapy; Drugs are often used in maximum tolerated doses.
6. Formerly cancers were treated with one drug at a time. Now, more commonly, a combination of 2 to 6 drugs is given in intermittent pulses to achieve total tumor cell kill, giving time in between for normal cells to recover. Synergistic combinations and rational sequences are devised by utilizing:
   a. Drugs which are effective when used alone.
   b. Drugs with different mechanisms of action.
   c. Drugs with differing toxicities.

d. Empirically by trial and error; optimal schedules are mostly developed by this procedure.
e. Kinetic scheduling.

Combined Surgical and Radiation Therapy

Radiotherapy has ability to eradicate well-oxygenated tumor cells at the periphery of the tumor; and surgery manages, (a) tumor masses with radiation resistant hypoxic cells and (b) when tumor involves the bone; thus combined surgical and radiation therapy can be used for better results with improvement in survival rate of patients in advanced tumors.

Radiation can be used pre-operatively or post-operatively. Preoperative radiation results in destruction of peripheral tumor cells, control of subclinical diseases and converting inoperable into operable lesions. Surgery prior to radiation can be used to remove bulk of tumor containing hypoxic cells. Preoperative radiation may result in delayed healing after surgery which could be critical, so post-operative radiotherapy is chosen in case of extensive carcinoma. Incidence of metastasis is also lower in postoperative technique. Carcinoma of the lips (Figs 14.18, 14.23 to 14.25) have been treated by surgical excision, radiotherapy and Chemotherapy.

OTHER HEAD AND NECK CANCERS

Malignant Neoplasm of Salivary Glands

The majority of tumors of salivary glands involve the parotid gland which are mainly benign mixed tumors. Tumors involving the submandibular or sublingual glands are mostly malignant. Most of the salivary gland tumors are spread by local infiltration or hematogenous spread.

The most common site of involvement is the posterior region of the hard palate. The tumor clinically present as a painless mass that may be associated with ulceration. Parotid tumor may lead to facial paralysis due to involvement of facial nerve. The treatment of choice for salivary gland tumor is surgical resection.

Nasopharyngeal Carcinoma

Nasopharyngeal carcinoma is caused by smoking, Epstein-Barr virus infection and childhood consumption of salted fish and preserved foods. The presenting symptoms of nasopharyngeal carcinoma are nasal bleeding, mass in neck and nasal obstruction. Other symptoms include pain, earache and limited jaw opening. Treatment of choice is radiation therapy or combination with chemotherapy. If lymph nodes are involved surgery is required.

Basal Cell Carcinoma

Basal cell carcinoma is a slow growing, locally destructive, ulcerative cancer with gradual invasion of underlying tissues. It may occur in the head and neck region. Exposure to sun is principal etiological factor.

Clinically, it appears as an indurated papule that may ulcerate. Basal cell carcinoma is treated by surgical excision or topical chemotherapy.

Malignant Melanoma

Melanoma is a malignant neoplasm arising from melanocytes. It presents as an area of altered pigmentation on the oral mucous membrane. The lesions appear as flat ulcerated lesion associated with bleeding; mostly occurring on the maxillary mucosa. Melanoma is an aggressive malignant disease and usually gets metastasized through lymphatics and hematogenous routes. The prognosis is poor.

Intraoral head and neck sarcoma: Intraoral sarcoma has poor prognosis and is very rare. Chondrosarcoma and osteosarcoma may involve the jaw. Treatment is surgical excision with chemoradiotherapy.

Malignancy in HIV positive patients: Immunosuppression makes HIV positive patients prone to malignancy.

Kaposi's Sarcoma (KS)

In acquired immunodeficiency syndrome (AIDS) patients most common malignant disease of head and neck region is Kaposi's sarcoma (KS). Non-Hodgkin's lymphoma may present with head, neck and oral lesions. The lymphoma have poor prognosis. In AIDS patients oropharyngeal squamous cell carcinoma can also occur. In KS there is multicentric neoplastic proliferation of endothelial cells.

The occurrence of KS is 55 percent in male homosexuals suffering from AIDS. KS is often the first sign of AIDS. KS is mostly seen in sexually transmitted AIDS patients. Hence KS is associated with sexually transmitted agents which is human herpes virus type 8 (HHV-8). KS is usually seen in attached mucosa of palate, gingiva and dorsum of the tongue but can occur anywhere in oral cavity. KS usually appear as blue purple or red purple discoloration and may ulcerate. The lesions of KS do not blanch with pressure. Initially KS is asymptomatic but gradually will cause discomfort in eating, speech and denture use. KS can also be seen on skin, lymph nodes, GI tract and other organs. In the differential diagnosis ecchymosis, vascular lesions and salivary gland tumors should be ruled out by the biopsy.

Malignant Oral Tumors

Treatment

Intralesional chemotherapy provide relief from local discomfort. Intralesional injection of vinblastine (0.2 mg/ml) after giving local anesthesia for several weeks provide relief from discomfort, mobility of teeth, reduction in tissue mass but persistence of discoloration for about 4 weeks. For further relief injection can be repeated.

Kaposi's sarcoma is radiosensitive. Fractional radiotherapy with total dose of 25 to 30 Gy over 1 to 2 weeks provide local comfort.

For multiple sites of KS systemic chemotherapy is required. To reduce angiogenesis cytokines may be used. The antiviral agents are also used for HHV-8 infection.

Vinblastine: It is mostly employed in Hodgkin's disease choriocarcinoma, lymphosarcoma, testicular malignany and Kaposi's sarcoma. It is also provide relief in Kaposi's sarcoma. Its dose is 0.1 to 0.15 mg/kg IV weekly × 3 doses.

PRETREATMENT DENTAL AND ORAL EVALUATION

Assessment of dental and oral conditions prior to cancer treatment is very necessary. The oral evaluation is needed to recognize those conditions that should be treated before cancer therapy for the following reasons:
a. To reduce the risk or severity of complications
b. To reduce the risk of infection
c. To minimize development of xerostomia

The pretreatment interference is directed at maintenance of dental and periodontal health, mucosal and bony integrity, salivary gland function and prevention of complications of treatment. The patient's history should emphasize on previous dental care, current dental and oral symptoms and condition of prosthesis, if any.

The head and neck examination should include intraoral mucosal examination, full periodontal probing, dental examination and examination of lymphadenopathy. Radiographic examination of teeth and periapical region; salivary examination for change in flow rate; and cultures and treatments for any infection are also necessary throughout the course of radiation therapy.

COMPLICATIONS OF CANCER TREATMENT

Radiotherapy is the common treatment therapy used in the management of oral cancer, but it may lead to chronic complications. These radiation reactions occur due to fibrosis in connective tissue and muscle and change in vascular supply and cellularity of tissues.

To reduce complications of radiotherapy Benzydamine HCl.

HCl Acetyl salicylic acid (ASA) and nonsteriodal analgesics in low dosage may be used.

Mucositis

Mucositis is the inflammation of the oral mucous membrane following radiotherapy. It occurs due to increased rate of epithelial growth and repair, resulting in epithelial thinning, erosion and ulceration. In mucositis, mucosa may appear white due to hyperkeratinization or red due to hyperemia. There may be pseudomembrane formation with ulceration. There may be edema following irradiation (Figs 14.27A and B).

Mucositis should be managed by use of coating agents and topical anesthetics for symptomatic relief of pain and ulcers. Diluting agents and lip lubricants should be used for hydrating. Analgesic agents like Benzydamine hydrochloride reduce the signs and symptoms of mucositis if used prophylactically throughout the course of radiation therapy.

Xerostomia

Exposure of salivary glands to radiation therapy results in acinar cell atrophy and necrosis, changes in vasculature and altered neurologic function. The saliva becomes thick and viscous. There is decrease in the salivary flow and changes in the composition of saliva also occur. Xerostomia also results in decrease in buffering capacity and acidity and secretory immunoglobulin. Pilocarpine, (a parasympathomimetic agent), Bethancecol and Anetholetricthione can be used to stimulate saliva secretion.

Radiation Caries

Xerostomia due to radiation therapy results in dental caries affecting the gingival third and tips of the teeth. The etiological factors are reduced saliva production resulting in loss of buffering capacity, loss of remineralization potential, increased acidity and change in bacterial flora.

Management of caries includes maintenance of oral hygiene, management of xerostomia and use of fluorides and remineralizing products besides restorations.

Osteoradionecrosis

Osteoradionecrosis is the necrosis of bone that has received high dose of radiation. Radiation therapy results in

110   Oral Medicine

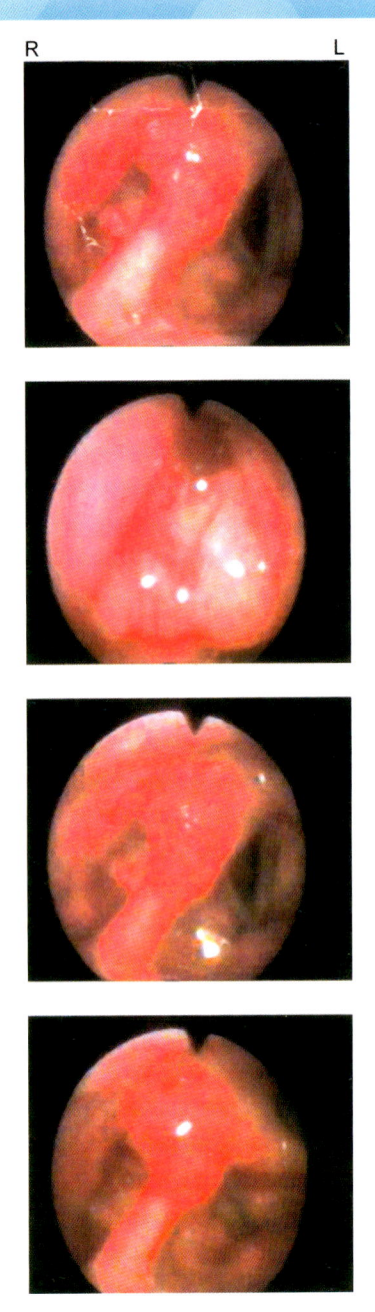

Fig. 14.27A: Videoendoscopy report-impression: Malignancy involving RT pyriform fossa. RT cord is fixed (T3) before irradiation

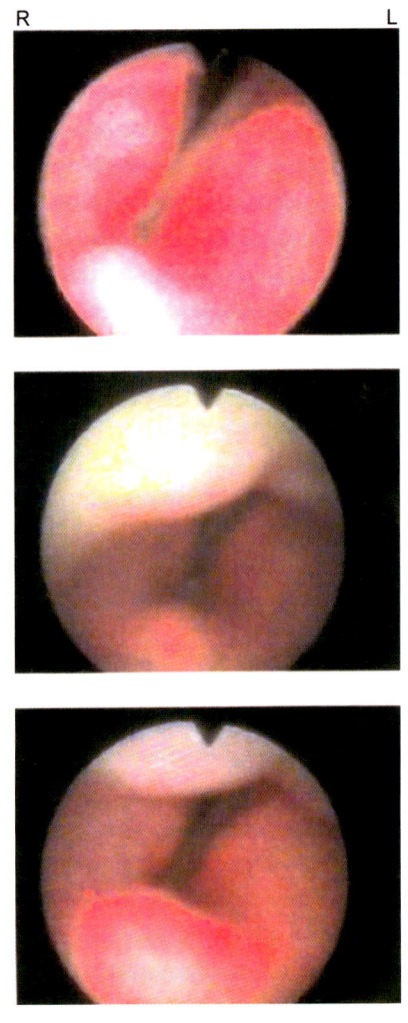

Fig. 14.27B: Videoendoscopy report. After irradiation edema is evident. Impression: FTC irradiated CA RT pyriform fossa. Flexible endoscopy reveals marked edema of the right arytenoid. RT cord is fixed

hypovascular, hypocellular and hypoxic tissue that is unable to repair or remodel effectively. Thus any injury or trauma such as dental extraction or surgical procedure results in impaired healing leading to necrosis. The mandible is most commonly involved than maxilla. The presenting signs and symptoms are pain and tenderness, bad taste, anesthesia and paresthesia, development of extraoral and oro-antral fistula, pathologic fractures and secondary infections.

The measures should be taken to prevent osteoradionecrosis from the beginning, when the radiotherapy treatment starts. Oral hygiene should be maintained and teeth with periodontal disease should be extracted. When the osteoradionecrosis develops, management includes avoiding use of dental appliance to reduce mucosal irritation, maintaining nutrition and stopping smoking and alcohol consumption. Hyperbaric oxygen therapy should be used as it increases oxygenation of tissue and promotes osteoblastic and fibroblastic functions.

Nutrition

Radiation therapy results in change of taste due to effect on the taste buds, xerostomia or secondary infections. The radiation reduces the acuteness of all tastes whether sweet, sour, salt or bitter. Zinc sulphate 220 mg, BD may be prescribed to patients experiencing taste disturbances.

Dentofacial Abnormalities

Radiation therapy in the head and neck region of children may affect the future growth and development of teeth and facial bones. Radiotherapy may lead to agenesis of teeth, agenesis of roots only, abnormal calcification and abnormal root structure. Growth of facial skeleton may also be affected and may lead to retrognathia, micrognathia, altered maxillary growth and asymmetric growth. Trismus may also occur due to fibrosis of muscles.

BIBLIOGRAPHY

1. Bansal Ajay. Tumor Markers. Impression 2006;(5)3.
2. Califano J, Westra WH, Koch W, et al. Unknown primary head and neck SCC: Molecular identification of the site of origin. J Natl Cancer Inst 1999;91(7):599-604.
3. Croce CM, Sozzi G, Huebner K. Role of FHIT in human cancer J Clin Oncol 1999;17:1618-24.
4. Dodd MJ, Miaskowski C, Shiba GH, et al. Risk factors for chemotherapy-induced oral mucositis: Dental appliances, oral hygiene, previous oral lesions and history of smoking. Cancer Invest 1999;17:278-84.
5. Epstein JB, Gorsky M. Topical application of vitamin A to oral leukoplakia: A clinical case series. Cancer 1998;83:629-34.
6. Epstein JB, Lunn R, Le N, Stevenson-Moore P. Periodontal attachment loss in patients after head and neck radiation therapy. Oral Surg Oral Med Oral Pathol Oral Radiol Endod 1998;86: 715-9.
7. Mao L, EI-Naggar AK, Papadimitrakopoulou V, et al. Phenotype and genotype of advanced premalignant head and neck lesions after chemopreventive therapy. J Natl Cancer Inst 1998;90(20):1545-51.
8. McCarthy GM, Awde JD, Ghandi H, et al. Risk factors associated with mucositis in cancer patients receiving 5-fluorouracil. Oral Oncol 1998;34:484-90.
9. Rishiraj B, Epstein JB. Basal cell carcinoma: What dentists need to know. J Am Dent Assoc 1999;130:375-80.
10. Schoelch ML, Sekandari N, Regezi JA, Silverman S Jr. Laser management of oral leukoplakias: A follow-up study of 70 patients. Laryngoscope 1999;109:949-53.
11. Sciubba JJ. Improving detection of precancerous and cancerous oral lesions: Computer-assisted analysis of the oral brush biopsy. J Am Dent Assoc 1999;130:1445-57.
12. Sonis ST, Eilers JP, Epstein JB, et al. Validation of a new scoring system for the assessment of clinical trial research of oral mucositis induced by radiation or chemotherapy. Cancer 1999;85:2103-13.
13. Sonis ST. Mucositis as a biologic process: A new hypothesis for the development of chemotherapy-induced stomatotoxicity. Oral Oncol 1998;34-39-43.
14. Sharma LM, Agnihotri PK, Rajan SY, Padmavathi BN, Guruprasad R. Gene therapy and its applications in Dentistry, JIAOMR 2006;18:1.
15. Uzawa N, Yoshida MA, Hosoe S, et al. Functional evidence for involvement of multiple putative tumor suppressor gene on the short arm of chromosome 3 in human oral squamous cell carcinogenesis. Cancer Genet Cytogenet 1998;107:125-31.
16. Van der Meij EH, Schepman KP, Smeele LE, et al. A review of the recent literature regarding malignant transformation of oral lichen planus. Oral Surg Oral Med Oral Pathol Oral Radiol Endod 1999;88:307-10.

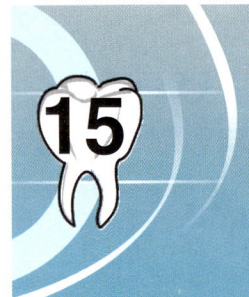

Diseases of the Tongue

STRUCTURE OF THE TONGUE

Tongue is a complex muscular structure situated in the floor of the mouth. At rest, the tip of the tongue and its lateral border approximate the edges of the teeth. The tongue is divided into small anterior portion (oral portion) and large posterior portion (base of the tongue). The surface of the tongue is covered with specialized mucous membrane from which different types of papillary projections are developed. These papillary projections are filiform, fungiform, and circumvallate papillae.

The filiform and fungiform papillae are found only on anterior two-thirds of the tongue. Filiform papillae modulate pressure sensations on the tongue and help in pushing food distally. Fungiform papillae bear taste buds and function as taste receptors. The anterior two-thirds of the tongue is free from mucous or serous glands except glands of Blandin and Nuhn, which are present directly under the tip of the tongue.

Circumvallate papillae are present at junction of anterior two-third and posterior third of the tongue. They contain large number of taste buds on their walls and clusters of serous glands (glands of von Ebner). Secretions from glands of von Ebner contain a lipoprotein lipase which helps in digestion of fat in neonates.

The bulk of the tongue is made up of four intrinsic and four extrinsic muscles. The tongue is supplied by right and left lingual arteries arising from external carotid arteries.

FUNCTIONS OF THE TONGUE

The tongue serves numerous functions in humans. The knowledge of these functions helps in diagnosis and management of local and systemic disorders affecting the tongue.

Ingestion

The coordinated muscular activity of the tongue and jaws, lips and cheeks helps in licking, sucking and chewing movements and propelling the food to the pharynx.

Suckling

The rhythmic compression of tongue and jaw of infant helps in discharging milk from mother's breast and thus helps in suckling.

Swallowing

Tongue helps in swallowing the food by sequential muscular activity in tongue and constrictor muscles of pharynx, which closes the epiglottis, allowing the bolus to enter into the esophagus, without regurgitation into nasal cavity or respiratory tract.

Respiration

Position of the tongue and the jaw along with lingual muscular tonicity, influences respiratory control.

Perception

The specialized mucous membrane and nerve supply of the dorsum of the tongue helps in perception of taste, pain, temperature and general sensation.

Jaw Development

Muscular pressure from the tongue is a contributing factor in the development of shape of mandibular arch. Increased tongue size as in case of acromegaly or tumor lead to spacing of teeth. Tongue thrusting is an important etiological factor in anterior open bite.

Phonation

Strength and control of lingual muscles along with lingual sensory system are required for accurate pronunciation, thus in this way tongue helps in speech.

EXAMINATION OF THE TONGUE

Routine Examination

Already described in chapter 6.

Specialized Examination Procedures

Cine Radiography

Cine radiography helps in diagnosing abnormalities of phonation, swallowing and other functions associated with congenital and surgically induced defects.

Isotopic Scanning Techniques

This technique helps in outlining the extent of lingual and other oral tumors.

Doppler Ultrasound

Doppler ultrasound is used to study the characteristics of arterial blood flow in the tongue.

Real-time Ultrasound

It is used to produce an image of cyst, abscess or other lesions of the tongue and to differentiate a vascular lesion from a fluid-filled cavity

Magnetic Resonance Imaging

MRI helps in providing details of lingual musculatures and extent of tumor infiltration.

Electromyography

Electromyography can be used to record electric activity generated in the lingual muscles which helps in understanding lingual muscular functions.

DISEASES OF MUCOSA OF THE TONGUE

Though the mucosa of the dorsal surface of the tongue is heavily keratinized, it may undergo inflammatory and degenerative processes. Changes in the surface of the tongue are usually due to secondary inflammatory changes that occur as a result of alterations in the microbial flora of tongue dorsum. Strawberry tongue is a classic sign of infection with Streptococcus pyogenes.

Changes in Tongue Papillae

Coated or Hairy Tongue

Hairy tongue is a condition characterized by overgrowth of the filiform papillae. The keratinized surface of filiform papillae gets desquamated through friction of the tongue with food, palate and upper anterior teeth and are replaced by new one. During painful oral conditions, the tongue movements are restricted due to which filiform papillae gets enlarged and become heavily coated with microorganisms. This gives the tongue a hairy or coated appearance which retains debris and pigments.

Hairy tongue may also be associated with use of local and systemic medications like antibiotics, oxidizing agents and chlorhexidine. Treatment of hairy tongue includes thorough cleaning and scraping of the tongue and application of keratolytic agents (see Figs 12.10 and 12.11).

Geographic Tongue (Benign Migratory Glossitis)

Geographic tongue is an idiopathic condition characterized by mucosal atrophy or desquamation of the filliform papillae situated on the superficial epithelium of the tongue. There is irregularly shaped, reddish area where atrophy and depapillation has occurred, surrounded by narrow zone of white area in which new papillae are regenerating.

The etiology of geographic tongue is not clearly known but it may be associated with various factors like nutritional deficiency, psychologic stress, allergy and local irritation. The lesions of geographic tongue are usually asymptomatic, but may clinically present as painful, burning and stinging lesions. Painful lesions of geographic tongue can be treated by application of topical local anesthetic agents (Figs 15.1 and 15.2). Rarely tongue lesions are accompanied with similar looking lesions on gingiva, palate and buccal mucosa with burning sensation. This is called ectopic geographic tongue. Both the conditions show annular, circinate and serpiginous lesions of the tongue. These lesions have slightly depressed atrophic lesions without filliform papillae and raised white borders in irregular areas giving appearance of the geographic tongue.

Loss and Atrophy of the Tongue Papillae
Nutritional Deficiencies and Hematologic Disorders

Nutritional deficiencies can produce various changes in the tongue. The most frequently occurring lesions of the tongue

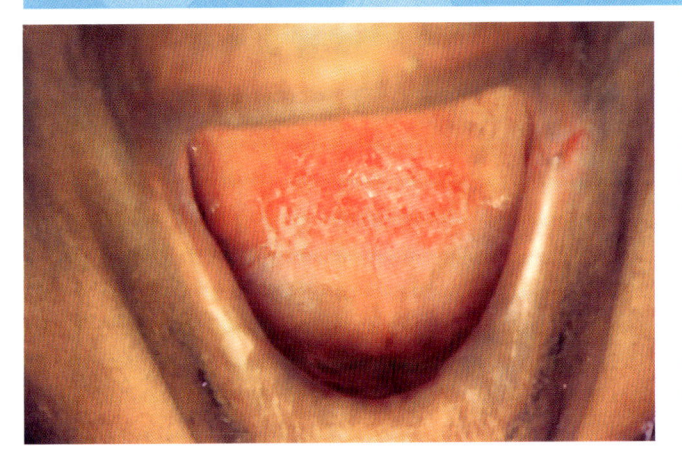

Fig. 15.1: Geographic tongue (severely affected)

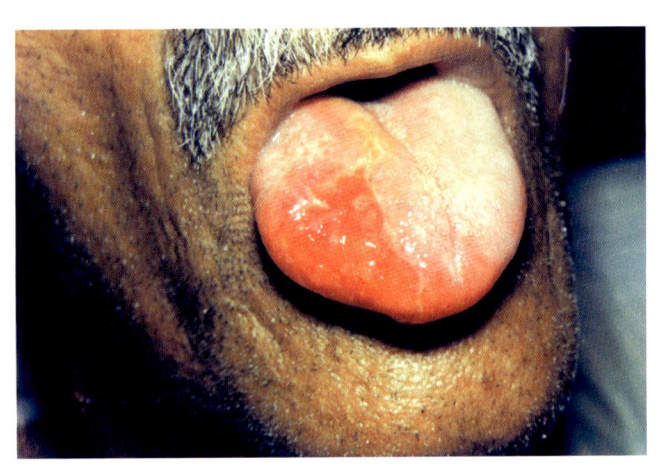

Fig. 15.2: Geographic tongue (mildly affected)

related to nutritional deficiencies are associated with vitamin B-complex deficiency, which clinically presents as loss of papillae, redness and painful swelling of the tongue. These signs and symptoms are also associated with iron deficiency. Deficiencies of these nutrients can be due to dietary deficiency or may result from malabsorption syndrome. Atrophic glossitis is the common term used to describe appearance of tongue in various nutritional deficiencies and hematological abnormalities. Purplish red colored tongue with edema and complete atrophy of papillae is seen in riboflavin deficiency.

Hematological disorders such as pernicious anemia and sideropenic anemia are caused due to nutritional deficiency. Deficiencies of vitamin B_{12} and folic acid leads to pernicious anemia. The most frequent oral symptom is burning and itching sensation in the tongue, atrophy of filiform and later the fungiform papillae, leading to complete atrophic, smooth, fiery red surface of the tongue.

Iron deficiency anemia (sideropenic anemia) also features atrophic glossitis. The tongue in iron deficiency anemia appears pale yellow and bald and has a glazed appearance. There is atrophy of the filiform papillae, beginning usually at the tip and lateral borders. The lesions may or may not be associated with pain (Fig. 15.3).

Median Rhomboid Glossitis

Median rhomboid glossitis is rounded or rhomboid-shaped erythematous area on the median portion of the dorsum of the tongue just anterior to circumvallate papillae. The affected area may be fissured or lobulated with absence of papillae.

Ulcerations and Traumatic Injuries on Tongue

Various physical and infectious agents acting on normal or diseased mucosa may lead to ulcerations of the tongue. Traumatic injuries along with oral microbial flora also contribute in the etiology of tongue ulcers. Traumatic injuries to the tongue may result from various factors. The mobility of the tongue and its proximity to the rough surface of the restorations, jagged and broken cusps of the teeth may cause ulceration of the tongue. Riga's ulcers on the tongue of the infants occurs on lingual frenum.

Aspiration by saliva ejector during dental procedures can cause ulceration and ecchymosis at the junction of the frenum and lingual folds. Similarly, the ventral surface and lateral borders of the tongue can be damaged by rotating burs and other dental instruments.

The ulceration at the tip of the tongue and lateral margins can be seen in recurrent aphthous ulcers, Behcet's syndrome and vesiculobullous lesions. Severe ulcers with bruising and

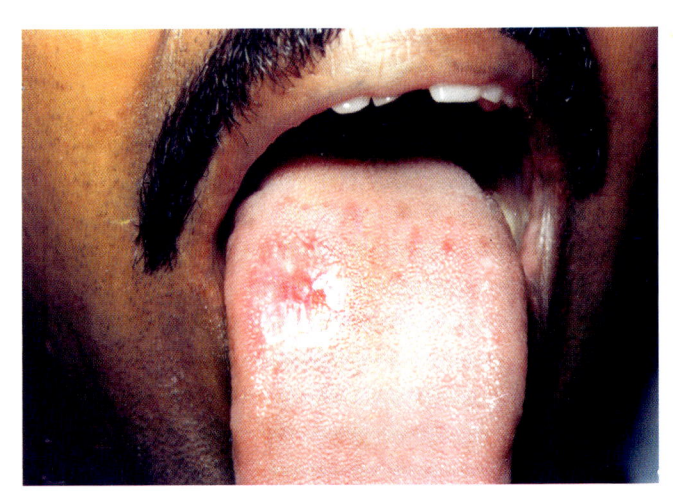

Fig. 15.3: Tongue of anemic male adult

laceration are caused by sudden biting trauma during epileptic seizure and in patients of brain damage with uncontrolled chewing and grinding movements.

The ulcerative lesions of the tongue are also seen in the infectious disease. Chronic ulcers located on the posterior ventral surface of the tongue can be seen in histoplasmosis, cryptococcosis, blastomycosis, mucormycosis and tuberculosis of the tongue. Dorsal and ventral surface and lateral margins of the tongue may be ulcerated in primary herpes simplex gingivostomatitis. Herpes zoster may produce a series of ulcers along the anterior third of the tongue on one side (Figs 15.4 and 15.5).

Superficial Vascular Changes

Superficial vascular changes which are seen on the tongue are as follows.

Lingual Varicosity

Lingual varicosities refers to dilatation of lingual veins on the anterior ventral surface of the tongue, around the submandibular and sublingual gland orifices and on the posterior pharyngeal surface of the tongue. They appear as purplish blue spots and firm nodules or ridges. Lingual varicosities are quite common in old individuals.

Petechial Hemorrhages

They are usually found on the ventral surface of the tongue in the patients of thrombocytopenia and hereditary hemorrhagic telangiectasia.

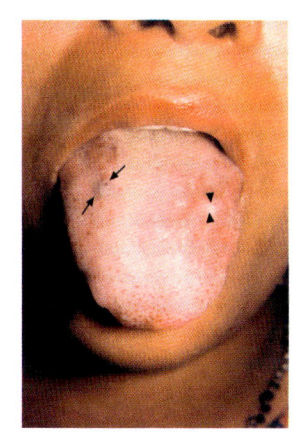

Fig. 15.4: Ulceration and traumatic injuries on dorsum of the tongue. Melanin pigmentation is present on the tip. Small hematoma (shown by arrows) and a small leukoplakic patch (shown by arrowheads) and bald areas are also present on the dorsal surface of the tongue

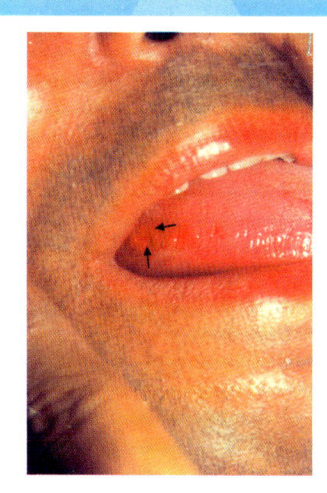

Fig. 15.5: Ulcer on the lateral border of the tongue (shown by arrows)

Syphilitic Interstitial Glossitis

In tertiary syphilis, tongue may be affected by interstitial glossitis. In syphilitic interstitial glossitis, non-ulcerating, irregular indurations develop on the tongue with accompanying ischemia, resulting in atrophy of tongue. The papillae are lost due to pathologic changes and subsequent irritation results in leukoplakic changes. It occurs predominantly in males and may transform into carcinoma of the tongue.

DISEASES OF BODY OF THE TONGUE

Infections

Ludwig's Angina

It is an infection involving submaxillary, submental and sublingual spaces originating from periapical abscesses of the mandibular molars. It results in painful swelling of the floor of the mouth and base of the tongue, which elevates the tongue upwards and leads to dysphagia, dysphonia and upper airway obstruction.

Actinomycosis of Tongue

Abscesses of the tongue may get infected by actinomyces species, when contaminated with calculus and tooth fragments. The tongue becomes enlarged, erythematous, nodular and very tender to touch.

Cysticercosis and Trichinosis

Cysticercosis and trichinosis are the diseases caused by encystment of larvae of Taenia solium and Trichinella spiralis respectively, in the muscles of the tongue. The signs and symptoms are muscleache, facial edema, fever and marked eosinophilia.

Amyloidosis of the Tongue

Amyloidosis is a disease characterized by extracellular accumulation of amyloid in the various organs and tissues of the body. Amyloidosis of tongue is of either AA or AL varieties, having amyloid deposits in mesenchymal tissues of the tongue.

The tongue in amyloidosis gets enlarged and develops yellowish nodules. The thickened tongue can affect mastication, dentition, deglutition and phonetics.

Angioneurotic Edema

Angioneurotic edema is a type of anaphylactic reaction representing a sudden hypersensitivity response. It is characterized by well circumscribed, localized edema involving the mucosa and subcutaneous tissues. It may affect the mucosa of the tongue, causing swelling of the tongue which may lead to occlusion of the airway.

It is caused by various antigenic stimuli like respiratory allergens, various drugs and medicaments, foods, such as egg, shellfish, bacterial antigens, cold and trauma to the tongue. Antihistaminics and sympathomimetic drugs provide symptomatic relief.

Neuromuscular Disorders

Oropharyngeal Dysphagia

It is caused by weakness of muscles of the tongue. The symptoms of oropharyngeal dysphagia are inability of the tongue to move the bolus into pharynx, regurgitation of fluid into nose, pharyngeal pain on deglutition and sensation of lump in the throat. Oropharyngeal dysphagia is mostly caused by neuromuscular disorder, it may also occur in patients with Plummer-Vinson syndrome and Sjogren's syndrome.

Tardive Dyskinesia

Tardive dyskinesia refers to involuntary movement of the tongue and facial muscles that develops as late complications of phenothiazine, reserpine and antipsychotic medications. Symptoms are rapid movement of tongue, lips and jaw.

Dystonia

Dystonia refers to hypertonicity of muscles resulting in impairment of voluntary functions. Dystonia involving the tongue may occur with levadopa therapy used for treatment of parkinsonism, and due to complications of chronic use of neuroleptic drugs. This condition can be treated by administration of benzotropine mesylate.

Weakness of the Tongue

Weakness of the tongue muscles can occur in number of diseases like multiple sclerosis, myositis, Duchenne's muscular dystrophy, myotonic dystrophy and hypoglossal palsy. The tongue becomes small and flaccid that cannot be extended and falls backward into the mouth blocking the airway.

Myasthenia Gravis

Myasthenia gravis is characterized by weakness and fatigue of voluntary muscles. Protrusive movements of tongue become weak which results in posterior collapse of tongue with airway obstruction. Other symptoms are poor control of saliva, dysphagia and regurgitation of food into the mouth.

Vascular Disease of Body of Tongue

The lingual arteries have high susceptibility of developing atherosclerosis. The disease increases with age and is common in patients of arteriosclerotic heart disease. The symptoms are pain, burning of tongue and loss of taste sensation.

SQUAMOUS CELL CARCINOMA OF THE TONGUE

Squamous cell carcinoma of the tongue is the most common carcinoma occurring in the oral cavity. About 60% of the tongue carcinoma occurs on the lateral borders of anterior two-third, and remaining arise from the ventral surface of the tongue. The dorsum of the tongue is rarely affected. Carcinoma of the tongue is usually seen in middle and later decades of life.

Etiological Factors

Tongue carcinoma is associated with following factors:
A. Tobacco, "Khaini" and alcohol use
B. Chronic dental trauma

Diseases of the Tongue

C. Infection with Candida albicans
D. Atrophic glossitis
E. Dietary deficiencies.

Clinical Features

Most of the carcinomas of the tongue clinically appear as ulcer or exophytic lesion. The most common presenting symptoms are local pain, pain on deglutition and sensation of lump in the neck. The tumor gets metastasized to submandibular and upper cervical lymph nodes.

Treatment

Early carcinoma of the tongue can be successfully treated by surgical excision or radiation. Advanced T_3 stage of lingual carcinoma can be treated by combined surgical and radiation therapy. Carcinoma of anterior two-third with lymph-node involvement is treated by radical neck dissection, partial mandibulectomy and intraoral dissection. Carcinoma of posterior tongue is mostly treated by radiation.

MISCELLANEOUS

Smoker's Glossitis

Excessive smoking usually cause two types of changes (A) Inflammatory changes which appear as reddish patches on the dorsum of the tongue. (B) Degenerative changes showing atrophy of the papillae and blackish degeneration of the papillae (Figs 15.6 and 15.7).

Fissured Tongue (Scrotal Tongue)

In fissured tongue many irregular fissured are present on the dorsal surface of the tongue ranging from 2 to 6 mm in depth. It is a benign condition and special treatment is required. Regular cleaning and brushing of tongue should be done because food or debris if remain in grooves may act as a source of irritation (Fig. 15.8).

Tongue with thick leathery coating in dehydrated and debilitated patient is called 'Earthy' tongue.

Hyperplastic Foliate Papillae of Tongue with Midline Fissure

This is benign condition. Hyperplasia of the foliate papillae may be due to some irritation. Midline fissure on the tongue is a developmental anoma and has no clinical significance (Fig. 15.9). 'Long and narrow' tongue as a result of hyperos-

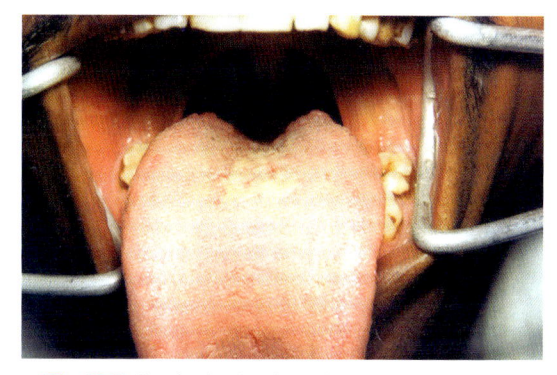

Fig 15.7: Smoker's glossitis—degenerative changes

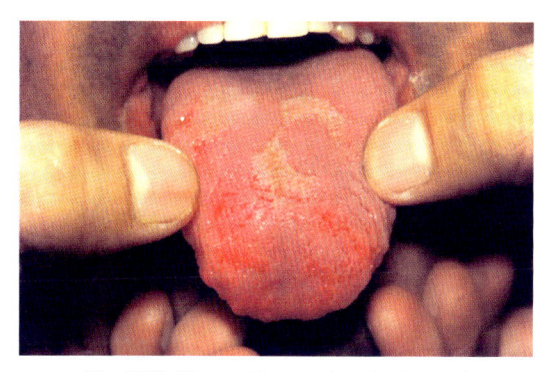

Fig. 15.8: Fissured tongue (scrotal tongue)

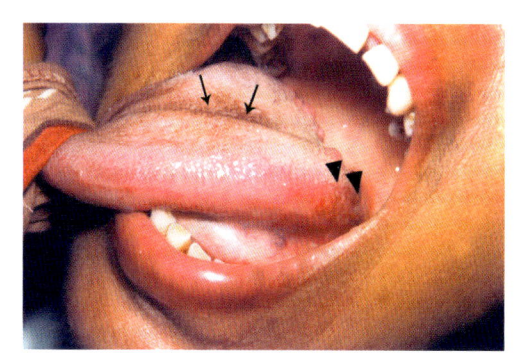

Fig. 15.9: Hyperplastic foliate papillae of tongue (shown with arrowheads) with midline fissure (shown with arrows)

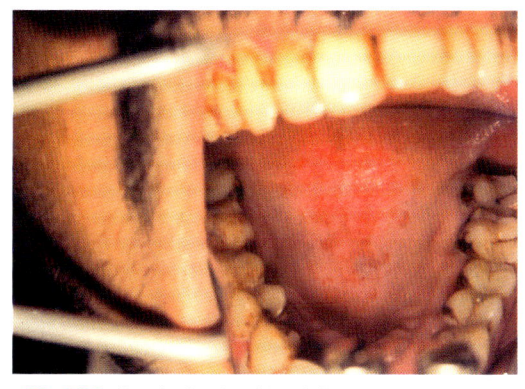

Fig 15.6: Smoker's glossitis—inflammatory changes

tosis and thickening of the mandible is seen in tuberous sclerosis.

vander woude's syndrome—Shows there are pits on the lower lip and cleft lip and/or cleft palate.

BIBLIOGRAPHY

1. Cohen PR, Kazi S, Grossman ME. Herpetic geometric glossitis. A distinctive pattern of lingual herpes simplex virus infection, South Med J 1995;88:1231.
2. Dunham ME, Austin TL. Congenital aglossia and situs inversus. Int J Pediatr Otorhinolaryngol 1990;19:163-68.
3. Flinck A, Paludan A, Matsson L, et al. Oral findings in a group of new-born Swedish children, Int J Paediatr Dent 1994;4:67-73.
4. Heymann WR. Psychotropic agent-induced black hairy tongue. Cutis 2000;66 (1): 25-6.
5. Morgan WE, Friedman EM, Duncan NO, et al. Surgical management of macroglossia in children, Arch Otolaryngol Head Neck Surg 1996;122:326-9.
6. Wolford LM, Cottrell DA. Diagnosis of macroglossia and indications for reduction glossectomy, Am J Orthod Dentofac Orthop 1996;110:170-7.

16

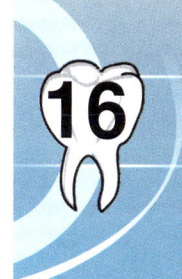

Diseases of Salivary Gland

There are three major pairs of salivary glands: parotid, submandibular and sublingual. They secrete a highly modified saliva through a branching duct system. There are also thousands of minor salivary glands situated throughout the mouth. They are called by their anatomic situations like labial, palatal and buccal. They are situated just below the oral mucosa and open in oral cavity by short ducts. All major and minor salivary glands produce saliva. Saliva is a highly complex mixture of organic, inorganic components and waters. The three major salivary glands are composed of acinar and ductal cells. Saliva is protein rich hypotonic fluid. The salivary secretion is controlled by sympathetic and parasympathetic neural input.

DIAGNOSIS OF ENLARGED SALIVARY GLAND OR SALIVARY MASS

Salivary tumors both benign and malignant are mostly asymptomatic growth. Infection, cystic involvement can cause pain. Tumor may arise from minor salivary glands, obstruct and involve nose or paranasal sinus.

Physical Examination of Salivary Glands

All the three pairs of major salivary glands are palpated. When gland is pressed or 'milked' clear saliva should come out from the orifices. The regional lymph nodes are palpated. Any mass observed on palpation is evaluated for ulceration and invasion of the adjacent structures. Pain is not dependable indicator for malignancy.

Parotid Gland

Tumors present as painless solitary mobile nodes or masses usually located at the tail of the gland. When there is any decrease in motor function, the facial nerve should be evaluated as the facial nerve passes through parotid gland. Usually malignancy causes facial nerve paralysis. Rarely infection and sudden rapid growth in benign tumor can also cause paralysis of facial nerve (Figs 16.1 to 16.4).

In malignant growth following will be present:
a. Multiple masses
b. Fixed mass involving surrounding tissues
c. Involvement of the regional lymph nodes—Bimanual palpation is done. By one hand intraorally and by other hand extraorally.
d. Pain is usually present on palpation.

Submandibular and Sublingual Glands

Benign tumors are mostly slow growing painless solitary mobile masses. The malignant tumors are mostly non-mobile and fixed to the surrounding structures and usually painful on palpation. They involve regional lymph nodes.

Minor Salivary Glands

Benign tumors of minor salivary glands are mostly small masses located on the palate. In malignant tumors usually the ulcerations of the overlying mucosa takes place.

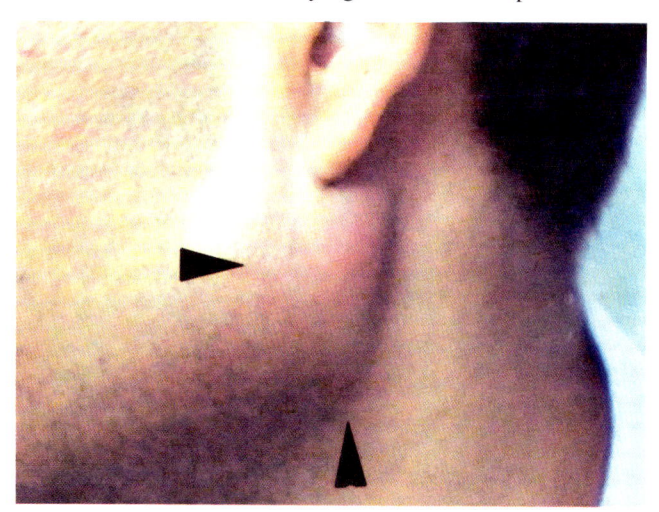

Fig. 16.1: Acute parotitis in male (shown by arrowheads) (*Courtesy* Dr Rohit Chandra, Noida)

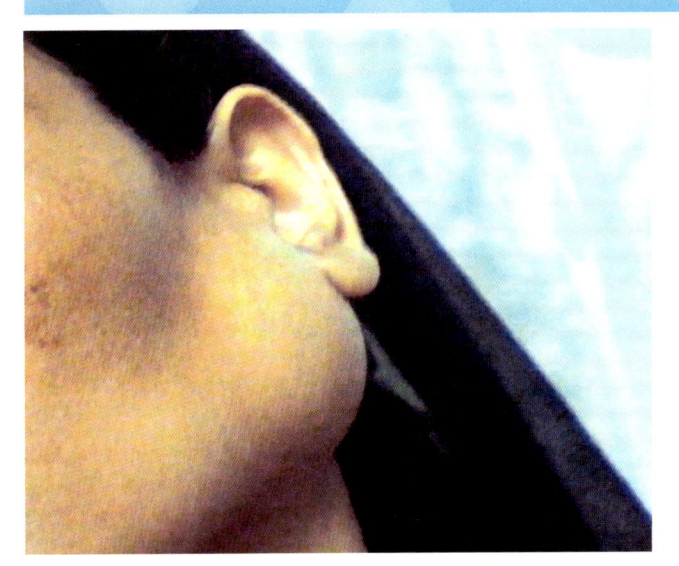

Fig. 16.2: Acute parotitis in female
(*Courtesy* Dr Rohit Chandra, Noida)

Differential Diagnosis

Many other lesions may be confused with salivary gland tumors. Glandular enlargement may take place in nutritional deficiencies, infections and inflammatory diseases. HIV positive patients may have cystic lymphoepithelial lesions which look like tumors. The malignant tumors of oral cavity like squamous cell carcinoma and melanoma can metastasize to the salivary glands and look like primary tumor of salivary glands. In the submandibular gland chronic sialadenitis may appear like tumor. Necrotizing sialometaplasia in minor salivary glands may be confused with squamous cell carcinoma.

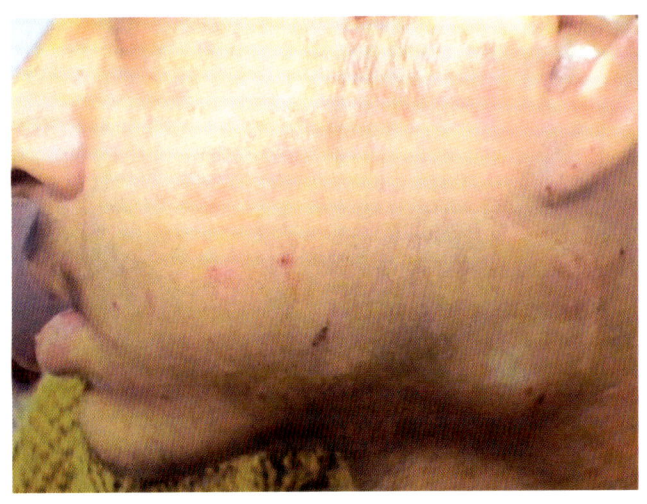

Fig. 16.3: Recurrent parotid tumor (*Courtesy* Dr Rohit Chandra)

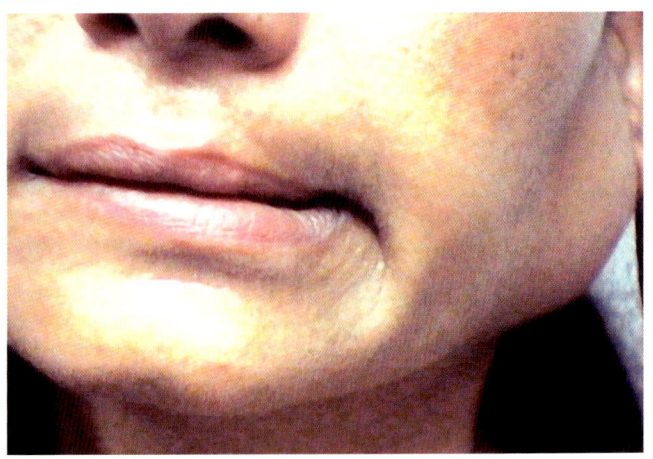

Fig. 16.4: Facial palsy due to tumor in the parotid gland
(*Courtesy* Dr Rohit Chandra)

DIAGNOSTIC PROCEDURES IN DRY MOUTH (XEROSTOMIA) EVALUATION

Xerostomia is not a disease but a symptom. It may be due to salivary gland dysfunction. Nonsalivary causes of oral dryness may be dehydration. There may be psychological conditions for dryness in mouth. Investigations should include the following:
1. Past and present medical history
2. Oral examination
3. Salivary function evaluation
4. Salivary imaging
5. Biopsy
6. Hematological examinations

Salivary gland dysfunction-symptoms
1. Decreased fluid in oral cavity-dryness in oral mucosa.
2. Difficulty in chewing, swallowing and speaking.
3. Pain-mild to moderate
4. Mucosa sensitivity to spicy, dry and rough food.

Medical History—Past and Present

The taking of medicines for malignancy or radiation in head and neck region may interfere with salivary gland function. In Sjogren's syndrome dryness at other mucous membrane openings like nose, eye, throat and vagina also takes place along with oral cavity.

EXAMINATION

Signs of dryness of oral cavity are poor oral hygiene, rampant caries, cracking, peeling, and atrophic lips and red and smooth oral mucosa and tongue. Palpation of salivary glands should be painless. If salivary glands are painful on palpation, infection or acute inflammation is present. There should be rubbery consistency without any hard nodule.

Collection of Saliva Sample

Whole Saliva

Unstimulated whole saliva is collected for general assessment. The flow rate of saliva varies with individual. The mixed saliva from all glands is called 'whole saliva'. Chewing of paraffin wax increases salivary flow for collection of "whole saliva". The flow rate is affected by position of patient, hydration, diurnal variation, and time since stimulation.

Saliva from Individual Gland

Saliva from parotid gland can be collected by Carlson-Crittenden collectors by gentle suction after placing them over the openings of the Stensen's ducts. Saliva from submandibular and sublingual glands is collected by 'segregator' which is an aspirating device. Stimulated saliva is collected by applying a sialagogue like citric acid to the dorsal surface of the tongue. The salivary flow rate is determined gravimetrically in mm per minute per gland, assuming that the specific gravity of saliva is 1 (i.e., 1 gm equals to 1 ml of saliva).

IMAGING OF SALIVARY GLANDS

Various imaging techniques are used for evaluation of salivary glands. Among them the important are plain film radiography, sialography, ultrasonography, radionuclide imaging, magnetic resonance imaging and computed tomography.

Plain Film Radiography

Radiographs of salivary glands can be taken by normal radiographic techniques. Sialoliths (stones) can be seen as radioopaque bodies usually oval in shape by plain film radiography. Parotid glands can be seen by lateral oblique, occlusal and anteroposterior (AP) views. To visualize the stones in the parotid gland opening an occlusal X-ray film is placed intraorally next to parotid gland opening like periapical film and X-ray tube is near the molar bone. Stones in the submandibular gland can be seen by panoramic, occlusal and lateral oblique views. For smaller or poorly calcified stones repeated radiographs with different angulations are required.

Sialography

Sialography of the salivary gland is its radiographic visualization after retrograde instillation of solution of contrast material into the duct.

Indications

A. Obstruction in salivary duct by a stone. Identification and localization of stone.
B. Stricture can be easily seen by sialography.
C. Autoimmune and radiation induced stone.
D. Delineating ductal anatomy.

Contraindications

A. Neoplasms are more clearly seen by cross-sectional imaging technique like MRI and computerized tomography.
B. Allergy to contrast media (most of the contrast media contain iodine, which may cause allergy).
C. Acute infection—Acute infection will spread by injection of contrast media.

Contrast Media (CM)

Advantage
Higher-viscosity water soluble contrast agents provide good visibility of ductal structures.

Disadvantages

A. Invasive
B. Risk of allergy due to presence of iodine in the dye
C. Functional efficiency cannot be determined and quantified.

Immediately after sialography, to promote salivary flow and flow out contrast media patient must do the following:
a. Repeatedly massage the gland
b. Chew sugar free lemon drops for one hour.

After one hour postsialography radiograph is done to check the complete outflow or resorption of the contrast media. If contrast media is still present patient should be recalled for follow up on the next day to check the presence of left over contrast media. If left over contrast media is still present patient is directed to massage the gland properly.

Ultrasonography

The submandibular and superficial part of parotid gland are easily and correctly visualized by ultrasonography but the deep portion of the parotid gland which is behind the mandibular ramus is difficult to visualize.

Indications

A. Guidance for biopsy
B. Growth and mass detection

Advantages

a. Ultrasonography can differentiate between the following:
   i. cysts
   ii. solid lesions
   iii. abscess in inflamed gland
   iv. stones
b. Noninvasive
c. Cost effective

Disadvantages

a. Chances of error due to observer's variability are present
b. Functional efficiency cannot be quantified
c. Morphologic information cannot be obtained
d. Deeper portions of the glands are not clearly visible.

Radionuclide Salivary Imaging (RSI), (Scintigraphy)

For evaluation and quantification of the function of the salivary glands scintigraphy with technetium (Tc) 99 m pertechnetate is a minimally invasive and dynamic diagnostic test. It can measure abnormalities, gland uptake and excretion. It is the only salivary imaging technique which can measure functional capabilities of the glands. After the injection of 10 to 20 mCi of Tc 99 m pertechnetate salivary imaging is carried out. Tc 99 m scans are interpretated visually and on clinical judgement. Quantification is done for research purposes.

Indication of Radionuclide Salivary Imaging (RSI), (Scintigraphy)

A. When sialography is not possible. Scintigraphy is indicated when patient cannot be evaluated by sialography due to (a) gland infection (b) iodine allergy. (c) inability to successfully connulate major duct:
B. In presence of tumor
C. When ductal obstruction is present
D. When sialolithiasis is present
E. When gland aplasia is present
F. When Bell's palsy is present
G. When Sjogren's syndrome is present

Advantages of RSI (Scintigraphy)

A. Functional efficiency of the gland can be quantified.
B. Can be used in the diagnosis of many diseases.
C. Results can be stored in computer for future use.

Disadvantages of RSI (Scintigraphy)

A. Radiation exposure
B. Quantification is very time consuming and difficult
C. No morphological information can be obtained.

Computed Tomography (CT)

CT images are produced by radiographic beams which can penetrate the tissues.

Indications of CT

1. CT is used for study of calcified structures.
2. To evaluate the salivary gland pathology and adjacent structures.

Advantages of CT

1. Can differentiate calcified tissues from soft tissues.
2. Can evaluate the salivary gland pathology and nearby structures like facial nerve, retromandibular vein, carotid artery and deep lymph nodes.
3. Osseous defects and sclerosis are clearly seen.
4. Pathology associated with sialoliths can be clearly seen.
5. Fluid filled masses like cyst can be distinguished from abscess and other pathologies.
6. Ultrafast CT and three-dimensional image CT sialography is more effective in seeing the defects and growths which are not clearly seen.
7. Ultrafast CT is useful for patients in which MRI is contraindicated.

Disadvantages of CT

1. Quantification of defects is not possible
2. Radiation exposure cannot be avoided
3. Intravenous iodine—containing contrast media is required.
4. Dental restorations may interfere with CT requiring repositioning of the patient to a semiaxial position.
5. Non-enhanced and enhanced CT images are routinely required for differential diagnosis.

Magnetic Resonance Imaging (MRI)

MRI uses nonionizing radiation from the radiofrequency (RF) bond of the electromagnetic spectrum: Different water concentration of the tissues permits MRI to distinguish between various types of the tissues. The absorption and then re-emission of the electromagnetic energy differ from tissue to tissue when exposed to a strong electromagnetic field. Net magnetization when analysed by radiofrequency provide an image. The images thus obtained are called T_1 and T_2 weighted images as per the rate constant with which magnetic relaxation or polarization takes place.

Indications of MRI

1. For differential diagnosis of soft tissue lesions of salivary gland.
2. For correct locations of adjacent soft tissue structures, facial nerve, carotid artery, retromandibular vein etc.
3. Preoperative evaluation of salivary gland tumors.

Advantages of MRI

1. No radiation hazard
2. Routinely no intravenous contrast media is required
3. Dental restorations provide negligible artifact
4. Provide excellent differential diagnosis for soft tissue pathologies
5. Can distinguish hard tissues with soft tissues.

For preoperative evaluation of salivary gland tumors MRI has become the imaging modality of choice as it can excellently differentiate between various soft tissues and provides multiplaner imagine.

Disadvantage of MRI

MRI is contraindicated in following patients:
(a) with pacemakers (b) with metallic implants anywhere in the body (c) patients who cannot remain in still position.

Biopsy of Salivary Glands

Major Glands

Biopsy of major salivary glands is usually done by extra-oral approach. For this fine needle aspiration is done, if it fails to provide adequate sample for diagnosis, an open biopsy procedure is done.

Minor Glands

Biopsy of a minor glands of the lower lip is a minimal operative procedure. After incision on the unvisible part of lower lip 6 to 10 minor gland lobules are removed just below the mucosa for examination. Minor glands biopsy is useful in diagnosis of amyloidosis.

Serological Assessment

Serum amylase is usually elevated in inflammation of salivary glands. The important contributor for the diagnosis of Sjogren's syndrome are the presence of nonspecific markers of immunity like antinuclear antibodies, rheumatoid factors, ESR and elevated immunoglobins.

Fine Needle Aspiration Biopsy (FNAB)

It is a simple, easy and effective technique for diagnosis of the solid lesions. Cells are aspirated from the lesion for cytological examination. FNAB can provide information if the lesion is benign or malignant.

Open Surgical Biopsy

Excisional biopsy is indicated in salivary gland tumors. This is both diagnostic and curative.

Imaging

Radiological examination of mandible and maxilla can detect the involvement of the adjacent bony structures with the tumors. CT and MRI both can show tumors but cannot definitely distinguish between benign and malignant.

STAGING

For staging of salivary gland tumors of parotid and submandibular glands tumor—node-metastasis (TNM) staging system is used. "T" shows tumor size and its extension, "N" shows nodal (lymph) involvement. "M" denotes metastases (Table 16.1).

Table 16.1: Staging for major salivary gland cancer

T_x	Primary tumor which cannot be assessed
T_0	No evidence of primary tumor
T_1	Tumor < 2 cm in greatest dimension
T_2	Tumor 2 to 4 cm in greatest dimension
T_3	Tumor 4 to 6 cm in greatest dimension
T_4	Tumor > 6 cm in greatest dimension

All the above categories have been subdivided: (a) no local extension, (b) local extension. Local extension is clinical/macroscopic invasion of skin, soft tissue, bone or nerve. Microscopic evidence alone is not considered local extension for classification purposes.

N_x	Regional nodes cannot be assessed
N_0	No regional lymph node metastases
N_1	Single ipsilateral node <3 cm in diameter
N_{2a}	Single ipsilateral node 3 to 6 cm in diameter
N_{2b}	Multiple ipsilateral node, none > 6 cm
N_{2c}	Bilateral or contralateral nodes, none > 6 cm
N_3	Metastasis in a lymph node > 6 cm

Contd...

Contd...

M$_x$ Presence of distant metastases cannot be assessed
M$_0$ No distant metastases
M$_1$ Distant metastases

Stage	T	N	M
Stage I	T$_{1a}$	N$_0$	M$_0$
	T$_{2a}$	N$_0$	M$_0$
Stage II	T$_{1b}$	N$_0$	M$_0$
	T$_{2b}$	N$_0$	M$_0$
	T$_{3a}$	N$_0$	M$_0$
Stage III	T$_{3b}$	N$_0$	M$_0$
	T$_{4a}$	N$_0$	M$_0$
	Any T (except T$_{4b}$)	NI	M$_0$
Stage IV	T$_{4b}$	Any N	M$_0$
	Any T	N$_2$N$_3$	M$_0$
	Any T	Any N	M$_1$

Adapted from the American Joint Committee for Cancer Staging and End Results Reporting: manual staging of cancer. Chicago 1988

SPECIFIC DISEASES AND DISORDERS

Developmental Disorders

Ectopic Salivary Gland

Ectopic salivary gland is a salivary gland tissue that develops at a place other than its normal position. They are most frequently found in the cervical region near the parotid gland or the body of the mandible. The ectopic salivary gland in the mandible is found posterior to the first molar and may have communication with the major salivary gland. Ectopic salivary gland may be present alone or in combination with other facial anomalies. Ectopic salivary gland occurring in the neck region are mostly found in the area of branchial cleft and branchial cleft cysts.

Agenesis, Aplasia and Atresia

Agenesis means absence of an organ due to nonappearance of its primordium in the embryo or imperfect development of a part or organ. Aplasia means congenital absence or defective development of an organ or tissue. Atresia means congenital absence of a normal opening or normally patent lumen. Total agenesis means total congenital absence. Total aplasia or congenital absence of the major salivary glands is very rare. Either one of the glands or group of glands may be missing, unilaterally or bilaterally. It may occur alone or in combination with other congenital anomalies. The major symptom is xerostomia.

Atresia is a congenital absence or occlusion of one or more ducts of major salivary gland. It may result in formation of retention cyst or may lead to xerostomia.

Diverticuli

Diverticuli are characterised by presence of extension from the wall of ductal system of one of the major salivary glands as small pouches or sacs. They may lead to repeated attacks of acute parotitis. Diagnosis is confirmed by sialography. Promotion of salivary flow through the duct by regularly milking by the patient is recommended.

Accessory Ducts

Accessory ducts are commonly occurring developmental anomaly in the salivary glands. They are mostly found in association with parotid gland. Accessory ducts are most frequently found superior and anterior to the normal Stensen's duct orifice. They do not require any treatment.

Darier's Disease

In darier's disease, there are abnormalities of the salivary duct. In this there are periodic strictures affecting the main ducts. There may be symptoms of occasional obstructive sialadenitis.

FUNCTIONAL DISORDERS

Sialorrhea (Increased Saliva Secretion)

Sialorrhea refers to excessive flow of saliva. It is associated with physiological factors such as in infancy and childhood during eruption of teeth. It may be one of the symptoms in diseases like herpetic gingivostomatitis, pemphigus vulgaris, mucous membrane pemphigoid, acute necrotizing ulcerative gingivitis (ANUG) and stomatitis. Various drugs that stimulate the parasympathetic nervous system also result in increased salivary flow.

Decreased or Arrested Saliva Secretion (Xerostomia)

Decreased or arrested salivary secretion is associated with various conditions like salivary gland aplasia, radiation therapy that results in loss of salivary gland function, and destruction and atrophy of the acinar tissue of the salivary gland in Sjogren's syndrome. Decreased salivary secretion is also seen in dehydration, emotional reactions, blockage of duct by calculus, acute or chronic infection of the salivary gland and with administration of various drugs that cause depression of parasympathetic activity.

Its major clinical manifestation is xerostomia, or dryness of the mouth. In xerostomia, oral mucosa and tongue appear dry. Pain, soreness and burning of mucous membrane are common symptoms. There may be dry, cracked, peeling and atrophic lips and fissuring at the corners of the mouth. Xerostomia interferes with eating and may lead to severe dental caries. Patients with xerostomia have difficulty in wearing artificial dentures because saliva which provides retention and stability by cohesion and adhesion is missing.

RADIATION INDUCED PATHOLOGY

Effects of External Beam Radiation

For head and neck tumors external beam radiation is the treatment. The salivary glands fall within the radiation field. Radiation doses of 50 Gy or more result in severe and permanent damage of salivary glands resulting into dryness of oral cavity. However the mechanism of destruction of salivary gland is not clear.

Clinical Features

Radiotherapy is done for 6 to 8 weeks at the rate of 2 Gy daily, for 5 days per week. At the end of 2 weeks of treatment dryness of oral cavity starts. Inflammation of oral mucosa (mucositis) also takes place. There is difficulty in speaking, swallowing and increased caries as the saliva secretion is very much reduced and it becomes thick and ropy. 'Radiation caries' along with candidiasis and sialadenitis occurs. 'Radiation caries' is a type of adult rampent caries. It develops after the radiation treatment. This is very rapidly advancing caries, usually involve the incisal and cervical part of the teeth even in meticulously clean mouths. In post radiation patients there is risk of osteonecrosis and tumors of salivary glands.

Treatment

Proper radiation planning and protection of salivary glands are must. Amifostine is a radioprotective agent approved by food and drug administration of USA. Amifostine preserves the salivary function and reduces dry mouth. The mechanisms of action involves scavenging of free oxygen radicals. Amifostine is dephosphorylated in the blood by alkaline phosphatase and free thiol metabolite is formed.

The thiol metabolite scavenges free oxygen species generated by radiation. Normal tissues are more vascular and have more alkaline phosphatase. Hence the concentration of the active thiol metabolite is higher in normal tissues than cancerous tissues. Therefore normal tissues are protected and not cancerous tissues.

Dose

Amifostine is intravenously injected 15 to 30 minutes before each fractioned radiation treatment.

Side Effects

Nausea, vomiting, hypotension, hypocalcemia, temporary unconsciousness. Proper care must be taken in cardio-vascular and cerebrovascular patients. Best will be to avoid such patients till further studies are under taken.

Effects of Internal Radiation Therapy

Radioactive iodine 131 (^{131}I) given to thyroid patients can cause permanent damage and fibrosis of salivary glands resulting in less salivary flow. But ^{131}I is less harmful than external beam radiation therapy.

Treatment

Chewing of sugar free lemon drops and gums is recommended to increase salivary flow to clear ^{131}I from salivary glands, as early as possible.

Management of Xerostomia

Cause of xerostomia must be investigated and ascertained. Proper treatment must be provided for salivary gland dysfunction and its underlying systemic disorder so that the root cause of xerostomia may be corrected permanently. Management of dry mouth can be divided into following four categories.

Preventive

Good oral hygiene and daily to once a week topical fluorides for caries prevention, depending on the severity of xerostomia. Use of fluoride tooth paste is recommended. Antifungal therapy to prevent mucositis. No alcohol should be taken as it increases dryness. Dental checkup every month should be carried out.

Symptomatic

Water sipping for the whole day and also with meals. Room humidifiers should be used. Use of moisturing cream and lotions and increase in environmental humidity is recommended.

Local Salivary Stimulation

Continuous chewing of sugarfree gums, lemon drops and mint drops is recommended.

Systemic

Saliva stimulators like pilocarpine hydrochloride, bromhexine, [Dose, adults 8 mg TDS, children 4 mg TDS (Tablet 8 mg Elixir 4 mg/5ml)] anetholetrithione and cevimeline hydrochloride are used in patients with xerostomia. Pilocarpine hydrochloride and cevimeline hydrochloride are systemic sialogogues (saliva stimulator) which are popularly used in USA. Before prescribing these sialogogues drugs medical advice must taken.

OBSTRUCTIVE DISORDERS

Mucocele

Mucocele refers to swelling caused by collection of saliva at the site of damaged or obstructed minor salivary gland duct. The commonest site of occurrence of this cyst is lower lip, but it may also be found on tongue, palate and floor of mouth.

Mucocele is of two types—(a) mucous retention cyst and (b) mucous extravasation cyst.

Mucous Retention Cyst

It develops due to obstruction of minor salivary gland duct, which leads to accumulation of saliva within the gland or its duct and formation of cyst-like lesion (Fig. 16.5).

Mucous Extravasation Cyst

Mucous extravasation cyst develops as a result of damage of minor salivary gland duct by trauma, which leads to extravasation and collection of saliva into the submucosal tissue, resulting in inflammation and formation of granulation tissue.

a. Etiology
   – Obstruction of the duct by sialolith formation
   – Crushing or perforation of duct due to trauma
   – Scarring of the duct after surgery
   – Absence of the duct
b. Clinical Features
   Mucous extravasation cyst occurs mostly on the lower lip as it is more often traumatized, whereas mucous retention cyst are usually found on the palate or floor of mouth. The appearance of mucocele depends upon its location. Superficial mucocele appear as small, thin-walled bluish lesions that rupture easily. Deep seated lesions are well-circumscribed swelling with an overlying normal appearing mucosa.

   Ranula is a special type of mucocele that specifically occurs in the floor of mouth, due to damage of a sublingual or submandibular gland duct. It may be present superficial or deep to the mylohyoid muscle and clinically present as soft, fluctuant, unilateral swelling.
c. Treatment
   Treatment of mucocele is done by surgical excision or marsupialization. Intralesional injection of corticosteroid solution may also be administered for treatment of ranula.

Sialolithiasis (Salivary Gland Stones)

Sialolithiasis is a condition characterized by formation or presence of calcified and organic masses (sialoliths) in the parenchyma or duct of salivary gland. The etiological factors responsible for sialolith formation are inflammation, local irritants or drugs resulting in stasis of salivary flow. About 80 to 90% sialoliths occur in submandibular gland, followed by 5 to 15% in parotid gland, and 2 to 5% in sublingual and minor salivary gland. Submandibular gland is more prone to develop sialoliths due to: (a) sharp curvatures of Wharton's duct which trap mucin plug or cellular debris, (b) higher calcium level in submandibular saliva and (c) dependent position of the submandibular gland that increases the risk of stasis.

Clinical Features

The main symptom of sialolithiasis is pain and swelling in the area of major salivary gland, especially before meals due to stasis of saliva. This stasis may result in infection, fibrosis and atrophy of salivary gland. In most chronic cases sinus tract, fistula and ulceration over the stone may also

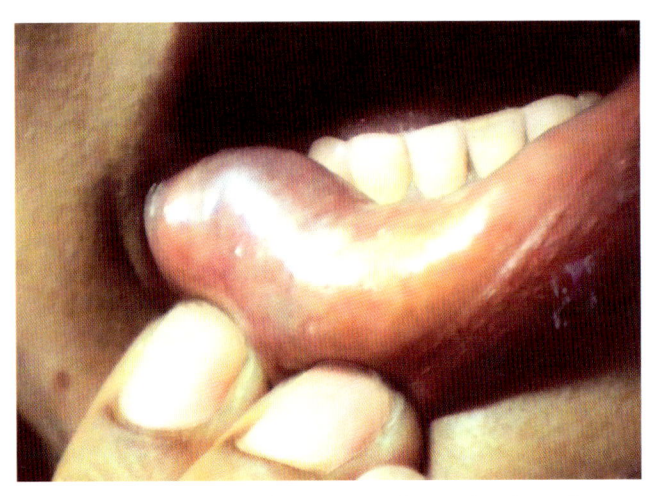

Fig. 16.5: Mucocele- (mucous retention cyst) on lower lip (*Courtesy* Dr. Rohit Chandra, Noida)

form. Sialoliths may produce asymptomatic, well-circumscribed freely movable swelling. Sialography, ultrasound and computerized axial tomography are the diagnostic methods of detecting calcified stones.

Treatment

Stones in the distal part of the duct can be removed manually. The larger and deeper stones require surgical removal. Infections secondary to the stasis should be treated by antibiotics. Lithotripsy (noninvasive treatment) can also be used for disintegrating sialoliths (Fig. 16.6).

INFLAMMATORY DISEASES (SIALADENITIS)

Inflammation of the salivary gland is called sialadenitis. It is characterized by pain and swelling of the affected gland with alteration of function. Inflammation is mainly due to bacterial or viral infection. It may also be secondary to allergic reactions or manifestation of systemic diseases. The parotid gland is affected most frequently. The rate of salivary flow is usually reduced with increase in turbidity and viscosity of saliva.

Bacterial Infections

Acute Bacterial Sialadenitis

Acute bacterial sialadenitis or acute suppurative parotitis is usually caused by *Staphylococcus aureus* or *Streptococcus viridans*. The disease is associated with decreased salivary flow in children or dehydrated and debilitated individuals. Disease occurs due to combined effect of development of antibiotic-resistant bacteria and increased use of drugs like diuretics, tranquilizers, antihistamines and anti-parkinsonian drugs which decrease salivary flow. Dehydration and poor oral hygiene are important contributing factors.

Clinical Features

Most of the cases of acute bacterial sialadenitis are unilateral. There is pain at the submandibular area and the angle of the mandible, which intensifies during opening of mouth. The affected gland on palpation appears enlarged and tender. The skin over the gland is red and warm. Discharge of purulent material from the salivary gland duct confirms the diagnosis. The symptoms are high fever, leukocytosis and other common symptoms of acute bacterial infection (Fig. 16.7).

Treatment

The electrolyte balance of the patient should be maintained by adequate hydration and intravenous fluids. Oral hygiene should be maintained by debridement and irrigation. Antibiotics should be prescribed after doing culture and sensitivity test.

Chronic Bacterial Sialadenitis

Chronic or recurrent bacterial sialadenitis can be seen in otherwise healthy children and adults. The disease in children commonly starts between the ages of 3 and 5 years.

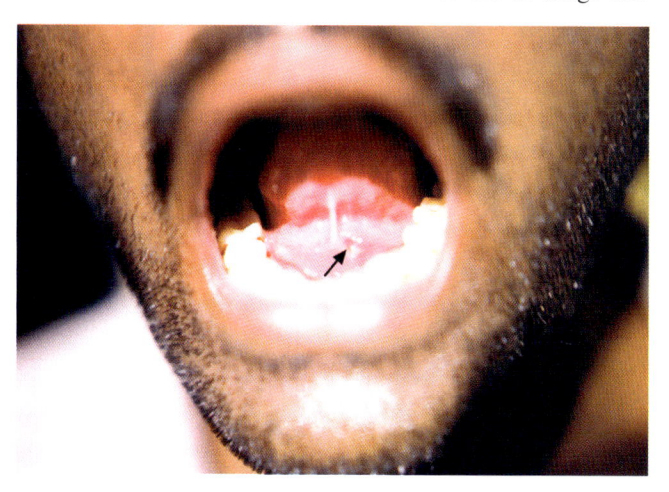

Fig. 16.6: Sialolithiasis- Arrow showing dilated opening of Wharton's duct of submandibular gland. The stone was extracted from the duct (*Courtesy* Dr Rohit Chandra, Noida)

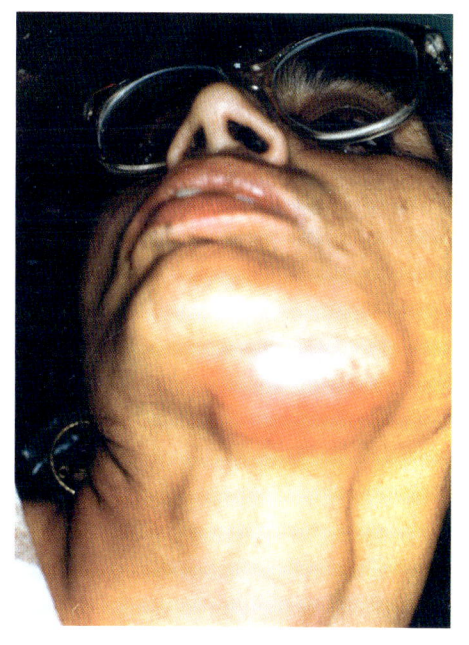

Fig. 16.7: Unilateral acute sialadenitis of a submandibular salivary gland (extra oral view)

Most of the cases of chronic sialadenitis in children disappear at puberty. The disease is mostly caused by *Streptococcus viridans*, *Escherichia coli* and proteus.

Clinical Features

The major sign is sudden onset of unilateral or bilateral swelling/s at the angle of the mandible. Purulent discharge comes out from salivary duct orifice. Mild pain and fever may be present. After several recurrences, salivary flow may be decreased due to fibrosis of parenchyma of the gland.

Treatment

Adequate hydration, sialagogues and antibiotics are included in conservative management of majority of the patients. Use of intraductal erythromycin and tetracycline; occluding the ductal system with a protein solution; and tympanic neurectomy are the other methods used in chronic cases.

VIRAL INFECTIONS

Mumps (Epidemic Parotitis)

Mumps is an acute contagious viral infection caused by a ribonucleic acid (RNA) Paramyxovirus. It mostly affects the salivary gland, but may also involve gonads, central nervous system, pancreas and thyroid gland. It predominantly occurs among children and young adults. The incubation period of infection is 2 to 3 weeks. It is transmitted by direct contact with droplets of saliva.

Clinical Features

The major sign of mumps is unilateral or bilateral swelling of the salivary gland without purulent discharge from salivary gland ducts. The parotid gland is mostly involved. Usually there is bilateral involvement of the parotid gland, but more commonly, second gland enlarges 24 to 48 hrs after the first. The enlarged glands are painful and tender.

The affected salivary gland enlarges continuously for two to three days and returns to normal size in seven days. The clinical symptoms start as fever, malaise and anorexia. There may be edema of skin overlying the gland and inflammation around the affected salivary gland duct.

Vaccination

Vaccination for prevention of mumps is done. The first dose is given at the age of 12 to 18 months and the second dose is given at the age of 4 to 6 years. In USA and Canada vaccination is compulsory and is monitored at the time of school admission.

Treatment

There is only supportive treatment for mumps. Best method for controlling the disease is vaccination by live attenuated mumps virus vaccine. Fatalities are rare and may be due to viral encephalitis, myocarditis and neuritis.

Cytomegalovirus (CMV) Infection

Etiology: Human CMV is beta herpesvirus. This virus only infects humans and may remain latent in human body. Its activation in healthy individuals does not produce any illness, but in immunocompromised persons its activation can be dangerous for life.

Transmission of virus is through urine, fomites, breast milk and respiratory secretions. Congenital infection and malformations may result from transplacental spread. Infection in newborn and young children can be fatal.

Clinical features: CMV mononucleosis occurs in young adults with acute febrile illness with enlargement of salivary glands. On the basis of elevated titer of antibody to CMV diagnosis is made. For healthy adult prognosis is very good. CMV end-organ damage has declined due to highly active antiretroviral therapy (HAART) for treating HIV infection. Diagnosis methods include culture, antigen detection and CMV deoxyribonucleic acid (DNA) detection.

Treatment: Symptomatical treatment is given to healthy patients. Aggressive treatment is required by immunocompromised patients like IV injections of ganciclovir, cidofovir or foscarnet.

HIV Infection

In HIV infected patients neoplastic and non-neoplastic salivary gland lesions frequently occur. AIDS related tumors are Kaposi's sarcoma and lymphoma. In "HIV salivary gland disease" (HIV-SGD) Sjogern's syndrome like phenomenon is seen which are xerostomia and benign salivary gland enlargement.

Clinical features: Salivary gland swelling with or without xerostomia is important symptom of HIV-SGD. Mostly parotid gland is involved. HIV-SGD must be distinguished by Sjogren's syndrome by salivary flow rates autoimmune serologies and ophthalmic evaluation. In HIV- associated benign lymphoepithelial hypertrophy multiple cysting masses are present. Major salivary glands when involved can be imaged with ultrasonography, CT or MRI.

Diseases of Salivary Gland

Treatment: Symptomatic for xerostomia, frequent sipping of water, chewing sugar-free gum, salivary substitute, sugar free candy sucking. Surgery is done for benign tumor of parotid gland. In HIV infected patients with parotid hypertrophy 8 to 10 Gy of radiotherapy is done. Radiotherapy increases xerostomia. Aspiration of cysts and tetracycline sclerosis is also done. For caries control topical fluoride application should be done.

On benign parotid enlargement surgical or laser excision is carried out for cosmetic purpose. Systemic anti HIV treatment augment radiation therapy. In big cystic lesions for tetracycline sclerosis, aspiration of cysts and injection of tetracycline solution into the cyst are carried out. This induces an inflammatory reaction and later on sclerosis.

Hepatitis C Virus (HCV) Infection

Etiology: HCV infect the cells of immune system and disrupt immunoregulation. HCV DNA is present in saliva of the patients having chronic hepatitis C infection. Such saliva is infective. HCV may be associated with Sjogren's syndrome.

Clinical features: Many extrahepatic manifestations like salivary gland enlargement and xerostomia without dry eyes may be present. In infected patients anti-HCV antibodies and HCV DNA is present.

Treatment: Symptomatic treatment is done as there is no specific treatment.

INFLAMMATORY AND REACTIVE LESION

Necrotizing Sialometaplasia

Necrotizing sialometaplasia is a benign self-limiting reactive inflammatory lesion that affects the minor salivary glands. The etiology of the disease is not clearly known but may be associated with ischemia of minor salivary gland due to trauma. The disease most frequently occurs in males, in fifth and sixth decades of life.

Clinical Features

Rapid onset: This lesion mimics malignancy. The lesion starts as an ulcerated nodule that is well-separated from surrounding normal tissue. There is an inflammatory reaction around the edge of the lesion. It mostly occurs on the palate, but may also be found on retromolar pad and lips.

Treatment

Treatment includes debridement of the lesion and saline rinse. The lesion is self-limiting and usually heals by secondary intention in about six weeks without recurrence. No specific treatment is required.

ALLERGIC REACTION OR DISEASE

Allergic Sialadenitis

Salivary glands may get enlarged as a result of allergic reaction to drugs or other allergens. The toxic or idiosyncratic reaction to drug causes decreased salivary flow resulting in secondary infection. In true hypersensitivity reactions, other signs of allergy like angioedema, skin rashes etc. may also appear.

The drugs like sulfisoxazole, phenothiazine, phenobarbital, ethambutol, isoproterenol, heavy metals and iodine-containing compound may as a side effect cause salivary gland enlargement. Allergic sialadenitis is a self-limiting disease, but if secondary infection is present, antibiotic therapy is necessary. Allergen must be avoided and hydration must be maintained.

GRANULOMATOUS CONDITIONS

Sarcoid Sialadenitis

Sarcoidosis is a chronic systemic granulomatous disease that usually involves the lungs, skin, liver, spleen, eyes and parotid gland. The disease predominantly occurs in third or fourth decades of life. In this T lymphocytes, mononuclear phagocytes and granulomas cause destruction of involved tissues. The etiology is still not clear.

Oral lesions are characterized by the involvement of oral mucosa and granulomatous invasion of the parotid gland. There is bilateral, firm, painless enlargement of salivary gland with decreased or absent salivation. Treatment of disease is usually asymptomatic. Corticosteroids are effective in acute stages. Chloroquine alone or with corticosteroids is also helpful.

Tuberculosis (TB)

Tuberculosis is chronic bacterial infection which leads to the formation of granulomas in the infected tissues. Usually lungs are involved. Other tissues like lymph nodes, salivary glands may be involved. TB patients may feel xerostomia with or without swelling of salivary glands. The affected salivary gland may have granuloma or/ and cyst (Fig. 16.8).

Treatment

Multidrug anti TB chemotherapy. Resistant patient may require surgery or laser intervention.

Oral Medicine

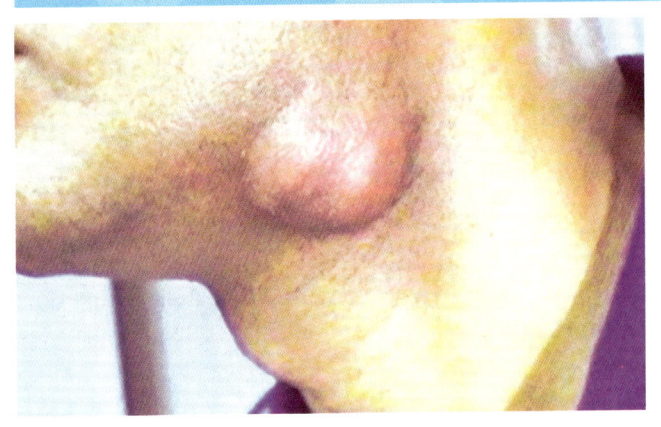

Fig. 16.8: Tubercular submandibular lymph node (*Courtesy* Dr. Rohit Chandra, Noida)

IMMUNOLOGICAL DISORDERS

Sjogren's Syndrome (SS) (Primary and Secondary)

Sjogren's syndrome is a chronic autoimmune disorder of exocrine glands associated with connective tissue diseases, neuropathy and lymphoproliferative disorders. It is of two types primary and secondary. Primary Sjogren's syndrome is characterized by involvement of lacrimal and salivary glands only. Secondary type also involves connective tissue diseases along with exocrine glands. Its etiology is obscure.

Clinical Features

The disease frequently occurs in middle aged and elderly women. Xerostomia is a major complaint in most of the patients. The oral manifestations are inability in chewing and swallowing, or wearing dentures; dry cracked lips and dry tongue and buccal mucosa. As there is dryness of mouth, secondary oral diseases such as candidiasis or increase in dental caries are relatively common.

There is dryness of eyes, pharynx, larynx and nose. Generalized manifestations of primary Sjogren's syndrome are polyneuropathy, renal involvement, pneumonitis and vasculitis. Other signs and symptoms of secondary type are associated with collagen diseases like rheumatoid arthritis, systemic lupus erythematosus, polymyositis and sclerosis. There may be diffuse enlargement of lymph nodes particularly of the cervical region in Sjogren's syndrome.

Treatment

There is no specific treatment. Treatment of Sjogren's syndrome is limited and directed mainly to minimizing secondary effects of decreased exocrine secretion by antibiotics, immunosuppressive drugs and corticosteroids.

Xerostomia can be treated by pilocarpine, methyl cellulose or other saliva substitutes. Lack of saliva is accompanied by an increase in caries, so use of topical fluoride is recommended. Proper oral hygiene should be maintained. Oral candidiasis can be managed by topical nystatin or cotrimazole.

Sialadenosis

Sialadenosis refers to non-neoplastic, non-inflammatory enlargement of salivary gland. The condition is predominant in women and the parotid gland is most frequently affected.

Clinical Features

The enlargement of salivary gland in sialadenosis is usually bilateral, recurrent and painless. The most common symptom is swelling of the preauricular portion of the parotid gland. There may be intraoral swelling in the sublingual and submandibular area when respective glands are involved. There may be edema of interstitial supporting tissues and atrophy of striated ducts. There is an alteration in the chemical constituents of saliva which is characterised by elevation of salivary potassium and decrease in salivary sodium (Figs 16.9 and 16.10).

Etiological Factors

Various conditions in which sialadenosis may occur are as follows.
a. Alcoholism
   Sialadenosis is associated with alcoholic cirrhosis and other types of cirrhosis.

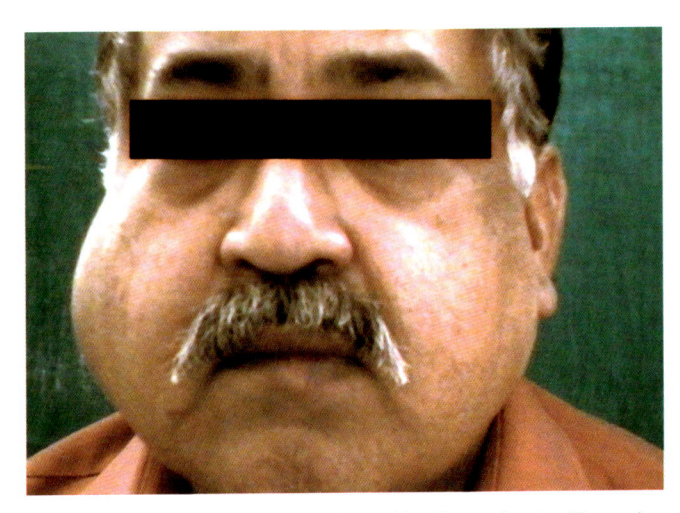

Fig. 16.9: Bilateral sialadenosis of parotid salivary glands. (Excessive formation of saliva) (*Courtesy* Dr Rohit Chandra, Noida)

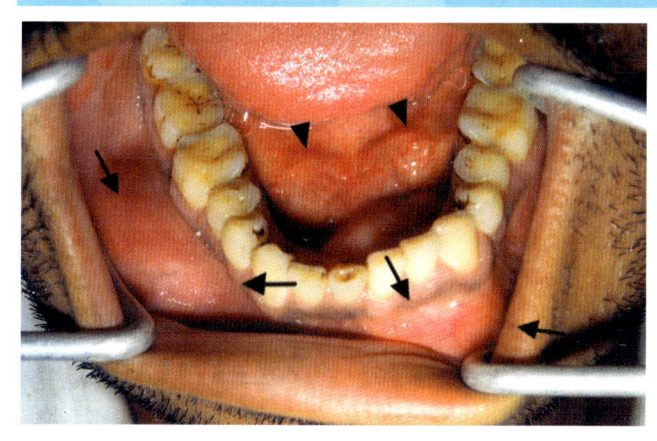

Fig. 16.10: Bilateral sialadenosis of sublingual gland (shown by arrowheads) and submandibular gland (shown by arrows) (*Courtesy* Dr Rohit Chandra, Noida)

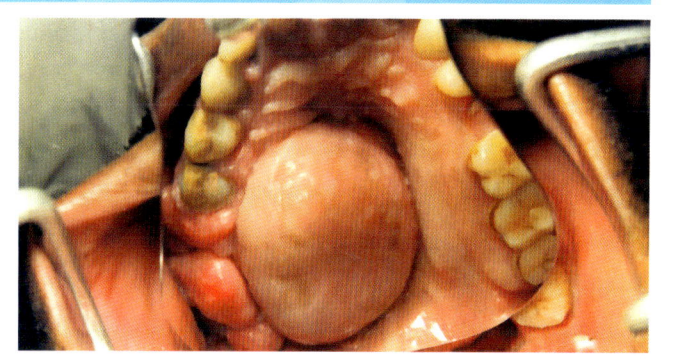

Fig. 16.11: Pleomorphic adenoma of palate

b. Hormonal Factors
   Sialadenosis may be seen in pregnancy, diabetes mellitus, menarche, menopause and after ovariectomy.
c. Other Diseases
   Repeated vomiting in anorexia nervosa, and pancreatic and renal diseases may cause sialadenosis.
d. Malnutrition
   In acute protein deficiency, there may be symmetric enlargement of the parotid gland.

SALIVARY GLAND TUMORS

Most of the salivary gland tumors arise in the parotid glands which account for 80% of the tumors. About 10 to 15% of tumors develop in submandibular gland and remaining develop in sublingual or minor salivary glands.

Benign Tumors

Pleomorphic Adenoma

It is the most common tumor of the salivary gland and may occur at any age. It is also called as mixed tumor because it contains both mesenchymal and epithelial elements. Parotid gland is the most common site for pleomorphic adenoma.
a. Clinical Features
   i. These tumors are painless, slow-growing, firm and mobile
   ii. In the parotid gland they usually occurs in posterior inferior aspect of the superficial lobe.
   iii. They most commonly occur on palate, followed by upper lip and buccal mucosa (Fig. 16.11).
b. Treatment
   The treatment of pleomorphic adenoma consists of surgical removal with adequate margins.

Oncocytoma (Acidophilic Adenoma, Oxyphilic Adenoma)

Oncocytomas are rare benign salivary gland neoplasms that contain oncocytes, the large granular acidophilic cells. This tumor mostly occurs in parotid gland and usually in sixth decade of life.
a. Clinical Features
   i. Oncocytomas are solid round tumors that may occur in any of the major salivary gland.
   ii. This tumor is commonly found in superficial lobe of parotid gland.
   iii. It is the second most common bilaterally occurring salivary gland tumor.
b. Treatment
   i. Treatment of choice for parotid gland tumors is superficial parotidectomy with preservation of facial nerve.
   ii. For tumors in the submandibular gland, removal of the gland is treatment of choice.
   iii. Removal of gland with normal portion of tissue is the treatment of choice for tumors in minor salivary glands.

Basal Cell Adenoma

Basal cell adenomas are painless and slow growing tumors. About 70% of basal cell adenomas occur in the parotid gland. Basal cell adenomas of the minor salivary glands mostly occur on the upper lip. Treatment of basal cell adenomas consists of conservative surgical excision with a margin of normal tissue.

Ductal Papilloma

Ductal papillomas are benign salivary gland tumors that arise from the excretory ducts, mostly of the minor salivary glands. There are three forms of ductal papilloma which are as follows:

a. *Simple ductal papilloma*: Simple ductal papilloma occurs as an exophytic lesion with a pedunculated base. The lesion often has a reddish color. The lesion is treated by local surgical excision.
b. *Inverted ductal papilloma*: Inverted ductal papilloma occurs in the minor salivary glands and clinically appear as submucosal nodule. Surgical excision is the recommended treatment.
c. *Sialadenoma papilliferum*: This type of lesion occurs mostly on palate and buccal mucosa and appears as painless exophytic mass. The lesion mostly occurs in males between the fifth and eighth decades of life. The lesion is treated by local surgical excision.

Myoepithelioma

Myoepithelioma is the benign salivary gland tumor that clinically appear as well-circumscribed asymptomatic slow growing mass. They mostly occur in the parotid gland and its most common intraoral site is palate. The treatment of myoepithelioma consists of surgical excision, including a border of normal tissue.

Malignant Tumors

Adenoid Cystic Carcinoma

Adenoid cystic carcinomas are the most common malignant tumors of the submandibular and minor salivary glands. The tumor usually occurs in the fifth decade of life with men and women being equally affected.
a. Clinical features
   i. Adenoid cystic carcinoma appear as firm unilobular mass in the gland.
   ii. The tumor is slow-growing and may be sometimes painful.
   iii. Intraoral adenoid cystic carcinoma may also exhibits mucosal ulcerations.
   iv. Tumor may get metastasized into the lungs
   v. Adenoid cystic carcinoma has a tendency to spread along the nerve sheaths and may cause facial nerve paralysis in few patients.
b. Treatment
   The treatment of choice for adenoid cystic carcinoma is radical surgical excision.

Mucoepidermoid Carcinoma

It is the most common malignant tumor of the salivary glands. It is also most common tumor of the parotid gland. The tumor usually occurs in the third to fifth decade of life with men and women being equally affected. Mucoepidermoid carcinoma consists of both epidermal and mucous cells, and according to ratio of epidermal cells to mucous cells can be classified into high grade or low grade tumor.
a. Clinical features
   i. The low-grade tumor is less aggressive and may undergo long period of painless enlargement.
   ii. High-grade form exhibits rapid growth and has high incidence of metastasis.
   iii. Pain and ulceration of overlying tissue may be present.
   iv. Patients may exhibit facial palsy, if tumor involves facial nerve (Fig. 16.4).
b. Treatment
   i. Treatment of low-grade mucoepidermoid carcinoma consists of superficial parotidectomy, if only superficial lobe is involved.
   ii. High grade lesions are treated by total parotidectomy. Postoperative radiation therapy may also be recommended if required.

Acinic Cell Carcinoma

Acinic cell carcinomas are mostly found in the parotid gland. The tumor predominantly occurs in women in the fifth decade of life.
a. Clinical features
   i. The lesions clinically appear as slow-growing masses and may be associated with pain
   ii. The common site of occurrence are superficial lobe and inferior lobe of the parotid gland.
b. Treatment
   Treatment of acinic cell carcinoma includes superficial parotidectomy, with facial nerve preservation. Total gland removal is the treatment of choice for tumor in the submandibular gland.

Carcinoma Expleomorphic Adenoma

It is a malignant tumor that arises within a pre-existing benign pleomorphic adenoma.
a. Clinical features
   i. These tumors are slow growing and may be present for 15 to 20 years before appearing clinically.
   ii. They occur mostly in untreated benign pleomorphic adenoma.
b. Treatment
   The treatment of carcinoma expleomorphic adenoma consists of surgical removal with post-operative radiation therapy.

BIBLIOGRAPHY

1. Bohuslavizki KH, Brenner W, Lassmann S. Quantitative salivary gland scintigraphy in the diagnosis of parenchymal damage after treatment with radioactive iodine. Nucl Med Commun 1996;17: 681-6.
2. Bowen EF. Cytomegalovirus reactivation in patients infected with HIV; the use of polymerase chain reaction in prediction and management. Drugs 1999;57(5):735-41.
3. Caplan CE. Mumps in the era of vaccines. Can Med Assoc J 1999; 160 (6): 856-66.
4. Escudier MP, Drage NA. The management of sialolithiasis in 2 children through use of extracorporeal shock wave lithotripsy. Oral Surg Oral Med Oral Pathol Oral Radiol Endo 1999;88:44-9.
5. Mandel SJ, Mandel L. Persistent sialadenitis after radioactive iodine therapy. Report of two cases. J Oral Maxillofac Surg 1999; 57:738.
6. Matsuda C, Matsui Y, Ohno K, Michi K. Salivary gland aplasia with cleft lip and palate. A case report and review of the literature. Oral Surg Oral Med Oral Pathol 1999;87(5):594-9.
7. Mehta M. Amifostine and combined-mobility therapeutic approaches. Semin Oncol 1999; 26(2 Suppl 7): 95-101.
8. Mermann GA, Vivino FB, Shnier D. Diagnostic accuracy of salivary scintigraphic indices in xerostomic populations. Clin Nucl Med 1999;24(3):167-72.
9. Mumps and mumps vaccine. A global view. Bull World Health Organ 1999;77(1):3-14.
10. Rice DH. Salivary gland disorders. Neoplastic and nonneoplastic. Otolaryngology for the internist. Med Clin North Am 1999; 83 (1): 197-221.
11. Shimizu M, Ussmuller J, Hartwein J. Statistical study for sonographic differential diagnosis of tumorous lesions in the parotid gland. Oral Surg Oral Med Oral Pathol Oral Radiol Endod 1999; 88:226-33.

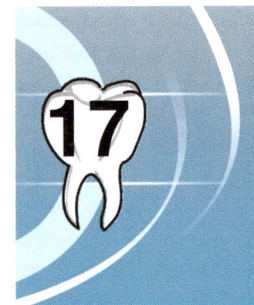

17 Temporomandibular Joint Disorders

INTRODUCTION

The causes of facial pain related to temporomandibular disorders (TMD) are now easily understandable due to advances in diagnostic devices. Technical advancement in magnetic resonance imaging (MRI), arthrography and arthroscopy have increased the clinician's ability to diagnose distinct temporomandibular joint (TMJ) disorders associated with facial pain and jaw dysfunction. TMD are more common in women between the ages of 20 to 50 years.

Treatment of facial pain is complicated by the interrelationship of temporomandibular disorders. Clinician may face difficulty in distinguishing that either the patient is experiencing pain only due to intracapsular disorder or due to myofacial pain disorder; or the patient is suffering due to combination of both disorders. Success in diagnosing and treating temporomandibular disorders depends on the clinician's ability to elucidate and assimilate data derived from patient's history, clinical examination and appropriate diagnostic tests.

FUNCTIONAL ANATOMY OF TMJ

TMJ is a ginglymodiarthrodial joint, which have hinge type and gliding movements with the bony parts enclosed and connected by a fibrous capsule. The temporomandibular joint is made up of mandibular condyle, the articular surfaces of temporal bone, the articular disc, and the joint capsule. The articular disc is a direct extension of superior portion of lateral pterygoid muscle. It is a fibrous plate which separates the joints into superior and inferior compartments. The disc is bound to lateral and medial poles of condyle.

Articular disc provides stabilization during condylar movement and shock absorption during mastication. The joint capsule consists of fibrous tissue that attaches to the articular eminence of the temporal bone and to the condyle. The capsule is lined by synovial membrane that helps in lubricating the joint.

The nerves innervating the joint are derived from branches of the auriculotemporal nerve, with branches of masseteric and posterior deep temporal nerves. The blood supply is provided by superficial temporal artery.

The condylar movements during function of the mandible are rotation and translation. The superior joint space is associated with anterior gliding movement and the inferior space is associated with rotation. Opening of the mandible is facilitated by contraction of lateral pterygoid muscles along with digastric, geniohyoid and mylohyoid muscles. Closing of the mandible is produced by masseter, medial pterygoid and anterior fibres of the temporalis muscles.

Lateral pterygoid muscle helps in protrusion, whereas retrusion is produced by contraction of posterior fibers of temporalis muscle. Lateral movement of the mandible occurs by contraction of lateral pterygoid muscles.

PATIENT HISTORY

The information obtained from patient's history is the most important aspect of a diagnostic process. The patient's description of the location, duration and characteristic of pain helps the clinician in differentiating the diseases with similar symptoms.

The process of history taking starts from the chief complaint, which reveals the problems in patient's own terms. Then history of present illness should be taken which provides chronological details of the disorders from onset of symptoms till present. Previous treatment for any disorder and their effect should be recorded. Information about the location of the pain and its characteristics should be obtained from the patient. The pain in myofacial pain dysfunction is described as a dull and unilateral ache which is intense on awakening. TMJ pain may be dull or sharp and usually increases with increasing function.

The patient should be interrogated about any previous illness, like rheumatoid arthritis and degenerative bone disease. History of any trauma to head and neck or injures to the side of the face and chin should be taken, as they are responsible for TMJ problems. Patients with facial pain should be asked about any headache, earache and neck or back pain they may have experienced. While taking family history, it is necessary to ask for any disease like rheumatoid arthritis, osteoarthritis and connective tissue disease in the family members.

The social history is also essential to determine any stress producing conditions at home or work, which may contribute in the etiology of myofacial pain.

EXAMINATION OF ARTICULATORY SYSTEM

The proper examination of the temporomandibular joint includes the following steps.

1. Visual Examination

Visual examination of the face helps in determining any gross asymmetry, any laceration or swelling over the joint area. Asymmetry may be due to trauma to the chin that results in TMJ ankylosis, abnormal facial growth, and abnormal opening pattern of the jaw.

2. Range of Movement

The maximum interincisal opening of the mandible without experiencing the pain should be measured. Normal range is usually between 35 to 50 mm. Any deviation of the mandible during opening should be recorded. The range of lateral mandibular movement is measured from the midline by having teeth in occlusion and then sliding jaw in both directions. Normal lateral range is usually 8 to 10 mm. Any pain during opening or lateral movement should be noticed.

3. Palpation of Joint

TMJ can be palpated by pretragus and intra-auricular palpation. During the palpation it is perceived that condyles move symmetrically with rotation and translation phases. If there is any unilateral problem, the mandible always deviates to the side with the limited condylar movement. These areas are also palpated for any tenderness, which signifies inflammation due to acute or chronic trauma.

4. Palpation of Muscles

The masticatory muscles are examined for any tenderness during palpation. The masseter muscle is palpated bimanually by placing a finger of one hand inside and another finger of another hand outside the mouth. The lateral pterygoids are palpated by placing a finger behind the maxillary tuberosity and the medial pterygoids are evaluated by running a finger in antero-posterior direction along the medial aspect of the mandible in the floor of the mouth.

5. Palpation of Lymph Nodes

Pain Provocation Tests

A. Clenching of teeth
B. Static pain test
C. Chewing of sugarless gum

6. Intraoral Examination

The clinical examination should also include evaluation of missing teeth, teeth contact relationship, and occlusion, periodontal and tooth decay status and condition of removable and fixed prosthesis. Any evidence of the oral habits, such as bruxism which may lead to occlusal wear and spasm of the masticatory muscles, should be noticed and recorded.

Jaw Jerk Reflex

It is like knee jerk reflex. In this stretching of the jaw closing muscles produce a reflex contraction of muscles by applying a downward tap on the chin (Figs 17.1 and 17.2).

Jaw Opening Reflex

It prevent injury to teeth and periodontium when suddenly some hard object which may cause damage comes between closing of teeth. In this mechanoreceptors in the mouth and nonreceptors triggers the jaw opening reflex.

Etiology of TM Disorders (TMD)

Main TMD are occlusal disharmony and psychological distress. Causes of TMD are as follows.
1. Emotional distress
2. Parafunctional habits (bruxing, teeth clenching, lip and cheek biting)
3. Laxity of the joint
4. Acute trauma
5. Prolonged hyperextension (long dental procedures, yawning, oral intubation for GA)
6. Musculoskeletal disorders

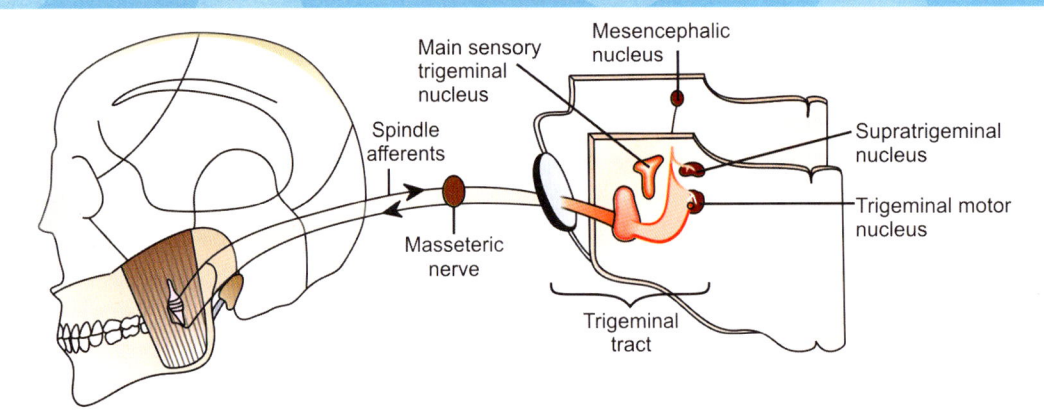

Fig. 17.1: Jaw closing or jaw jerk reflex. Muscle spindle in a jaw closing muscles are stretched by taping the chin

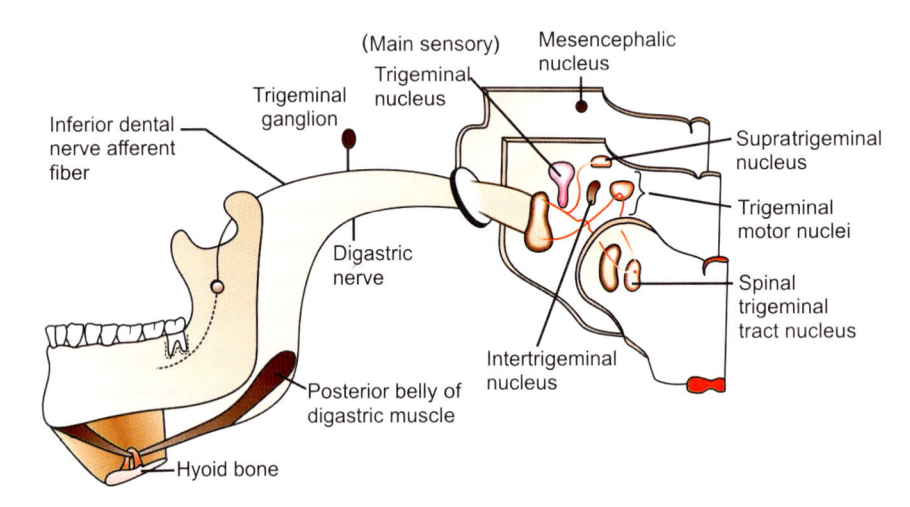

Fig. 17.2: Jaw opening reflex. Mucosal receptors with afferent fibers terminating in the trigeminal spinal tract nucleus are excited by stimulation of intraoral receptive fields

DIFFERENTIAL DIAGNOSIS

Before the treatment of temporomandibular disorder is started, it is essential to exclude other disorders that may present similar symptoms. Differentiating the disorders can be made easier by determining the stimulus, location and characteristic of the pain. The differential diagnosis of facial pain related to temporomandibular disorders includes the following.

A. Dental disorders
B. Salivary gland disorders
C. ENT disorders
D. Psychogenic disorders
E. Cystic degeneration of condyle—Ely's cyst
F. Trigeminal neuralgia
G. Elongated styloid process—Eagle's syndrome
H. Angina pectoris
I. Multiple sclerosis.

DIAGNOSTIC AIDS FOR TMJ DISORDERS

Various technical aids that facilitate the diagnosis of TMJ disorders are the following:
1. Plain radiography
2. Computed tomography
3. Magnetic resonance imaging (MRI)
4. Arthrography
5. Arthroscopy
6. Electromyography

MYOFACIAL PAIN DYSFUNCTION SYNDROME (MPDS)

It is a dysfunction of masticatory apparatus related to painful, self-perpetuating spasm of the masticatory muscle. The muscle spasm may be due to stress resulting in habitual clenching and grinding of teeth, which leads to muscle fatigue and subsequently spasm of masticatory muscles. The muscles most commonly involved in MPDS are lateral pterygoid and masseter muscle. Occlusal interferences, deep overbite-overjet relationship and posterior bite collapse may also be the predisposing factors for MPDS.

The signs and symptoms of myofacial pain dysfunction syndrome are as follows:

a. Unilateral, dull pain in ear or preauricular region which gets intense on awakening in the morning.
b. Limitation or deviation of the mandible during opening of the mouth.
c. Tenderness of the muscles of mastication.
d. Clicking or popping sound in temporomandibular joint (Tables 17.1 to 17.5).

Table 17.1: Diagnostic classification of temporomandibular disorders (TMD) accepted by American academy of orofacial pain (AAOP)

Diagnostic category of disorders	Diagnosis
1. Cranial bones and mandible	Congenital and developmental disorders: aplasia, hypoplasia, hyperplasia and dysplasia (e.g. 1st and 2nd branchial arch anomalies, hemifacial microsomia, Pierre Robin syndrome, Treacher Collins syndrome, condylar hyperplasia, prognathism, fibrous dysplasia) Acquired disorders (neoplasia, fracture)
2. Temporomandibular joint	Arthritis (osteoarthritis, osteoarthrosis and polyarthritis), Ankylosis (fibrous, bony), Deviation in form, Disk displacement (with reduction, without reduction); Dislocation, Inflammatory conditions (synovitis, capsulitis) Neoplasia
3. Masticatory-muscle	Myofacial pain, Myositis, Spasm Protective splinting, contracture

In 1996 National Institutes of Health Conference on TMD therapy concluded the following:
1. Most of the TMD patients should be treated initially by noninvasive and reversible therapies.
2. Permanent change in occlusion should be avoided.
3. Surgical intervention should be done in patients showing evidence of pathology or evidence of internal derangement of TMJ as source of pain and dysfunction and in whom conservative treatments have failed.
4. For the management of chronic pain relaxation and cognitive-behavioral therapies are effective.

Table 17.2: Diagnosis of temporomandibular disorders

Diagnostic group	Diagnosis
1. Muscle and facial disorders	Myalgia, muscle contracture, bruxism (myositis), spasm, splinting, habit of forceful jaw closure and hypertrophy.
2. TMJ disorders	Osteoarthritis, arthralgia, polyarthritis (inflammatory), articular disease (traumatic), incoordination of articular disc and condyle, restricted actions of articular disc and condyle, dislocation.
3. Mandibular mobility disorders	TMJ Ankylosis, muscular tissue fibrosis, intracapsular adhesions, TMJ hypermobility
4. Maxillomandibular growth disorders	Atrophy/dystrophy/ hypertrophy of masticatory muscles, tumor of masticatory muscles, tumor of maxilla or mandible, tumor of condyle, hypoplasia or hyperplasia of maxilla or mandible or condyle

Table 17.3: Diagnostic terms, characteristics and clinical findings for temporomandibular disorders

Diagnostic terms	Characteristics	Clinical finding
1. Osteoarthritis	Degenerative condition accompanied by secondary inflammation	Crepitus, deviation to affected side, pain with function due to inflammation, and point tenderness on palpation
2. Myofacial pain	Regional dull aching pain and presence of localized tender spots in muscle and tendon which reproduce pain when palpated	Dull regional pain localized tenderness
3. Myositis, delayed onset	Painful condition due to overuse that results in interstitial inflammation	Increased pain due to mandibular movement, on set following prolonged or unaccustomed use (up to 48 hours afterward)
4. Myositis, generalized	Constant, acutely painful and generalized inflammation and swelling	Usually acute pain in localized area, localized tenderness, increased pain due to mandibular move-

Contd...

Oral Medicine

Contd...

Diagnostic terms	Characteristics	Clinical finding
		ment, limited range of motion, due to pain and swelling. Onset following injury or infection
5. Synovitis or capsulitis	Inflammation of the synovial lining or capsular lining	Localized pain at rest exacerbated by function, limited range of motion due to pain
6. Deviation in form	Painless mechanical dysfunction or altered function	Faulty or compromised joint mechanics reproducible joint noise, structural bony abnormality or loss of normal shape
7. Disk displacement with reduction	Abrupt alteration or interference of the disk-condyle structural relation during mouth opening and closing	Pain if present is precipitated by joint movement Reproducible joint noise, during opening and closing mandibular movements displaced disk that improves its position during jaw opening. Pain (when present) precipitated by joint movement, no restriction in mandibular movement.
8. Disk displacement without reduction	Altered or misaligned disk-condyle structural reaction	Pain precipitated by movement, limited mandibular opening, straight-line deviation to the affected side on opening, limited laterotrusion to the contralateral side, displaced disk without reduction. Pain precipitated by forced mouth opening, pain with palpation of the affected joint, ipsilateral hyperocclusion
9. Osteoarthrosis	Degenerative noninflammatory condition of the joint. Structural changes of joint surfaces	Crepitus, deviation to the affected side on opening. Structural bony change (subchondral sclerosis, osteophyte formation) and joint-space narrowing
10. Protective muscle splinting	Restricted or guarded mandibular movement due to avoiding pain caused by movement of the parts	Severe pain with function but not at rest
11. Contracture	Chronic resistance of a muscle to passive stretch, due to fibrosis of the tendon, ligament and muscle fibers	Limited range of motion

Table 17.4: Term, definitions and clinical findings for temporomandibular disorders

Term	Definitions	Clinical findings
1. Arthralgia	Pain and tenderness in joint capsule	Pain in one or both joint sites, pain in joint during maximum opening, pain in joint during lateral excursion
2. Osteoarthritis	Inflammatory condition within the joint	Arthralgia and coarse crepitus or imaging
3. Osteoarthrosis	Degenerative joint disorder	Absence of arthralgia and Coarse crepitus
4. Myofacial pain	Pain of muscle origin including pain associated with localized areas of tenderness to palpation in muscle	Pain or ache in jaw, temples, face, preauricular area, or inside ear at rest or during function and pain on palpation in muscle sites
5. Myofacial pain with limited opening	Limited opening due to muscular pain	Myofacial pain, pain-free unassisted mandibular opening of less than 40 mm and a maximum assisted opening of equal to or more than 5 mm greater than the pain-free unassisted opening
6. Disk displacement with reduction	Disk is displaced from its position between the condyle and eminence to an anterior and medial or lateral position but is reduced in full opening usually resulting in a noise	Click on both vertical opening and closing
7. Disk displacement without reduction, with limited opening	Disk is displaced from normal position between condyle and fossa to an anterior and medial or lateral position	Limitation of opening. Maximum unassisted opening equal or less than 35 mm

HISTORY TAKING FOR EVALUATING A PATIENT FOR TEMPOROMANDIBULAR DISCOMFORT

1. What discomfort do you have?
2. Do you have pain in front of the ear, in the face and temple areas? When, where and what type of discomfort?
3. Do you get headaches, earaches, neckache or cheek pain if yes, when?
4. When is pain at its worst?
5. Do you experience pain when using the jaw for opening wide, yawning, chewing, speaking or swallowing?

6. Do you experience joint noises if yes when? Type of noise, clicking, popping or crepitus.
7. Does your jaw ever lock or get stuck (locking in the open position or locking in the closed position) unilateral or bilateral?
8. Does your jaw motion feel restricted if yes when?
9. Do you experience pain in the teeth if yes, which teeth?
10. Have you had an abrupt change in the way your teeth meet together?
11. Does your bite feel uncomfortable, when and how?
12. Have you had any jaw injuries, when? Describe the extent of injury.
13. Have you had treatment for the jaw symptoms? If so, describe it and what was the effect?
14. Do you have any other muscle, bone or joint problem?
15. Do you have pain in any other part of the body?
16. Do you have or did you have dizziness, nausea, fullness or ringing in the ears, diminished hearing, facial swelling, redness of the eyes, nasal congestion, altered sensation such as numbness, tingling, or burning, altered vision and muscle twitching, if yes when and for how long?

Table 17.5: Physical examination for temporomandibular dysfunction

Examination	Findings
Inspection	Facial asymmetry, swelling, and hypertrophy of masseter and temporal-muscle. Jaw opening pattern
Assessment of range of jaw movement	Between mandibular and maxillary incisal edges. Maximum opening in mm with comfort, with pain, and with clinician assistance. Maximum lateral and protrusive movements in mm
Palpation examination	Temporomandibular joints. Main masticatory muscles. Neck muscles and accessory muscles of mastication. Parotid and submandibular areas. Lymph nodes draining the area.
Provocation tests	Static pain test (mandibular resistance against pressure). Pain in the joints or muscles with teeth clenching. Reproduction of symptoms with chewing (wax, sugarless gum)
Intraoral examination	Signs of parafunction (cheek or lip biting, accentuated linea alba, scalloped tongue borders, tooth mobility occlusal wear.

Home Care Instructions to Patient of TMD

a. Eat soft foods in small pieces with little mouth opening.
b. Do only limited movements of the jaw.
c. Avoid stress on jaw.
d. During yawning support the lower jaw by providing mild pressure under the chin with back of the hand.
e. Keep the jaw relaxed to avoid teeth contact.
f. Do not clench the teeth.
g. Avoid unnecessary teeth contacts except chewing and swallowing.
h. Do not tense jaw muscles.
i. Application of moist warm compresses over TMJ areas (on the sides of the face and temple areas) for 10 to 20 minutes twice daily.

Treatment

The initial treatment modalities for the myofacial pain dysfunction syndrome, include the following:

A. Patient may be prescribed topical anaesthetic agent which anesthetizes the involved area and allows the patient to stretch the muscles in spasm.
B. Injecting the local anaesthetic agent in the spasmodic area may help in breaking the spasm.
C. Non-steroidal anti-inflammatory drugs can be prescribed to relieve the pain.
D. Diazepam or alprazolane can be prescribed to relieve anxiety and relax the muscles.

If pain and dysfunction persist even after the above treatment, the following treatment modalities can be tried.

Occlusal splints: A full coverage maxillary occlusal splint made up of soft acrylic (like soft denture liner) helps in decreasing the symptoms of MPDS.

Biofeed back: When the patient is unable to control stress and anxiety; biofeedback system can be used which enables the patient to gain control over the bodily functions such as bruxism.

Physiotherapy: Application of ice alternately with moist heat, ultrasound, short-wave diathermy and laser may help in resolving muscle related pain.

TENS: Transcutaneous electric nerve stimulation is successfully used in treating chronic pain.

Acupuncture: Brief intense stimulation using needles in acupuncture therapy helps in relieving pain.

Hypnosis and psychologic counseling may be used as supplement to other treatment for long-term myofacial pain.

INTRACAPSULAR DISORDERS OF TEMPOROMANDIBULAR JOINT

Intracapsular disorders of the temporomandibular joint include diseases of the bony or soft tissue structure of TMJ itself. These may be following:

Inflammatory Disorders

Rheumatoid Arthritis

Rheumatoid arthritis is an inflammatory joint disease. It involves the temporomandibular joint in about 40 to 80% of the patients. The disease starts as vasculitis of the synovial membrane, which progresses to chronic inflammation followed by formation of granulation tissue. The cellular infiltrate spreads from the articular surface and causes erosion of the underlying bone. In juvenile rheumatoid arthritis micrognathia and anterior open bite are observed.

Clinical features: Rheumatoid arthritis usually affects both the joints. Pain and restriction of mouth opening are the most common symptoms. Other symptoms are stiffness, crepitus sound, swelling and tenderness in the TMJ region. Radiographic changes in TMJ associated with rheumatoid arthritis reveal narrow joint space, destructive lesion of the condyle and restricted condylar movements.

Treatment: Rheumatoid arthritis of TMJ is treated mainly by anti-inflammatory drugs. Patient should take soft diet and follow exercise program to increase mandibular opening. Intra-articular steroids can be used in patients with severe symptoms.

Psoriatic Arthritis

Psoriatic arthritis is the combination of psoriasis and polyarthritis occurring in the patients with psoriatic skin lesions and pitting of nails. About 5 to 7% of the patients of psoriasis develop arthritis.

Clinical features: The signs and symptoms of psoriatic arthritis of temporomandibular joint are same as in rheumatoid arthritis, except that there is unilateral involvement of joints in psoriatic arthritis. On examination restricted mouth opening, slight swelling over TMJ areas, deviation of mandible to the side of the pain and tenderness over the joint is observed. Radiograph shows erosion of the condyle and glenoid fossa.

Treatment: The conservative treatment includes soft diet, physical therapy and administration of salicylates. Severe disease can be treated by methotrexate. Methotrexate 2.5 to 15 mg once a week orally controls inflammation for upto 2 years. It is a immuno-suppressant drug. Surgery is indicated when there is disabling restriction of mandibular movement and unmanageable TMJ pain.

Degenerative Joint Disease

It is a non-inflammatory process characterized by degeneration of the articular soft tissue and remodelling of underlying bone. The disease process starts with thinning and fibrillation of the articular cartilage which breaks during joint function, leading to sclerosis of underlying bone.

Etiology: It is a response of joint to chronic microtrauma due to natural wear of TMJ associated with age or increased forces in parafunctional activity. Degenerative joint disease can be categorised as primary or secondary. Primary disease is of unknown origin, often asymptomatic and is usually seen in older individuals. Secondary type usually results from trauma.

Clinical features: The symptoms of degenerative joint disease of TMJ are unilateral pain over the condyle, crepitus, restricted mouth opening and feeling of stiffness. On examination there may be tenderness on palpation and deviation of the mandible to the painful side. Radiographic appearance reveals narrow and irregular joint space, osteophytic formation and flattening of articular surfaces.

Treatment: Degenerative joint disease of TMJ is managed by conservative treatment which includes NSAIDS, soft diet, rest and occlusal splints of soft acrylic for free movement of the mandible. Chronic pain or pain of increased intensity due to internal derangements in the TMJ can be treated by mandibular protrusive splint. Surgery is indicated if pain persists and degenerative joint changes exist.

Traumatic Disorders

Fractures

Fracture of the condylar head and neck usually results from trauma to the chin region. Condylar fracture can occur either as unilateral or bilateral. Bilateral condylar fracture may lead to anterior open bite. The condylar fracture may result in pain and edema over the TMJ region and deviation of mandible to the affected side on opening.

In majority of cases, fractured condyle gets displaced medially and anteriorly. Treatment includes mobilization of the mandible. Undisplaced, intra-capsular fractures are left untreated.

Ankylosis

Ankylosis of jaw refers to fusion of the condyle to the temporal bone. The common causes of the TMJ ankylosis are trauma, infection and prolonged immobilization following condylar fracture. Ankylosis is common in children because of high osteogenic potential and less development of joint disc.

Clinical features are restricted jaw movement, deviation of the mandible to the affected side while opening, and facial asymmetry. Ankylosis can be treated by surgical procedures like gap arthroplasty.

Dislocation

Dislocation of the mandible refers to the condition when the condyle gets displaced anterior to articular eminence. Dislocation of the mandible occurs due to muscular incoordination in widely opening the mouth during eating or yawning. It mostly occurs in old females.

The major complaint of the patient with dislocation is inability to close the jaw and pain due to spasm of muscle. The condyle can be repositioned by the dental surgeon without the use of muscle relaxant or anesthetics, by putting downward pressure with the thumbs in the restromolar areas. As the condyles will go to their places with a sudden jerk, the thumbs should be wrapped up with a gauge bandage to prevent being bitten by the teeth, due to their sudden forceful closure.

INFECTIONS

Septic Arthritis

Septic arthritis of temporomandibular joint is mainly caused by blood-borne bacterial infections. It may also be caused by the extension of infection from adjacent sites like parotid gland, middle ear and maxillary molars. The primary causative agent of septic arthritis of TMJ is Gonococcus, Streptococcus, Pneumococcus and Staphylococcus may also lead to infection of the joint. Large and tender cervical lymph nodes are found in septic arthritis

Clinical features: The major symptoms of septic arthritis of TMJ are severe pain on movement and inability to occlude the teeth. On examination there is redness and swelling in the region of affected joint. Cervical lymph nodes on the side of infection become large and tender, which is a distinguishing feature of septic arthritis from other TMJ disorders. Septic arthritis of TMJ in children may lead to ankylosis and facial asymmetry.

Treatment: Treatment of septic arthritis of temporomandibular joint includes surgical drainage and antibiotics.

Synovial Chondromatosis

Synovial chondromatosis is a disorder characterized by occurrence of osteocartilaginous nodules in the synovial membrane. It is of unknown etiology, but may be associated with trauma.

Clinical Features

The most common symptoms of synovial chondromatosis are pain, restricted mandibular movement and slow progressive swelling in the pretragus region. TMJ locking, clicking and crepitus may also be present.

Treatment

Treatment of synovial chondromatosis includes removal of loose calcified bodies and affected synovial membrane.

Developmental Disorders

The developmental disorders affecting the temporomandibular joint may result in anomalies like condylar hypoplasia and hyperplasia. Agenesis and bifid condyle are rare developmental defects. Trauma or infection may lead to condylar growth disturbances.

Condylar Hyperplasia

Condylar hyperplasia refers to over-development of the condyle. It is usually unilateral and occurs after puberty. Condylar hyperplasia leads to deviation of mandible to the affected side, limited mouth opening and facial asymmetry.

Condylar Hypoplasia

Condylar hypoplasia is characterized by short wide ramus and shortening of body of the mandible and antigonial notch. There is elongation of the body of mandible and flattening of face on the opposite side. Deviation of the mandible to the affected side and facial asymmetry are also found in condylar hypoplasia.

Management of developmental disorders involves surgical correction to prevent facial asymmetry.

Disc Displacement

In some cases acute or chronic trauma to the temporomandibular joint may displace condyle in the posterosuperior direction and stretches the posterior attachment of the articular disc. This results in forward displacement of the disc. In this condition well innervated, highly vascular retrodiscal tissue gets intervened between the condyle and articular surface when the mandible is at rest. When the condyle moves anteriorly into its normal relationship with disc, during mandibular opening, a clicking sound is produced. Similar clicking sound is produced during closing of the mouth as the condyle slips back on the retrodiscal tissue.

There may be pain during the TMJ clicking and mandibular dysfunction due to disc displacement. Painful clicking of TMJ can be treated by conservative treatment which includes nonsteroidal anti-inflammatory drugs, soft diet and maxillary flat plane hard acrylic full coverage appliance. Chronic pain or pain of increased intensity can be treated by wearing mandibular anterior repositioning appliance 24 hours a day for four to eight weeks.

BIBLIOGRAPHY

1. Chen Y-J, Gallo LM, Meier D, et al. Individual Oblique-Axial Magnetic Resonance Imaging for Improved Visualization of Mediolateral TMJ Disc Displacement. J orofac Pain 2000;14: 128-139.
2. Clark GT, Seligman DA, Solberg WK, Pullinger AG. Guidelines for the examination and diagnosis of temporomandibular joint disorders. J. craniomandible disorder 1989;3:7-14.
3. Davies S, Gray R. The pattern of splint usage in the management of two common temporomandibular disorders. Part II: The stabilization splint in the treatment of pain dysfunction syndrome. Br Dent J 1997;183:247-51.
4. Deepa L Raut, Mody RN. Radiographic evaluation of cervical vertebrae. Carpal, Metacarpal bone and mandibular third molar during adolescence and in young adults. JIAOMR 2006;18:1.
5. Emshoff R, Redisch A, Bosch R, Ganer R. Effect of arthrocentesis and hydraulic distension on the temporomandibular joint disk position. Oral Surg Oral Med Oral Pathol Oral Radiol Endod 2000;89:271.
6. Epker J, Gatchel R, Ellis E. A model for predicting chronic TMD. Practical application in clinical settings. J Am Dent Assoc 1999;130:1470-5.
7. Hekkenberg RJ, Piedade L, Mock D, et al. Septic arthritis of the temporomandibular joint. Otolaryngol Head Neck Surg 1999;120: 780.
8. Hincapie JW, Tobon D, Diaz-Reyes GA. Septic arthritis of the temporomandibular joint. Otolaryngol Head Neck Surg 1999;121;836.
9. Hwang S-J, Haers PE, Zimmermann A, et al. Surgical Risk factors for Condylar Resorption After Orthognathic Surgery. Oral Surg Oral Med Oral Pathol Oral Radiol Endod 2000;89:542-552.
10. Mohl ND The Anecdotal Tradition and the Need for Evidence-Based Care for Temporomandibular Disorders, J Orofac Pain 1999;13: 227-231.
11. National Institutes of Health. Management of temporomandibular disorders. NIH technology assessment statement 1996.
12. Nebbe B, Major PW, Prasad NGN. Female Adolescent Facial Pattern Associated With TMJ Disk Displacement and Reduction in Disk Length. Part I. Am J Orthod Dentofacial Orthop 1999;116: 168-176.
13. Nussenbaum B, Roland PS, Gilcrease MZ, Odell DS. Extrarticular synovial chondromatosis of the temporomandibular joint. Pitfalls in diagnosis. Arch Otolaryngol 1999;125:1394.
14. Paesani D, Sales E, Martinez A, Isberg A. Prevalence of temporomandibular joint disk displacement in infants and young children. Oral Surg Oral Med Oral Path Oral Radiol Endod 1999;87:15-9.
15. Pettengill C, Crowney MR Jr, Schoff R, Kenworthy CR. A pilot study comparing the efficacy of hard and soft stabilizing appliances in treating patients with temporomandibular disorders J Prosthet Dent 1998;79:165-8.
16. Pharoah MJ. The Prescription of Diagnostic images for Temporomandibular Joint Disorders. J Orofac Pain 1999;13:251-254.
17. Raphael K, Marbach J, Klausner J. Myofacial pain-clinical characteristics of those with regional vs. widespread pain. J Am Dent Assoc 2000 ;131:161-71.
18. Ross RB (Univ of Toronto). Development Anomalies of the Temporomandibular joint. J Orofac Pain 1999;13:262-272.
19. Sato S, Sakamoto M, Kawamura H, Motegi K. Disc position and morphology in patients with nonreducing disc displacement treated by injection of sodium hyaluronidase. Int J Oral Maxillofac Surg 1999;28:253.
20. Strobl H, Emshoff R, Krezy A. Calcium pyrophosphate dihydrate crystal deposition disease of the temporomandibular joint. Oral Surg Oral Med Oral Pathol Oral Radiol Endod 1998;85:349.
21. Takahashi T, Nagai H, Seki H, Fukuda M. Relationship between joint effusion, joint pain, and protein levels in joint lavage fluid of patients with internal derangements of the temporomandibular joint. J Oral Maxillofac Surg 1999;57:1187.
22. Tang EK, Jankovic J. Treating severe bruxing with botulinum toxin, J Am Dent Assoc 2000;131:211-6.
23. Zarb GA, Carlsson GE. Temporomandibular Disorders. Osteoarthritis. J Orofac Pain 1999;13:295-306.

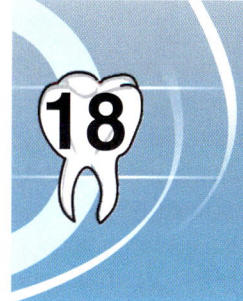

Orofacial Pain and Abnormalities of Taste

INTRODUCTION

The International Association for the Study of Pain (IASP) has defined pain as "An unpleasant sensory and emotional experience associated with actual or potential tissue damage, or described in terms of such damage". In short the pain is an unpleasant sensation associated with actual or potential tissue damage. Pain is subjective. Pain may be in absence of tissue damage or any pathophysiological cause, this may be due to psychological reasons.

Patients complaining of orofacial pain are common in dental practice. Majority of these patients have identifiable cause for their pain, for which there is adequate treatment. But in some cases, patients experience pain even after the treatment. Management of these patients requires considerations of pathophysiologic processes like infections, inflammatory, traumatic, metabolic, neurogenic and psychiatric disorders.

Some patients may experience pain even without any physical abnormality. Problems of this type usually concentrate on chronic sensory abnormality, such as atypical facial pain, glossodynia and burning mouth syndrome.

PAIN-RELATED TERMINOLOGY

- *Allodynia*: Allodynia is a condition in which nonpainful stimuli produce pain.
- *Hyperpathia*: Hyperpathia is a condition characterised by increased sensitivity, increased reaction to stimuli, imperfect identification and localization of stimuli and delayed sensation.
- *Causalgia*: Causalgia is a syndrome comprising allodynia, burning pain and hyperpathia caused due to traumatic nerve lesion.
- *Hyperalgesia*: Hyperalgesia is an increased response to pain stimuli.
- *Hyperesthesia*: Hyperesthesia is an increased sensiti-vity to stimulus that does not produce pain.
- *Hypoalgesia*: Hypoalgesia is a condition in which pain response to normal pain stimulus is decreased.
- *Hypoesthesia*: Hypoesthesia is a diminished sensitivity to stimulus.
- *Neuralgia:* Neuralgia is a pain in the course or distribution of nerve.
- *Neuropathy*: Neuropathy is alteration in function or pathologic change in a nerve.
- *Dysesthesia*: Dysesthesia is an impairment of sensation short of anesthesia or an unpleasant abnormal sensation produced by ordinary stimuli.
- *Central pain*: Central pain is a pain associated with a lesion of the central nervous system.
- *Anesthesia dolorosa*: Anesthesia dolorosa is a pain in an area of sensory loss after an injury to a nerve root or cranial nerve.

CLASSIFICATION OF OROFACIAL PAIN

1. Pain due to Diseases of Oral Cavity

A. Odontalgia
   - Pulpitis
   - Periapical pathology
   - Fractured tooth
   - Dentin defect
B. Periodontal abscess
C. Dental impaction
D. Cysts and tumors
E. Mucocutaneous diseases
F. Salivary gland diseases
G. Atypical facial pain
H. Glossodynia

2. Pain of Musculoskeletal Origin

A. Temporomandibular joint disorders
B. Myofacial pain dysfunction
C. Cervical sprain

D. Fibromyalgia
E. Eagle's syndrome.

3. Neuralgia

A. Primary trigeminal neuralgia (idiopathic)
B. Secondary trigeminal neuralgia (traumatic or CNS lesions)
C. Geniculate neuralgia (cranial nerve VII)
D. Glossopharyngeal neuralgia (cranial nerve IX)
E. Superior laryngeal neuralgia (cranial nerve X)
F. Occipital neuralgia (upper cervical spinal nerve)
G. Herpes zoster
H. Post herpetic neuralgia.

4. Vascular Pain

A. Migraine with aura
B. Migraine without aura
C. HEADACHE
   a. Cluster headache
   b. Tension-type headache
   c. Mixed headache
D. Cranial arteritis
E. Hypertensive vascular changes.

5. Generalized Pain Conditions

A. Peripheral neuropathy
B. Central pain
C. Causalgia
D. Post-traumatic pain.

6. Psychogenic Pain

A. Delusional
B. Hysterical

7. Orofacial Pains (OFP) or Pathologies which Resemble the Toothache

A. Trigeminal neuralgia
B. Trauma and/or tumor invasion of nerves (Trigeminal Neuropathy)
C. Maxillary sinusitis (pain is felt in maxillary posterior teeth)
D. Atypical odontalgia
E. Atypical facial pain
F. Cluster headache
G. Myofacial pain of masticatory muscles.

EVALUATION OF PAIN

Accurate measurement of pain is as important as classification of pain. Pain is a subjective experience so it is very difficult to measure it objectively. Measurement of pain can be helpful in determining treatment and evaluating the results of treatment. Though pain cannot be measured directly, there are few methods which enable the patients to express their pain more meaningfully. Various pain measurement methods are as follows:

1. Subjective or verbal pain reports
2. Unidimensional tools
   A. Visual analog scale
   B. Category scale
   C. Numeric rating scale
3. Multi dimensional tools
   A. McGill pain questionnaire
   B. Brief pain inventory.
4. Miscellaneous—Gnathodynamometer a device to evaluate the intensity of pain through biting force of the tooth. (For details refer chapter 7 of Textbook of Endodontics with MCQs by Satish Chandra and Shaleen Chandra).

ASSESSMENT OF PATIENT WITH OROFACIAL PAIN

The history, physical examination and diagnostic studies help in identifying the pathologic changes responsible for pain. When the treatment for presupposed diagnosis is not successful, further evaluation is necessary. Until a correct diagnosis is made, symptomatic relief should be provided.

History

The history of pain should include the intensity, quality, location, onset and duration of the pain. The patient's physical and emotional health at the time of pain and its effect on patient's work and social activities should be mentioned. The effect of rest, exercise, eating, mental distress, heat and cold on pain should be determined.

A complete past medical history should be taken, as some chronic pains are associated with systemic illness. The patient should be interrogated about medication use.

In history taking of pain the following must be noted. Intensity, location, mode of onset, timing, quality and type of pain, duration of pain, events at onset, when and how pain increases or decreases, course of symptoms, associated symptoms and previous treatments and their effects.

Physical Examination

Physical examination of the patient helps in identifying pathologic changes responsible for pain and determining the diagnosis. The head and neck examination should include the following.

Intraoral Examination (IOE)

It includes inspection and palpation of oral mucous membrane and dentition. Teeth are examined for dental and periodontal disease, fracture or faulty restoration. Tooth should be percussed for any pain associated with pulpitis and periapical or periodontal diseases. Floor of the mouth should be palpated for any mass or tenderness.

Range of Motion

Range of motion is evaluated for such movements that may produce pain. The examination is done by extension, flexion and rotation of the neck and mandible. Any pain or deviation of the movement should be recorded.

Tests of Sensory Discrimination

It is done with a sterile pin or needle by depressing in the skin gently in those areas innervated by trigeminal nerves, cervical spinal nerves and cranial nerves VII, IX and X. If the stimulation produce pain; the location and quality of the sensation should be noted.

Following orofacial symptoms may show chances of following serious diseases given in the brackets.
A. Trigeminal neuralgia in male below 50 years of age and in female below 40 years of age (multiple sclerosis)
B. Diffuse mandibular pain on the left side (Cardiac ischemia)
C. Sudden onset of severe headache in adults with unexplained nausea and vomiting (Intracranial tumor)
D. Severe earache, changed sensation in the area supplied by the mandibular nerve and trismus with deviated midline (tumor in the infratemporal fossa).

Headache and orofacial pain may be present in the following diseases.
A. Deficiency of vitamin B complex with folic acid
B. Iron deficiency anemia
C. Paget's disease
D. Hyperthyroidism
E. Metastatic disease.

Severe pain in head and neck is usually present in the following.
A. Acute pulpitis
B. Impacted third molars
C. Lesions of the jaw bones, ear, nose and oral cavity
D. Carious exposed teeth
E. Neuralgias of head, face and neck
F. Craniofacial pain of musculoskeletal origin.

Diagnostic Studies

Various diagnostic methods used for evaluating the pain are as follows.
A. *Temperature intolerance*: It helps in identifying dental diseases which evoke pain. Heat intolerance suggests pulpal diseases and cold intolerance suggests dentinal pathology.
B. Craniofacial imaging
C. Psychologic evaluation
D. Diagnostic local anesthetic blocks
E. Acetone and phentolamine test.

SPECIFIC OROFACIAL PAIN CONDITIONS

Neuralgia

Neuralgia is characterized by severe, recurrent, intense and shooting pain along the course or distribution of a nerve usually cranial or upper cervical spinal nerves.

Follow-up, repeated examinations and testing: Orofacial symptoms may come only with time. With time, follow-up, repeated examination and testing more than 50% of the unexplained orofacial pain problems are solved. Ever developing new imaging techniques may reveal pathogenesis of the undiagnosed OFP symptoms.

Trigeminal Neuralgia (TN)

It is characterized by severe, paroxysmal pain in one or more branches of trigeminal nerve. It may be primary or secondary. There is 'trigger zone' in the area supplied by the nerve on the mucous membrane or skin. Light touch of this zone precipitates the pain. Usually sites of 'trigger zone' are corner of the lips, eating, speaking, shaving, showering or exposure to wind can trigger an episode of pain. Intra oral 'trigger zone' can be confused with dental disorder.
a. *Primary trigeminal neuralgia*: Primary trigeminal neuralgia or idiopathic trigeminal neuralgia or tic douloureux is an extremely painful disorder involving maxillary or mandibular division of the trigeminal nerve.

The pain is usually initiated by minor tactile stimuli to skin at specific sites around the face (trigger zone). The pain is recurrent, lancinating and unilateral which lasts for seconds to minutes and then completely disappears by itself.

The pain occurs more frequently in women of 50 to 70 years of age. The etiology of primary trigeminal neuralgia is not clearly known, but it may be caused due to compression of trigeminal ganglion by adjacent atherosclerotic arteries and degeneration and demyelination of trigeminal ganglion and dorsal root ganglion.

b. *Secondary trigeminal neuralgia*: Secondary trigeminal neuralgia is caused due to peripheral nerve injury, intracranial trauma or central nervous system lesions. Extracranial or intracranial tumor, vascular malformation or degenerative changes may evoke secondary trigeminal neuralgia.

Diagnosis: Diagnosis is based on the (a) history of shooting pain along the nerve course (b) precipitation by touching the 'trigger zone'. The examination may precipitate the shooting pain. In about 10% of TN patients the cause may be underlying detectable pathology. Therefore MRI of the brain should be done to rule out etiological tumors, vascular malformations and multiple sclerosis. In primary TN pathology is obscure and the secondary TN is due to some pathology in vessels along the course of the nerve or the ganglion or the brain.

c. *Treatment*: Mostly primary or secondary trigeminal neuralgia can be treated by medication, alcohol injection and surgery. In secondary TN, etiological factor must be removed for permanent treatment.

   i. *Medication*

The drugs commonly used in treatment of trigeminal neuralgia are anticonvulsant drugs such as carbamazepine, baclofen, and phenytoin sodium. Carbamazepine is prescribed in initial dose of 200 mg/day which is, if require, can be further increased to 800 to 1200 mg/day in divided doses. Patients taking carbamazepine must have periodic hematologic laboratory investigations done as rarely serious blood dyscrasias may occur. Baclofen and phenytoin are less efficacious alternatives. Baclofen is prescribed in 50 to 80 mg/day in divided doses. It can be used in combination with carbamazepine. Phenytoin sodium may also provide relief in trigeminal neuralgia. Its recommended dose is 400 mg/day. Gabapentin, a new anticonvulsant, has few side effects but is not as reliable as carbamazepine.

Other drugs include phenytoin, lamotrigine and pimozide. If pain do not reoccur for 3 months, the drugs can be gradually withdrawn.

   ii. *Alcohol injections*: Two ml of absolute alcohol mixed with 0.5 ml of 2% local anesthetic solution when injected at the mandibular foramen as mandibular injection in case of TN of mandibular nerve gives relief for about 6 to 9 months. Alcohol causes necrosis of the nerve giving relief for about 6 to 9 months. In about 6 to 9 months nerve again regenerates. Local anesthetic is added as the injection of alcohol is very painful. After every 6 to 9 months alcohol injections can be repeated but it has been observed that with subsequent injections as the injections are repeated the duration of pain relief gradually decreases from 6 to 9 months to 5 to 8 months and like wise. As alcohol causes necrosis of the surrounding tissues along with the nerve a course of analgesics and antibiotics is prescribed for 5 to 7 days along with alcohol injections.

   iii. *Surgery*: When the pain is not responding to medications and alcohol injections or it is due to serious anatomic lesions. Surgery can be carried out for treatment of trigeminal neuralgia. Various surgical procedures are as follows.

Intracranial procedures
- Microvascular decompression
- Radiofrequency thermocoagulation of trigeminal ganglion
- Surgical or laser removal of the pathology.

Peripheral neuroablative procedure

Neurectomy is performed and about 2 cm or more long nerve piece is cut away and removed. If only cutting is done the nerve will regenerate within 3 to 6 months, hence longer piece of the nerve is removed. If the nerve is removed from bony canal the space between the two cut ends of the nerve in the bony canal is filled and sealed with bone wax to delay the regeneration of the nerve thereby reoccurrence of neuralgic pain.

Geniculate Neuralgia

Geniculate neuralgia is a rare paroxysmal neuralgia resulting from herpetic inflammation of the geniculate ganglion and nervus intermedius of cranial nerve VII. Pain most frequently occurs in ear but may sometimes involve soft palate and anterior portion of the tongue.

There may be some degree of facial paralysis due to involvement of motor root. Acyclovir 200 mg five times a day for 10 to 14 days reduces the duration of pain. High dose steroid therapy for two to three weeks can be prescribed for the treatment of inflammatory neural degeneration.

Glossopharyngeal Neuralgia (GPN)

Glossopharyngeal neuralgia is a neuralgia of ninth cranial nerve. It is a rare condition. The patient experiences pain in the region of distribution of glossopharyngeal nerve which are ear, posterior tongue, pharynx and retromandibular area. Pain is initiated by chewing, talking and swallowing. The most common cause of glossopharyngeal neuralgia is compression of ninth cranial nerve by vascular abnormalities and intraoral or extraoral tumors.

Differential diagnosis: The application of topical anesthetic to the pharyngeal mucosa eliminates pain of GPN. By this it can be differentiated from other neuralgias. It can be successfully treated by carbamazepine or baclofen. GPN may occur with TN when there is a common central lesion.

Occipital Neuralgia

Occipital neuralgia is an uncommon neuralgia associated with sensory branches of the cervical plexus, mostly in the neck and occipital region. It mostly results from trauma followed by a neoplasm, infection or aneurysm involving the affected nerve.

Mode of treatment includes corticosteroids, neurolysis or blocking the nerve with alcohol with local anesthetic injection.

Postherpetic neuralgia (PHN): About 15 to 20% of *herpes zoster* cases involve the trigeminal neuralgia. Due to the *herpes zoster* infection of the maxillary and mandibular divisions, lesions as well as orofacial pain occur. The chronic burning pain accompanied by sensory deficiency persist after the lesions heal (Fig. 10.3).

Management: The treatment may be topical and systemic medicines and surgery depending on the severity of the symptoms. For topical treatment and short term relief lidocaine or analgesics like capsaicin may be used.

The chronic burning pain is reduced by tricyclic antidepressant such as amitriptyline, dose 50-200 mg /day (preparations AMILINE, QUIETAL, TRYPTANOL, 10, 20, 75 mg Tab) nortriptyline 50-150 mg /day (preparations SENSIVALI, 25 mg Tab), doxepin 25-150 mg/day (preparation SPECTRA, DOXEPIN, EXIPEACE, DOXETAR 10, 25, 75 mg Cap/Tab) and desiprimine. In aged patient gabapentin is given. Episodes of shooting pain can be relieved by carbamazepine or phenytoin. PHN can be prevented and its severity can be reduced by antiviral drugs like famciclovir, and antidepressant drug like tricyclic along with the course of systemic corticosteroids during the acute phase.

Pain Due to Diseases of Oral Cavity

Pain in the intraoral cavity is mostly caused by dental diseases. Pain is relieved by providing appropriate dental treatment, so careful examination of periodontal and periapical diseases, caries, pulpal disease, faulty restoration or occlusal trauma is necessary.

Sometimes pain can also be referred from nearby structures. For example, pain can be referred from maxillary sinus to maxillary teeth, malar and zygomatic area of the face or vice versa. Sialoadenitis, polymyositis, rheumatoid arthritis, lupus erythematosus and scleroderma may cause orofacial pain.

Pain of Musculoskeletal Origin

Pain of musculoskeletal origin is characterized by deep, dull, depressing pain which is not well localized and increases with muscle function. It can be primary or secondary. Primary musculoskeletal pain arises in myofacial pain, dysfunction syndrome, fibromyalgia, and rheumatoid arthritis.

Secondary musculoskeletal pain results from traumatic, inflammatory, infectious, metabolic, neoplastic and immunologic disorders. Pain of musculoskeletal origin also arises in Eagle's syndrome which is characterised by deep, dull pain in the oropharynx and posterior auricular region. It is caused due to calcification of the stylohyoid ligament or elongated styloid process.

Vascular Pain

Pain arising due to vascular disorders is commonest of chronic head and neck pain. Pain is characterized as dull, pressing or throbbing which may be well localized or diffuse. The most common vascular pain disorder is migraine.

Migraine

Migraine is a vascular disorder characterized by unilateral pain in the head. This pain usually begins before the age of 40 years and rarely begins in older individuals. Migraine headache can be divided into migraine with aura and migraine without aura. Aura is defined as subjective symptoms at the onset of or just before a migraine headache.

Migraine with aura: Migraine with aura is characterized by subjective symptoms which appear before the onset of migraine headache. These symptoms are unilateral numbness and weakness, visual disturbance and speech difficulty. Pain is moderate to severe which occurs unilaterally in the temporal or orbital region.

Migraine without aura: Pain in migraine without aura is unilateral, mild to moderate and pulsating. It occurs behind the eye or temporal region and lasts for 4 to 72 hours. Pain is aggravated by physical activity and visual or auditory stimulation, and is associated with nausea, vomiting or photophobia.

Cluster Headache (CH)

Cluster headache is of sudden onset, unilateral, usually in the periorbital and maxillary area. Pain occurs in bouts or clusters having long intervals in between. The condition is associated with lacrimation, nasal blockage and conjunctival reddening. This headache occurs predominantly in males between the ages of 20 to 50 years. Pain is triggered by consuming small amount of alcohol. Most of the patients of cluster headache are smokers and alcohol abusers. Pain occurs one to three times a day and lasts for minutes to few hours. Pain may disappear for several months or years and then again reappear. Some patient show violent behavior during attack in contrast with migraine patients, who lie down in dark room and prefer to sleep.

Tension-Type Headache

It is the most common type of headache. The pain is deep and bilateral, occurring between the occipital and frontal region. The pain becomes worse with progression of the day and lasts for hours to days. Trigger points are usually observed in pericranial and cervical region.

Mixed Headache

Mixed headache shows both the features of migraine and tension type headache. It usually develops in older individuals who had previously suffered from migraine or tension type headache.

Traction Headache

This headache is associated with a brain tumor and is caused due to increased intracranial pressure. The pain can be localized over the site of tumor or can be generalized.

Cranial Arteritis

Cranial arteritis refers to obstruction of the artery due to inflammation. The arteries commonly involved are temporal arteries. This condition is characterized by deep, aching and throbbing pain with burning sensation over the artery. Pain may radiate to face, neck, maxilla or mandible. Blindness may develop in 50% of the patients.

Carotodynia

Carotodynia refers to facial pain associated with carotid body tumor or carotid aneurysm. The pain is characterised by a tender, throbbing or swollen carotid artery on the affected side. The pain is exaggerated by head movement, mastication and deglutition.

Prevention of Migraine

Migraine headache can be prevented by beta-blockers such as propranolol or nadolol. The usual dose is 60 to 80 mg daily to prevent migraine. Acute attacks of migraine can be treated by calcium channel blockers such as verapamil hydrochloride and nifedipine. The usual dose of verapamil is 40 to 160 mg TDS oral and of nifedipine is 5 to 50 mg BD/TDS/oral/ sublingual. Dihydroergotamine can be administered intramuscularly or intravenously to stop migraine attack.

Migraine is caused by vasoconstriction of intracranial vessels, followed by vasodilation.

Management
1. Determine common food triggers.
2. Drugs
    A. For prevention – Propranolol, verapamil and TCAs
    B. Drugs for interception of migraine are ergotamine and sumatriptan. These drugs can be given orally, nasally, rectally and parentally. These drugs cause hypertension and other c.v. complications parentally. To manage difficult cases which do not respond to safer drugs phenelzine can be used. Cluster headache (CH) can be intercepted by breathing 100% oxygen. Other drug which can prevent attacks is ergotamine. For shorter period methysergide can be given as its prolonged use cause pulmonary and cardiac fibrosis.

Cluster headache can be managed by prednisolone, 20 mg four times a day for 7 days followed by decreasing the dose by 20 mg every 2 days or any other cortisone (dose to be adjusted according to the potency of the salt). Lithium

Carbonate 600 to 1800 mg/day, oral can be used for preventing cluster headache. Mixed headache can be treated by tricyclic antidepressants in combination with vasoactive medications.

Generalized Pain Conditions

Central Pain

This pain occurs due to an injury to the central nervous system. The pain is spontaneous and may be evoked by stimuli which is normally harmful. Central pain can be observed in thalamic pain syndrome.

Thalamic pain syndrome is characterized by continuous pain opposite to the thalamic lesion, which can affect the orofacial region and may cause hypoesthesia, paresthesia or paralysis of facial and masticatory muscles.

Post-Traumatic Neuropathic Pain

Orofacial pain can also occur after an injury to the head, neck, face and cranial nerves. Post-traumatic pain may include different pain variants such as hyperpathia, hyperalgesia and anesthesia dolorosa. The cause for this type of pain is improper peripheral nerve regeneration, neuroma formation and scar tissue formation at the site of injured nerve.

Trigeminal nerve injuries may be caused by facial trauma, surgeries like impacted tooth, cysts and tumors removal, osteotomies or genioplasties. There nerve injury may cause numbness, pain with a trigger zone, or burning pain. Serious damage may cause degeneration of neural fibers. Total nerve section (neurotmesis) cause permanent nerve damage. In peripheral nerve injury pain may persist or may only response to touch. Nerve damage may cause anesthesia, paresthesia (feeling of pins and needles), allodynia or hyperalgesia.

Management: Depending on the nature of injury and severity of pain the management of neuropathic pain may be (a) nonsurgical (b) surgical (c) combination of both.

Nonsurgical management includes the following:
1. Systemic corticosteroids in the first week of injury.
2. Tricyclic antidepressants like amitriptyline, nortriptyline and doxepin.

Complex regional pain syndrome–1 (CRPS-1) [Reflex sympathetic dystrophy (RSD)]: CRPS-1 and RSD are the terms used to describe the condition which consists of localized pain, motor and sweat abnormalities, and trophic changes in the muscles and skin. The most usual symptoms are allodynia, hyperesthesia, spontaneous chronic burning pain, tenderness, sweating, cutaneous atrophy, motor dysfunction and the involved skin become edematous and erythematous.

Treatment: Multidisciplinary treatment including physical therapy, nerve blocks and drug therapy. Successful results have been obtained by blockade of regional sympathetic ganglia or blockade of regional veins intravenously with guanethidine, reserpine or phenoxybenzamine with local anesthetic.

ATYPICAL OROFACIAL PAIN

Atypical orofacial pain is a persistent facial pain that does not follow any anatomic pattern. It does not fulfill the criteria for other types of facial pain. It is not included in the etiological categories of facial pain and does not respond to any treatment. It is a psychiatric disorder for which the dental surgeon cannot make any specific dental or medical diagnosis.

The most common clinical feature of atypical facial pain is the patient's inability to describe the quality and location of the pain. The pain is described as deep, dull and poorly localized. The pain persists daily and starts from one side of the face which is not associated with objective signs or organic diseases. Psychosomatic disorder is the most significant etiological factor regarding atypical facial pain as it is commonly associated with depression. Middle-aged females are more commonly affected than males. Atypical facial pain should be managed with antidepressants and psychotherapy. For reducing or eliminating pain amitriptyline, nortriptyline, doxepin, gabapentin and clonazepam are effective.

ATYPICAL ODONTALGIA (AO)

Atypical odontalgia is a variant of atypical facial pain or psychogenic pain. The patient describes pain in a single tooth or group of teeth that does not show any abnormality on percussion, thermal or electric test or radiographic examination. This type of pain does not respond to any treatment, either endodontic therapy or extraction of the tooth and persists at site of extraction or transfers towards adjacent tooth.

Atypical odontalgia is predominant in middle-aged females. The pain usually starts after a dental procedure. It is associated with emotional and mental problems. Atypical odontalgia can be treated by antidepressant medication and psychotherapy. For reducing or eliminating pain amitriptyline, nortriptyline, doxepin, gabapentin and clonazepam are effective.

GLOSSODYNIA

Glossodynia is a psychogenic condition, found particularly in middle-aged patients with a normal tongue. The patient complains of pain and burning sensation in the tongue and oral cavity which has no detectable cause. The condition may be of psychosomatic, local or systemic origin. A number of factors may be responsible for glossodynia.

These factors are as follows.
1. *Local irritants*: Sharp margins of teeth, calculus, restorations, ill-fitting appliance and dentures, and heavy smoking.
2. *Allergic reactions*: Allergy to metallic restoration, denture base material, drugs, particular food, toothpastes and mouth washes.
3. *Muscular tension*: Muscular tension as in myofacial pain dysfunction syndrome and oral muscular habits may cause glossodynia.
4. *Systemic diseases*: Glossodynia can be observed in systemic diseases and deficiency states such as pernicious anemia, Plummer-Vinson syndrome and pellagra. It may also occur in diabetes mellitus either due to diabetic neuropathy or oral candidiasis.
5. *Neurologic factors*: Neuropathy of lingual nerve due to damage to the nerve may cause abnormal sensation in the tongue.

BURNING MOUTH SYNDROME

Burning mouth syndrome can be described as intraoral pain disorders that is not associated with clinical signs. The major symptoms in this disorder are burning, itching or pain in the oral mucosa. It is associated with various etiological factors such as nutritional deficiency, hormonal disorders (menopause, diabetes), xerostomia, psychosomatic disorders and oromucosal lesions such as geographic tongue, lichen planus and aphthous stomatitis. It is seven times more common in females than males. Burning mouth is more common in between 3 to 12 years after menopause.

The burning can be constant or intermittent. Increased salivation by eating, drinking and chewing of candy and gum decreases burning.

Treatment of Glossodynia and Burning Mouth Syndrome

Treatment includes the following:
A. Removal of local oral irritants
B. Treatment of muscular tension by muscle relaxants such as diazepam, correction of malocclusion and fabrication of night guard.
C. Application of topical analgesics such as 0.5% aqueous diphenhydramine alone or in combination with 0.5% dyclonine to the affected area.
D. Treatment of systemic diseases.
E. Surgical correction of the lingual nerve by removing scar tissue, or neuroma at the site of damaged lingual nerve.
F. Low doses of TCAs such as amitriptyline and doxepin or clonazepam (a benizodiazepine derivative).
G. If the etiology is parafunctional oral habits a splint covering the teeth and palate may be useful.

ABNORMALITIES OF TASTE

Classification of Taste Disorders

Gustatory-Olfactory Confusion

a. Upper respiratory tract infection
b. Industrial dust and air pollutants

Secondary Dysgeusias and Parageusias

a. Bacterial fermentation of dental plaque
b. Inflammed secretions from salivary glands
c. Metallic dysgeusia
d. Medications and particular food

Transport Disorders

a. Salivary hypofunction and xerostomia
b. Blocked taste bud nerves

Sensorineural Taste Disorders

a. Inherited disorders
b. Damage to taste nerves
c. Loss of taste buds

Lesions Affecting Central Pathways of Taste

a. Brain tumor
b. Trauma to head
c. Multiple sclerosis
d. Epilepsy
e. Cerebrovascular lesions

Metabolic Disorders

a. Diabetes mellitus
b. Hormonal disorders
c. Hepatic disease

Pregnancy

Idiopathic Taste Abnormality

Age-related Changes of Gustatory Function

Taste Loss in Anosmic Patients (Gustatory-Olfactory Confusions)

Upper Respiratory Tract Infection

Patients suffering from upper respiratory tract infection may experience taste loss or complain that the food does not taste as earlier. Such problem may be associated with decreased transport of volatile substance to olfactory receptors due to inflammation of sinus mucosa.

Industrial Dusts and Air Pollutants

Individuals exposed to industrial dust and air pollutants may complain of gustatory and olfactory loss. Industrial dusts such as chromium may cause mucositis of nasal passage and necrosis of nasal septum, which results in olfactory damage.

In both the above cases patient is actually suffering from olfactory disorder, but due to gustatory-olfactory confusion, may experience taste loss.

Secondary Dysgeusias and Parageusias

Secondary dysgeusia and parageusia occur in individuals with otherwise normal gustatory function. These taste disorders occur due to introduction of substances with an unpleasant or unusual taste.
A. Unusual or unpleasant taste may be produced in the mouth due to bacterial fermentation in dental plaque and retained food, poor oral hygiene, poorly cleaned bridges or dentures, gingivitis and periodontitis.
B. Secretions from inflamed, sclerosed and partially occluded salivary glands may produce abnormal excessive sweet, salty and even putrid taste in the mouth.
C. Crevicular fluid and inflammatory transudates in periodontitis, gingivitis, wounds and extraction socket may result in dysgeusic symptoms.
D. Iodine containing medications and ingredients in processed foods, such as saccharine, cyclamate and garlic may cause stimulated dysgeusia.
E. Bacterial or fungal metabolic products from coated tongue, periodontal pockets and pseudomembranous mucositis result in dysgeusias.

Transport Disorders

These are true taste disorders caused due to interference in the transport of gustatory stimuli to the taste receptor membrane.

Salivary Hypofunction and Xerostomia

Sensation of taste arises from direct stimulation of taste bud receptors by the substances dissolved in saliva. In patients with decreased salivary flow, the concentration of taste stimuli and salivary electrolytes reaching the cell membrane is greatly reduced. In xerostomia, there may be damaged taste bud cells or they may undergo regressive changes which cause alteration in perception of taste.

Blocked Taste Bud Pores

Salivary hypofunction and radiotherapy to the head and neck may result in overgrowth of bacteria and yeasts which lead to blockage of taste bud pores by microbial elements. This phenomenon causes taste loss in these patients. Edentulous patients wearing an upper denture may also complain of taste loss because some of the palatal taste receptors get occluded by the upper denture. Decreased touch and pressure sensation and retention of food particles and plaque on the surfaces of the denture also cause loss of taste.

Sensorineural Taste Disorders

Inherited Disorders

Inherited disorders associated with abnormal taste sensation are as follows:

Familial dysautonomia: Familial dysautonomia is characterised by absence of vallate and fungiform papillae. The children suffering from this disorder also exhibit excessive sweat and mucous production, hypersalivation and oral self-mutilation.

Pseudohypoparathyroidism: Patients suffering from this syndrome experience decreased sensitivity for taste stimuli.

Aglycogeusia: It is a congenital abnormality of taste buds in which patient is unable to differentiate between sugar solution and water.

Damage to Taste Nerves

Trauma to the lingual nerve: Lesions of the lingual nerve result from trauma to the nerve during extraction of mandibular molar teeth, removal of stone from submandibular gland duct, jaw fracture and laceration of the ventral surface of the tongue during dental procedures. This nerve carries sensory and gustatory fibers to the anterior third of the tongue, so any damage to this nerve results in the impairment of the sense of taste or decreased sensitivity for taste stimuli.

Trauma to the glossopharyngeal nerve: Trauma to the glossopharyngeal nerve may result during tonsillectomy and removal of pharyngeal tumors. This may lead to temporary decrease in the sensitivity for taste stimuli.

Trauma to chorda tympani nerve: Chronic inflammation and tumors of the middle ear, temporal bone and parotid gland and middle-ear surgery may cause damage to the chorda tympani nerve which results in unilateral anterior third dysgeusia. Salivary dysfunction on the affected side is also seen in trauma to the chorda tympani nerve.

Intracranial lesions of VII, IX and X nerves: Neoplasms, granulomas, aneurysms and infectious processes within the skull may affect the VII, IX and X cranial nerves. This may result in appearance of symptoms of dysgeusia.

Loss of taste buds and taste bud functions: Glossitis, lichen planus, leukoplakia, leprosy, salivary hypofunction and xerostomia are associated with atrophic and regressive changes affecting the taste buds. Radiation therapy for head and neck tumor leads to stomatitis. All these conditions lead to hypogeusia and parageusia.

Medications such as captopril, metronidazole, amphotericin B, penicillamine and chlorhexidine are associated with taste dysfunction. Use of tobacco specially smokeless tobacco is also associated with diminished taste sensation.

Lesions Affecting Central Pathways of Taste

Brain Tumor and Cerebrovascular Lesions

Vascular lesions and tumors of the brain may cause neurologic abnormalities in the orofacial region. Such lesions are associated with dysgeusic symptoms accompanied by pain and other sensory loss. Syndromes such as Wallenberg's syndrome, Dejerine-Roussy syndrome and tertiary-neurosyphilis that results from CNS lesions are associated with taste dysfunction.

Trauma to the Head

Head trauma and postneurosurgery patients may experience hypogeusia or ageusia. The symptoms of post-traumatic ageusia or hypogeusia may appear late as long as 4 months after injury. Damage to the temporal lobe by penetrating wound in the side of the head may lead to combined loss of olfactory and gustatory sensations.

Multiple Sclerosis

Multiple sclerosis is a chronic neurologic disease associated with demyelination of axons within the central nervous system. Demyelination of gustatory nerves passing through the pons or medulla may result in unilateral or bilateral ageusia.

Metabolic Disorders

Taste dysfunction can also be found in various metabolic disorders such as diabetes mellitus, hypothyroidism and hyperthyroidism, adrenal insufficiency, jaundice and hepatitis. Reasons and symptoms of taste abnormality commonly present are as follows.
A. Increased intake of salt and lowered taste threshold in adrenal insufficiency.
B. Taste loss following treatment with antithyroid drugs.
C. Specific food aversion and preferences in patients with hepatic disease.
D. Reduction in taste sensitivity for glucose in patients with impaired glucose tolerance.

Idiopathic Taste Abnormality

Idiopathic dysgeusia refers to taste abnormality for which no specific diagnosis can be made. But such type of dysgeusia improves with zinc supplementation, so it may be associated with defective taste bud function secondary to zinc deficiency.

BIBLIOGRAPHY

1. Lunardi G, Leandri M, Albano C, et al. Clinical effectiveness of lamotrigine and plasma levels in essential and symptomatic trigeminal neuralgia. Neurol 1998; 50:1192.
2. Morello CM, Leckband SG, Stoner CP, et al. Randomized double-blind study comparing the efficacy of gabapentin with amitriptyline on diabetic neuropathic pain. Arch Intern Med 1999;159:1931-7.
3. Rowbatham M, Harden N, Stacey B, et al. Gabapentin for the treatment of postherpetic neuralgia. A randomized controlled trial. JAMA 1998;280:1837-42.
4. Vickers ER, Cousins MJ, Walker S, Chisholm K. Analysis of 50 patients with atypical odontalgia. Oral Surg Oral Med Oral Pathol Oral Radiol Endod 1998; 85:24-32.
5. Watson CP, Vernich L, Chipman M, Reed K. Nortriptyline versus amitriptyline is postherpetic neuralgia. A randomized trial. Neurology 1998; 51:166-71.
6. Woolf CJ, Mannion RJ. Neuropathic pain. Aetiology, symptoms, mechanisms and management. Lancet 1999;353:1959-64.

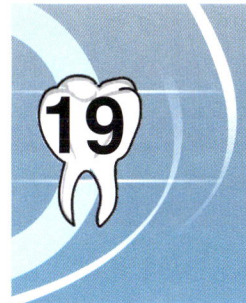

Cardiovascular Diseases Related to Oral Medicine

INTRODUCTION

Maximum people die of cardiovascular diseases (CVD), among all the diseases, all over the world. CVD includes high or low blood pressure, congestive heart failure (CHF), coronary artery disease (CAD), Congenital cardiovascular defects and cardiac stroke. Cardiac diseases are associated with increased risk in performing dental procedures. Infection of dental and oral origin may cause endocarditis; and any minor or major operations in oral region of patient with heart disease may lead to cardiac emergencies. There is a need for proper knowledge and identification of these cardiac diseases and dental surgeons must take precautionary measures while treating them.

HYPERTENSION

About 10% of world population above the age of 40 years has hypertension. In large cities of developed countries this percentage is 20% and in rural, backward and tribal people this percentage is 2%. Therefore like dental caries the percentage of hypertension also increases with civilization. Most of the rural people do not know that they have hypertension. Only 20 of 30% hypertension patients in large cities of developed countries know that they have hypertension and keep it under control by drugs. Therefore dental surgeon has to take all precautions against undetected hypertension in the patients. In spite of many benefits of adrenaline in local anesthetic solution many dental surgeons prefer to use LA solution without adrenaline to avoid problem of severe palpitations in patients after LA.

Hypertension refers to elevation of systemic arterial blood pressure. It is the most important risk factor for coronary heart disease. The systolic pressure of over 130 mm Hg and diastolic pressure above 90 mm Hg is considered to be hypertension. Hypertension can be classified into two types.

Primary or Essential or Idiopathic Hypertension

In this type, the cause is unknown. It is mostly found in those individuals who are working under stress, tension, hurry and worry.

Secondary Hypertension

Secondary hypertension, is that in which there is some organic etiology. It may be caused due to renal diseases, vascular changes associated with atherosclerosis, adrenal cortical hypofunction or central nervous system lesion.

Hypertension can be again categorized as follows:
a. STAGE I Mild hypertension-systolic BP 130 to 149 mm Hg or diastolic pressure of 90 to 99 mm Hg
b. STAGE II Moderate hypertension-systolic BP 150 to 169 mm Hg or diastolic pressure of 100 to 109 mm Hg
c. STAGE III Severe hypertension-systolic BP 170 to 189 mm Hg or diastolic pressure of 110 to 119 mm Hg
d. STAGE IV Very severe hypertension-systolic BP more than 190 mm Hg or diastolic pressure more than 120 mm Hg.

Clinical Features

The symptoms presenting hypertension are recurrent or persistent headache, general discomfort or uneasiness, shortness of breath, bleeding from nose and dizziness. Oral manifestations are occasionally present such as odontalgia and hyperemia or congestion of dental pulp due to increased blood pressure.

Management

Management of hypertension is important. It increases mortality rate. Management of hypertension includes two methods.

Non-drug management: Non-drug measures include change in lifestyle such as doing sufficient exercise, weight control,

control on alcohol and stoppage of smoking, dietary sodium restrictions, and avoiding stress, tension, hurry and worry.

Pharmacologic management: Drugs recommended for management of hypertension are diuretics or beta-blockers. Other suitable drugs are calcium antagonists, ACE inhibitors, alpha beta blockers and alpha-receptor blockers.

Oro-dental Considerations

Hypertensive patients have an increased rate of preoperative mortality. Treatment of hypertension reduces over all mortality rate.

A. Blood pressure apparatus (stethoscope and sphygmomanometer) should be present in dental clinic to determine the blood pressure in patient with known or having signs and symptoms of hypertension, to ensure that there is no risk from the stress of dental procedure.
B. Dental patient with elevated blood pressure requires careful evaluation in treatment planning, premedication, selection of an anesthetic (without adrenaline) and short durations of operative procedures.
C. A high concentration of adrenaline in the local anaesthetic solution is contraindicated in hypertensive patients.
D. Antihypertensive drugs such as diuretics, alpha adrenergic and ganglionic blocking agents can cause orthostatic hypotension or fall in blood pressure due to sudden change of posture from a supine position to an upright position, which may lead to fainting.
E. Antihypertensive drugs that act on central nervous system may cause a dry mouth.
F. Methyldopa, a centrally acting Alpha$_2$—Agonist may cause ulcerations on the oral mucous membrane.
G. Calcium channel blockers such as nifedipine and diltiazem may cause gingival enlargement.

Rapid Control of Hypertension

For rapid control of hypertension before orodental treatment nifedipine (DEPIN) 5 mg soft capsule is punctured and discharged sublingually. Usually within 15 minutes hypertension comes under control.

CORONARY HEART DISEASE (CHD)

Coronary heart disease or ischemic heart disease is caused by decreased or inadequate blood supply to the heart. This insufficiency of the blood supply results in two types of heart diseases, angina pectoris and myocardial infarction.

Causes of Coronary Heart Diseases are as follows:

A. Coronary atherosclerosis
B. Aortic valvular disease
C. Coronary embolism
D. Coronary arterial spasm
E. Dissecting aneurysm
F. Vasculitis
G. Carbon monoxide poisoning
H. Tachycardia
I. Acute anemia

Risk Factors For Coronary Heart Disease

A. Hypertension
B. Diabetes
C. Smoking
D. Increased serum cholesterol level
E. Left ventricular hypertrophy
F. Family history of coronary disease

Two types of coronary heart diseases are, angina pectoris and myocardial infarction.

Angina Pectoris

Angina pectoris is a short acting chest pain or discomfort that results due to imbalance between the oxygen demand and oxygen supply to heart muscles. It is most common in individuals of 45 to 65 years of age.

Clinical features: The attack of angina occurs after physical exertion or emotional stress. Patient experiences crushing pain and discomfort in substernal region which may radiate to left shoulder, arm, neck or jaw. Pain is of short duration lasting for few seconds to few minutes.

Treatment: The patients of angina should take following steps to decrease coronary risk factors:
a. Reducing weight
b. Cessation of smoking
c. Low cholesterol diet
d. Exercising
e. Controlling diabetes or hypertension

Short-acting drugs such as sublingual nitroglycerine can be administered for an acute attack. For long-term prevention, long-acting nitrates such as isosorbide dinitrate tablets are administered. Beta-adrenergic blocking agent alone or in combination with nitrate is also effective in angina pectoris.

Oro-dental considerations: Stressful dental procedures such as time consuming and difficult extractions should be avoided in patients with angina pectoris as it can precipitate anginal attack on the dental chair. If patient experiences an anginal attack, a nitroglycerine tablet should be kept immediately under the tongue. In such patient in dental clinic only emergency procedures should be performed in consultation with and preferably in presence of a cardiologist. Other procedures should be carried out in a hospital where full cardiac set up is present to meet out any emergency.

Myocardial Infarction

Myocardial infarction is characterized by angina-like pain that remains for more than half an hour and is not caused by exertion. In myocardial infarction there is death of cardiac muscle tissue caused by coronary insufficiency.

Clinical features: Pain in myocardial infarction is severe and lasts for more than 30 minutes. The other symptoms which may accompany pain are nausea and vomiting, pulmonary edema with difficulty in breathing, irregular pulse and tachycardia and shock with pallor. Myocardial infarction may result in cardiac arrest.

Treatment: Treatment of myocardial infarction consists of relieving the pain by administering morphine sulphate in early stages of disease and complete mental and physical rest during period of recovery. Oxygen and anticoagulants are also administered.

Management of Patient with Coronary Heart Disease in Dental Clinic

Patients with coronary heart disease have decreased ability to withstand stressful conditions, so they require a special management in dental clinic. Dental procedure may intensify existing cardiovascular disease.

Premedication: Rapid acting oral benzodiazepines can be prescribed to patients before treatment. A 5mg dose of diazepam should be given 1 hour before the dental procedure to minimize stress occurring in waiting room and on the dental chair. Patient susceptible to attack of angina should be administered isosorbide dinitrate sublingually.

Use of local anesthesia: Local anesthetic agents should be properly administered in the patients of cardiovascular disease. Complete anesthesia is necessary in these patients to minimize uneasiness and release of endogenous epinephrine. The procedure for administration of local anesthetic agents, especially aspiration before injection should be carried out carefully. Normal concentration of vasoconstrictor used in dental local anesthetic agent can be administered to cardiac patients without any risk, but the total anesthetic solution should not be more than 5 ml. If more anesthetic solution is required then it should be without vasoconstrictor.

Other considerations: Patients with cardiovascular disease should be given shorter appointments and less extensive traumatic procedures should be carried out. If patient develops chest pain, breathlessness, pallor or irregular pulse during the dental procedure, the procedure should be stopped immediately and cardiologist/physician should be consulted.

VALVULAR HEART DISEASE

Mitral valve disease: It may be (a) mitral valve prolapse (MVP) (b) mitral regurgitation (MR) and mitral stenosis (MS).

Oro-dental Considerations

Prophylactic premedication with antibiotic must be given to all patients (a) with valvular heart disease (b) undergone mitral or aortic valve repair or replacement (c) with prior history of infective endocarditis (d) with mitral stenosis or (e) with aortic regurgitation.

CONGESTIVE HEART FAILURE

Congestive heart failure refers to inadequacy of the heart to pump enough blood to meet the metabolic demands of the body.

Causes

1. Cardiac valvular lesions
2. Coronary artery disease
3. Hypertension
4. Hyperthyroidism.

Clinical Features

1. Breathlessness following moderate exertion
2. Cyanosis of lips, tongue and oral mucosa
3. Pulmonary edema with chronic productive cough
4. Pitting edema of lower extremities
5. Hepatic enlargement and ascites
6. Anorexia and vomiting may also be present

Treatment

The treatment of congestive heart failure includes rest, restriction of salt and fluid intake and administration of drugs such as diuretics and digitalis.

Dental Considerations

Dental surgeon should watch for early signs of congestive heart failure like cyanosis and ankle edema in patients before carrying out dental treatment. Patients with no risk of developing cardiac decompensation may undergo any dental procedure. Patients more prone to congestive heart failure require consultation between dental surgeon and patient's physician/cardiologist before carrying out the dental procedure.

CARDIAC ARRHYTHMIA

Cardiac arrhythmia refers to abnormality in the pulse rate or abnormal rhythm of the heart. Precipitating factors of cardiac arrhythmia are stress and anxiety. Arrhythmia may lead to myocardial infarction, angina, pulmonary edema and congestive heart failure.

Treatment

Some arrhythmias can be treated by mild sedatives. Serious or life-threatening dysrhythmias require antiarrhythmic drugs such as propranolol, verapamil, quinidine, procainamide or lidocaine. Severe arrhythmias can be corrected by implantation of cardiac pacemaker.

Dental Considerations

The dental treatment of patient with abnormal pulse rate should be carried out after consultation with the patient's physician. Beta-blocker can be administered prophylactically to inhibit the effect of epinephrine in local anesthetic agent or LA without adrenaline should be used. If patient loses consciousness due to decreased heart rate, vigorous thumping on the precordium may help in the situation. Dental surgeon dealing with a patient with cardiac pacemaker should consult the patient's cardiologist before starting the treatment.

RHEUMATIC FEVER AND RHEUMATIC HEART DISEASE

Rheumatic fever is a disease of childhood that mostly occurs between six to sixteen years of age. It is caused by group A beta hemolytic streptococcal infection. This infection causes lesions in the joints, heart, nervous system and subcutaneous tissues.

Clinical Features

Rheumatic fever comes on one to three weeks after the streptococcal infection. The initial symptoms of rheumatic fever are acute carditis, rheumatic arthritis and subcutaneous nodules. The patient complains of sore throat and 100 to 102° F body temperature. Erythematous skin eruption known as erythema marginatum is commonly present.

Rheumatic arthritis is characterised by red, tender and painful joints. Small, painless subcutaneous nodules are present on extensor surface of wrists and ankles. Rheumatic fever leads to permanent cardiac lesions in 25 to 50% of the patients and in majority of the cases mitral valve is affected.

Diagnosis

Diagnosis of rheumatic fever is made on the basis of clinical presentation and laboratory investigations. Diagnosis can be made with the help of "Jones criteria for diagnosis of Rheumatic fever" which include five major and four minor criteria.

Major criteria
a. Carditis
b. Arthritis
c. Erythema marginatum
d. Chorea
e. Subcutaneous nodules

Minor criteria
a. Fever
b. Arthralgia
c. Increased erythrocyte sedimentation rate
d. Prolonged PR interval in ECG

Presence of two major or one major and two minor criteria with positive throat culture for group A streptococcus provides sufficient evidence for the diagnosis of rheumatic fever.

Treatment

Treatment of rheumatic fever consists of bed rest, sedation, non-steroid anti-inflammatory drugs and corticosteroids.

Prevention

Patients who have suffered from rheumatic fever have 50% chances of its recurrence so they should take antibiotic prophylaxis until 20 to 30 years of age which includes 1.2 million units of benzathine penicillin injection intramuscularly once in a month. Before oral surgery patient with rheumatic heart disease should be given amoxicillin or any other suitable antibiotic.

CONGENITAL HEART DISEASE

The incidence of congenital heart diseases is approximately 0.5% of live births. The common anomalies of heart are pulmonary stenosis, artrial and ventricular septal defects, coarctation of the aorta, right ventricular hypertrophy and persistent ductus arteriosus.

Coarctation of Aorta

Coarctation of the aorta is characterized by narrowing of the aortic arch distal to origin of the left subclavian artery. Due to this abnormality, the blood pressure in the head and upper extremities is higher than that in lower extremities. The presenting symptoms are cardiac symptoms, arterial pulsations of neck, weakness or cramps of the legs and headache. There may be development of cerebral aneurysms with hemorrhage.

Oral Manifestations

The increased blood pressure in head and neck region may cause enlargement of the mandibular arteries and its branches supplying the individual teeth. Pulp may become congested and highly vascular that occupies a maximum portion of the crown and root in patients with coarctation of the aorta.

Tetralogy of Fallot

Tetralogy of fallot is a congenital heart defect that includes ventricular septal defect, pulmonary stenosis, dextroposition of aorta and right ventricular hypertrophy. Oral manifestations are cyanosis of the oral mucosa, fissured and edematous tongue, marginal gingivitis and delayed eruption of deciduous and permanent teeth.

INFECTIVE ENDOCARDITIS [SUBACUTE BACTERIAL ENDOCARDITIS (SABE)]

Infective endocarditis is a bacterial disease that involves heart valve or the endothelial surface of the heart. Endocarditis of dental origin is caused by bacteria of low virulence that subacutely affect a previously damaged endocardium resulting in sub-acute bacterial endocarditis. It is most common in patients with rheumatic or congenital heart diseases and vascular defects.

Infective endocarditis has dental significance because the oral microorganisms get released into the blood stream during dental surgical procedure which can cause endocarditis.

Clinical Features

The presenting symptoms are low-grade fever, loss of weight, weakness, dyspnea, anorexia and muscular and joint pain. Petechial hemorrhage in oral mucosa and conjunctiva may occur in 20 to 40% of the patients. Release of infectious emboli of vegetative lesions present on cardiac valves may occur and these may get lodged in organs such as brain, kidney, lungs and spleen.

Diagnosis

Subacute bacterial endocarditis is suspected in patients with valvular heart disease, fever for more than one week, anemia and embolic phenomenon. The diagnosis is confirmed by positive blood culture report and echo-cardiography that detect the presence of valvular vegetations.

Treatment

The patients of endocarditis can be treated by administration of following medicines (a) 2 million units of penicillin G intravenously every four hours for four weeks. (b) ampicillin, Dose–0.25 to 2 gm oral/i.m./i.v. every 6 hours, Children (c) Amoxicillin, Dose–0.25 to 1gm TDS oral (d) Cloxacillin Dose–0.25 to 0.5 gm orally every 6 hours; for severe infections 0.25 to 1gm injection IM or IV (e) Cephalosporins. Surgery can be carried out in those patients with fungal endocarditis, who do not respond to medications.

Prevention

Patients should be asked about a history of valvular defects, rheumatic fever, a heart murmur or mitral valve prolapse. If history of endocarditis is known to be present, all the dental surgical procedures should be carried out under prophylactic antibiotic therapy.

Cardiac Conditions in which Endocarditis Prophylaxis is Recommended are as follows:

a. Previous bacterial endocarditis
b. Rheumatic heart disease with valvular involvement
c. Prosthetic heart valves
d. Congenital cardiac diseases
e. Surgically constructed systemic pulmonary shunt

Dental Procedures in which Endocarditis Prophylaxis is Recommended are as follows:

a. Dental procedures that may induce gingival or mucosal bleeding
b. Incision and drainage of infected tissue
c. Surgical procedures involving maxillary sinus or respiratory mucosa
d. Intraligamentary infections

The following prophylactic regimen is usually recommended.

Adults: Amoxicillin 3 gm orally one hour before dental procedure and 1.5 gm six hours after initial dose.

Children: Amoxicillin 50 mg/kg body weight one hour before dental procedure and 25 mg/kg body weight six hours after the initial dose or ampicillin or cloxacillin or cephalosporin.

Patients allergic to amoxicillin and above drugs: Patients who are allergic to amoxicillin and above drugs are given erythromycin stearate 1 gm or erythromycin ethylsuccinate 800 mg orally two hours before dental procedure, then half the dose six hours after initial dose.

CAVERNOUS SINUS THROMBOSIS

It is a condition characterized by formation of thrombus in the cavernous sinus and its communicating branches. Infections from the upper lip, face and nasal cavity reach the cavernous sinus through the angular veins, which may give rise to cavernous sinus thrombosis.

Clinical Features

The cavernous sinus thrombosis may lead to edema, exophthalmos and ecchymosis of the eyelids and sclerae, papilledema and edema of conjunctiva. Other symptoms are headache, vomiting and paralysis of external ocular muscles.

Dental Considerations

The majority of cases of cavernous sinus are of dental origin arising from infections in the third molar region. Infection may also reach from other teeth or the surrounding tissues through the pterygoid plexus and emissary veins.

Acute infections in the molar region should be carefully treated to prevent cavernous thrombosis. Prophylactic antibiotic therapy should be prescribed before carrying out any surgical procedure in the areas of face draining into the veins that communicate with cavernous sinus.

PERMANENT PACEMAKERS

Permanent pacemakers are used in various cardiac diseases. These diseases include the following:
1. Heart failure
2. Symptomatic heart block and bradycardia
3. Brady-tacky syndrome
4. Carotid hypersensitivity
5. Neurocardiogenic syncope
6. Hypertrophic cardiomyopathy

Dental surgeon should not use any electrical or battery operated devices inside the body of patient in which pace maker or metallic implants has been fitted. Before undertaking any treatment for cardiac patient cardiologist of the patient should be consulted.

BIBLIOGRAPHY

1. American Heart Association. 2001 Hear and stroke statistical update. Dallas (TX): American Heart Association 2000.
2. Ardekian L, Gaspar R, Peled M, et al. Dose aspirin therapy complicate oral surgery procedures. J Am Med Assoc 2000;131:331.
3. Cambell JH, Alvarado F, Murray RA. Anticoagulation and minor oral surgery: Should be anticoagulation regimen be altered? J Oral Maxillofac Surg 2000;58:131.
4. Demystifying Medical Complexities. Wahl, MJ (Christiana care Health Services, Wilmington, Del). Calif Dent Assoc J 2000;28: 510-18.
5. Glick M. Screening for risk factors for cardiovascular disease: A review for oral health care providers. J Am Dent Assoc 2002;133: 291-300.
6. Hyman DJ, Pavlik VN. Characteristics of patients with uncontrolled hypertension in the United States. N Engl J Med 2001;345:479.
7. Izzo JL, Levy D, BlackHR. Importance of systolic blood pressure in older Americans. Hypertension 2000;35:1021.
8. Lip GYH. Target organ damage and the prothrombotic state in hypertension. Hypertension 2000;36:975.
9. Periodontal Disease and coronary Heart Disease Risk. Hujoel PP, Drangsholt M, Spiekerman C, et al. JAMA 2000;284:1406-10.
10. Roberts HW, Mitnitsky EF. Cardiac risk stratification for postmyocardial infarction dental patients. Oral Surg Oral Med Oral Pathol Oral Radiol Endod 2001;91:676.
11. Sun P, Dwyer KM, Merz C, et al. Blood pressure, LDL cholesterol, and intima-media thickness. A test of the "response to injury" hypothesis of atherosclerosis. Arterioscler Thromb Vasc Biol 2000; 20-2005.
12. Suwaidi JA, Hamasaki S, Higano ST, et al. Long-term follow up of patients with mild coronary artery disease and endothelial dysfunction. Circulation 2000;101:948.
13. The third report of the National Cholesterol Education Program (NCEP) Expert Panel on Detection, Evaluation, and Treatment of High Blood Cholesterol in Adults (Adult Treatment Panel III). Bethesda (MD): NCEP/ National Heart, Lung and Blood Institute/ National Institutes of Health 2001.
14. Todd DW, Roman A. Outpatient use of low-molecular weight heparin in an anticoagulated patient requiring oral surgery: Case report, J Oral Maxillofac Surg 2001;59:1090.
15. Vasan RS, Larson MG, Kannel WB, Levy D. Evolution of hypertension from non-hypertensive blood pressure levels: Rates of progression in the Framingham Heart Study. J Am Coll Cardiol 2000;35:292A.

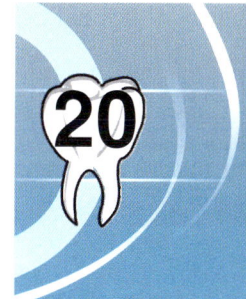

Diseases of Respiratory System Related to Oral Medicine

Respiratory infections are usually seen in dental patients. Anatomic proximity of respiratory system and almost common medicaments interplay between oral and respiratory infections. There is a direct association between oral and respiratory pathogens.

INFECTIONS OF UPPER RESPIRATORY TRACT

Acute Rhinitis

It is an acute infection of upper respiratory tract caused by viruses. It is also called as 'common cold'. The viruses responsible for acute rhinitis are rhinovirus, respiratory syncytial virus, coxsackievirus and para influenza viruses. Rhinoviruses are usually transmitted by respiratory droplets and close person-to-person contact. The infection spreads from one person to another through aerosol droplets. The incubation period is of 2 to 5 days. During winter season infection by these viruses is quite common.

Clinical Features

The common symptoms of acute rhinitis are sneezing, secretion from nose, nasal obstruction and sore throat. Few patients may also complain of headache, cough and fever. Two or three days after the onset of disease, the nasal secretions becomes thicker and purulent. Complications of common cold are sinusitis and lower respiratory tract infections.

Effect on oral health: Small round erythematous macular lesion may appear on the soft palate. These macules may be due to virus infection or a response of lymphoid tissue. There may be enlargement of lymphoid tissue specially at the lateral borders of the base of the tongue.

Treatment

Treatment of common cold includes administration of antihistamines and sympathomimetic amines. Antihistamines help in decreasing nasal secretions. Sympathomimetic amines can be given topically or systemically to relieve nasal congestion. Non-steroidal anti-inflammatory drugs are used to manage pain and pyrexia. Oral decongestants relieve congestion. Antihistaminics and decongestants create oral dryness. Long term use of corticosteroid sprays promote growth of oral candidiasis.

Pharyngitis and Tonsillitis

Pharyngitis and tonsillitis refer to infection of the mucosa and lymphoid tissue in the pharynx and tonsils respectively. The microorganisms responsible for pharyngitis and tonsillitis are parainfluenza virus, rhinovirus, coxsackie virus, Herpes-simplex virus and Epstein-barr virus. Bacteria such as Streptococcus pyogenes may also sometimes be the etiologic agent.

Clinical Features

Sore throat and difficulty in swallowing are the common symptoms of pharyngitis. If the etiological agent is virus, symptoms of common cold may also be present. Complication of acute tonsillitis is peritonsillar abscess which is characterized by painful enlargement of tonsils and dysphagia. The infection may also extend to deeper structures of neck resulting in erosion of large arteries.

Treatment

Pharyngitis and tonsillitis caused by virus are treated by analgesics, decongestants and antihistaminics. If the disease is of bacterial origin, treatment includes administration of penicillin or erythromycin (in patients allergic to penicillin). Oral cephalosporins also give good results.

Sinusitis

Sinusitis is an inflammation of the mucosa of the paranasal sinuses. It is caused by bacterial or viral infection and often occurs as a complication of acute rhinitis. The maxillary sinus is mostly involved. The organisms commonly involved are *Staphylococcus aureus*, *Streptococcus pneumoniae*, *Streptococcus pyogenes* and *Haemophilus influenza*.

Sinusitis may be categorized as follows:
a. Acute sinusitis-few days to three weeks duration
b. Subacute sinusitis- three weeks to three months duration
c. Chronic sinusitis- more than three months duration

Clinical Features

The common symptoms of acute sinusitis are headache, increased temperature, malaise, pain in the region of involved sinus and edema and redness beneath the eyes. Patient may get referred pain in the maxillary posterior teeth. The patient with chronic sinusitis may experience headache in the morning which gradually disappears afterwards due to drainage of the sinuses in upright position. Physical examination will reveal sinus tenderness and purulent nasal discharge. The nasal mucosa appear edematous and erythematous.

Treatment

The initial step in the management of sinusitis is administration of antibiotics. Amoxycillin is the drug of choice or if the patient is allergic, erythromycin or cephalosporin can be prescribed. Sympathomimetic drug should be used to provide drainage from maxillary sinus. In case the patient is not responding to antibiotic therapy, he or she should be referred to otolaryngologist for drainage of the sinus by surgical methods. Corticosteroid nasal drops may be used for few days.

Dental Considerations

The roots of maxillary premolars and molars are situated very close to maxillary sinus. Abscesses of the maxillary premolar and molar may sometimes open into the maxillary sinus which give rise to maxillary sinusitis. The maxillary teeth in close proximity to the infected sinus may feel elongated, painful and sensitive to percussion. Due to maxillary sinusitis there may be feeling of dull pain in the maxillary premolars and molars or vice versa which will disappear after treating the etiological factor; which may be maxillary sinusitis or pulpal and periapical or/and periodontal infection in the teeth. Very often symptoms of maxillary sinusitis disappear after root canal treatment of the affected maxillary posterior teeth. Dull pain of maxillary posterior teeth disappear by treating maxillary sinusitis. For correct diagnosis radiography with different angles and CT are important.

Laryngitis

Laryngitis refers to inflammation of the mucous membrane of the larynx. Laryngitis may be classified as follows.

Acute Laryngitis

Acute laryngitis occurs due to excessive use of vocal cords, irritation due to excessive smoking or as a complication of acute rhinitis and other inflammation of nose and throat.

Chronic Laryngitis

Chronic laryngitis occurs as a result of carcinoma of larynx and rarely in syphilis or tuberculosis.

Clinical features: Hoarseness of voice is a common feature in laryngitis. The throat becomes dry and sore. In acute laryngitis the symptoms usually subside with resting of the voice. In chronic laryngitis hoarseness may extend for months. The patient may experience pain and difficulty in swallowing in tuberculous laryngitis.

Management: Mild laryngitis is selflimiting with rest to larynx within 3 to 7 days without any medicine. In severe and prolonged laryngitis short course of oral corticosteroid hasten recovery.

DISEASES OF LOWER RESPIRATORY TRACT

Chronic Obstructive Pulmonary Diseases

Chronic obstructive pulmonary disease is a condition characterized by difficulty in breathing caused by obstruction of air flow due to chronic bronchitis or emphysema

Chronic Bronchitis

Chronic bronchitis is characterized by cough and hypersecretion of mucus. Chronic bronchitis is diagnosed if productive cough is present for at least three months in a year during two consecutive years. Patient may also experience dyspnea on slight exertion. Chronic bronchitis is mostly caused by smoking. Inhalation of air contaminated by dust or noxious gases of combustion and recurrent infections may also be the etiological agents.

Emphysema

Emphysema refers to distension of the alveolar spaces due to presence of air. Clinical manifestation is breathlessness on exertion due to combined effect of reduction of alveolar surfaces for gas exchange and collapse of smaller airways. Emphysema is usually the result of chronic bronchitis.

Clinical features: The main clinical features of chronic obstructive pulmonary disease are mucus producing cough, wheezing and dyspnea on exertion. These symptoms may become severe in upper respiratory tract infections. Sometimes patient only complains of dyspnea without cough or wheezing if he/she exhibits emphysematous changes prior to chronic bronchitis.

Treatment: The management of chronic obstructive pulmonary disease includes the following:
a. Patient should stop smoking and wear face mask to protect against air pollution and occupational inhalants. Dental surgeon and auxillaries must use face masks specially when trimming acrylic appliances.
b. Bronchospasm which is common in chronic obstructive pulmonary disease can be relieved by administration of bronchodilators such as beta-adrenergic agonists or an anticholinergic agent.
c. If infection of upper respiratory tract is also present, antibiotic therapy should be prescribed.

Dental considerations: Patients with chronic obstructive pulmonary disease have difficulty in breathing. So, before carrying out any dental procedure in which there is need of rubber dam which partially obstructs the oral airway, the dental surgeon should make sure that the nasal passage are capable of supplying the patient's respiratory needs.

Inhalation analgesics or anesthetics should be given in supervision of anaesthesiologist.

Asthma

It is an inflammatory disease of lungs characterized by reversible airway obstruction. There is narrowing of the bronchial airways due to smooth muscle spasm, mucosal edema and excessive mucus in the lumen of the airways.

Etiology

The etiological factors for asthma are as follows:
a. The attack of asthma is mostly induced by airborne allergens such as dust, mites, pollens, animal oral and nasal discharge and cockroach antigens.
b. Inhaled irritants such as cigarette smoke and cold air are also the etiological agents for asthmatic attack. The most common and serious ingested allergen is aspirin.
c. Respiratory infections usually of viral origin may stimulate asthmatic attack.
d. Some patients may have asthmatic attack after physical exercise.
e. Emotional states such as anxiety and nervousness may also be the inciting factor in asthma patient.

Clinical Features

Wheezing, coughing and dyspnoea are the common symptoms in asthmatic attack. In severe cases there may be tachycardia and central cyanosis.

Treatment

The following treatment modalities are followed in the management of asthma.
a. The first line of treatment includes use of bronchodilator such as beta-adrenergic agonist.
b. Inhaled corticosteroids such as betamethasone or triamcinolone alone or in combination with inhaled bronchodilators are also prescribed.
c. Other drugs administered are theophylline preparations, tranquilizers and systemic corticosteroids.
d. In acute asthmatic attack, emergency treatment includes inhalation of salbutamol or terbutaline and infection of aminophylline intravenously.
e. Avoidance of allergens, irritants and other known triggers is essential for control of asthma.

Dental Considerations

Specially when attending an asthmatic patients keep all emergency drugs handy. Usually asthmatic patients are allergic to many drugs and materials. Any time asthmatic attack can take place. The following are the guidelines for dental treatment of asthmatic patients.
a. In all asthmatic patients history should be taken carefully about allergy. Medicines and materials likely to create allergy must be avoided. Even doubtful medicines and materials should also be avoided.
b. The dental materials which may precipitate an attack must be avoided. For example dental materials without methyl methacrylate must be used. If acrylic appliances are must they must be completely cured before insertion in the oral cavity. Only heat cured acrylic should be used.
c. To reduce the risk of an asthmatic attack such patient should be given appointment in the late forenoon or afternoon.
d. Stress reducing techniques like conscious sedation should be used. Conscious sedation should be done with hydroxyzine to avoid bronchoconstrictions.

e. Medicaments causing bronchospasm and reduce respiratory functions such as barbiturate and narcotics should be avoided.
f. Asthmatic patients should bring their beta-adrenergic inhaler with them to the dental clinic. Every time mouth should be rinsed after using inhaler.
g. Inhalation anesthetics or analgesics should be avoided in asthmatic patients as they can stimulate asthmatic attack.
h. Emergency drugs to control acute asthmatic attack should be available in dental clinic.
i. Use of inhalational corticosteroids can cause oral and pharyngeal candidiasis hence precautions should be taken like use of antifungal medicines.
j. Fluoride supplements should be given to all asthmatic patients specially those using β_2 (Beta two) agonists.
k. In the patients having severe asthma methyl methacrylate should be avoided as it may cause an attack.
l. All those materials and drugs which may precipitate an attack must be avoided.
m. Sodium metasulfite used as a preservative in LA may precipitate an attack in asthmatic patients hence such LA solution should be avoided.
n. Suction tips should be placed in such a way so as to avoid to elicit cough reflex.
o. Rubber dam should be placed in such a way so that it does not cause any hinderance or difficulty in comfortable breathing.
p. Keep oxygen and other emergency drugs and bronchodilator handy in case of an attack.
q. Good oral hygiene must be maintained to prevent gingivitis and periodontitis.

Management of an acute asthmatic attack: If an asthmatic attack takes place to an asthmatic patient in the dental clinic following steps should be taken.
a. Stop all dental procedures
b. Remove all intra oral devices.
c. Make sure the airway is open and place the patient in a relaxed and comfortable position.
d. Administer oxygen and β_2-agonist.
e. If the condition do not improve, inject subcutaneously epinephrine (1:1000 concentration, 0.01mg/kg of body weight, up to a maximum of 0.3 mg)
f. If the condition do not improve call for medical emergency assistance and the physician of the patient.

Pneumonia

Pneumonia or pneumonitis refers to inflammation of the lung parenchyma. The majority of cases of pneumonia are caused by virus.

Bacteria, fungi and protozoa may also cause pneumonia.

Clinical Features

Pneumonia of viral and mycoplasmal origin exhibits mild symptoms such as cough with or without production of sputum, mild fever and difficulty in breathing. Fever, cough with purulent sputum and pleuritic chest pain are the features of bacterial pneumonia.

Treatment

a. Pneumonia of mycoplasmal origin can be treated by erythromycin and tetracycline.
b. Viral pneumonia is managed by supportive treatment.
c. Bacterial pneumonia is treated by antibiotic therapy.

Tuberculosis

Tuberculosis is an infectious disease of lungs caused mainly by *Mycobacterium tuberculi*. Other mycobacterium species that may cause tuberculosis are *M. avium* and *M. intercellulare*. Pulmonary tuberculosis is mostly transmitted from infected individual to others by inhalation of air droplets of sputum less than 8 micron in diameter. Tuberculosis is also called as 'acid fast infection'. Scrofula refers to tuberculous involvement of cervical lymph nodes.

Clinical Features

a. Weight loss
b. Chronic cough
c. Evening rise in temperature
d. Fatigue
e. Anorexia
f. Hemoptysis
g. Night sweats

Treatment

The treatment of tuberculosis includes:
a. Rest and good nutrition
b. Antitubercular drug therapy which consists of four drugs-Isoniazid, rifampicin, pyrazinamide in combination with either ethambutol or streptomycin.

Oral Manifestation

Oral lesions in tuberculosis are relatively rare and are seen in patients with advanced disease. Oral tuberculosis lesions may result from contact of infected sputum with oral tissues subjected to chronic irritation or inflammatory response. Oral lesions that may be seen in tuberculosis are as follows:

a. Small tubercles or nodules on the lips especially at corners of mouth that breakdown to form ulcers.
b. Painful ulcers on palate, check and lateral margin of tongue
c. Deep central ulcers occur on dorsum of the tongue with thick mucous material in base of ulcers.
d. Tuberculosis may also involve salivary glands, periapical dental granuloma and may result in tuberculous periostitis.

Treatment of Oral Lesions

All sources of irritation of mucosa and tongue should be eliminated. Oral lesions should be managed by local palliative therapy along with systemic treatment of tuberculosis. Good oral hygiene should be maintained.

Dental Considerations

As pulmonary tuberculosis is mostly spread by aerosolized droplets, dental surgeon may get infected by inhaling infectious droplets from dental patient suffering from tuberculosis. If a patient with past history of tuberculosis seeks any dental treatment, dental surgeon (after providing emergency treatment) should contact patient's physician to ensure that patient had taken full course of antitubercular therapy.

Though infected patient becomes non-infectious after two to three weeks of antitubercular therapy, dental treatment, except emergency treatment, should be carried out when the sputum culture is negative (usually in three months). Infection control measures such as mask, gloves, glasses and gowns should always be used. Use of ultrasonic scalers and high speed handpiece should be minimized to avoid aerosolization.

OTHER RESPIRATORY DISEASES

Sarcoidosis

Sarcoidosis is a granulomatous disease of unknown etiology, especially involving the lungs with resulting interstitial fibrosis. It leads to bilateral pulmonary hilar adenopathy and pulmonary infiltration.

Clinical Features

The predominating symptoms of sarcoidosis are fever, weight loss and fatigue. In some cases disease is asymptomatic which is detected on routine chest radiograph by the presence of hilar adenopathy.

Oral Manifestations

Oral lesions in sarcoidosis consist of painless submucosal nodules with a normal overlying mucosa. Intraosseous lesions in maxilla or the mandible may also be present.

Treatment

Treatment of sarcoidosis includes administration of corticosteroids. Oral lesions are managed by high doses of corticosteroids several times a day in the beginning which is gradually decreased over a period of weeks to a maintenance dose of once a day.

Wegener's Granulomatosis

It is a granulomatous disease of blood vessels resulting in necrosis of tissue. It initially involves the nose and the paranasal sinuses gradually extending to lower respiratory tract, joints, kidneys and nervous system. The disease affects the individuals of forty-five to sixty years of age.

Clinical Features

The predominating symptoms of Wegener's granulomatosis are nasal stuffiness with chronic discharge which may be tinged with blood.

Oral Manifestations

Oral structures such as tongue, gingiva, palate and oropharynx are commonly involved in Wegener's granulomatosis. There is swelling, inflammation and ulceration of the involved oral tissues. The inflammation begins in the interdental papilla which spreads into the remaining gingiva and periodontium. The gingiva become enlarged with petechial hemorrhage and appears granular. There may be alveolar bone loss with tooth mobility.

Treatment

Wegener's granulomatosis is treated by administration of cyclophosphamide-prednisone combination. The drug therapy is continued for one year after complete subsidence of symptoms. Patients unable to tolerate cyclophosphamide can be prescribed azathioprine.

Midline Granuloma

Midline granuloma is a chronic progressive destructive disease affecting the midline structures of the face. It is of unknown etiology. The disease mostly occurs in males of 20 to 50 years of age.

Clinical Features

The early symptoms of midline granuloma are nasal blockage and discharge. With the advancement of the disease skin of the nose and maxillary area is involved which leads to progressive loss of facial tissue.

Oral Manifestations

There is localized destruction of tissue in the midline of the face which leads to perforation of the hard and soft palate and other structures in close proximity to the midline of the nose. Few patients may exhibit oral mucosal, gingival or palatal ulcerations.

Treatment

Radiation therapy is the treatment of choice for midline granuloma. Secondary infections can be controlled by antibiotic therapy.

Cystic Fibrosis

Cystic fibrosis or mucoviscidosis is an autosomal recessive inherited disorder of mucus producing exocrine glands. The disease prominently affects the lungs and pancreas.

Clinical Features

The typical feature of cystic fibrosis is increased viscosity of the mucus. In pancreatic involvement, the pancreatic and bile ducts get blocked resulting in deficiency of pancreatic enzymes. Symptoms usually appear in childhood and include poor growth despite good appetite, but due to malabsorption and large frequent stools.

Pulmonary involvement consists of obstruction of bronchioles due to mucous plugs which may result in chronic bronchitis, bronchiectasis and respiratory infection. Symptoms are cough and rapid breathing.

Treatment

The treatment of cystic fibrosis includes the following:
a. Addition of pancreatic extract to the diet to correct pancreatic deficiency
b. Use of nebulizers with agents to decrease viscosity of pulmonary secretions.
c. The chronic lung disease can be treated by antibiotic therapy. The drugs commonly used is tetracycline and other broad spectrum antibiotics.

Oral Manifestations

Tetracycline staining of teeth is commonly seen in patients of cystic fibrosis. Patient may manifest hypoplasia or hypomineralization of the enamel, but there is low incidence of dental caries.

Severe Acute Respiratory Syndrome (SARS)

Severe acute respiratory syndrome is a highly infectious atypical pneumonia. It was first reported in the patients in North America, Europe and Asia. According to World Health Organization on April 18, 2003; 3461 cases and 170 deaths from SARS has been reported from 25 countries.

Etiological Agent

The disease is caused by unrecognized strain of coronavirus. The known viruses of this family generally cause cold and cough.

Mode of Transmission

The SARS usually spreads through droplet or air transmission. It may also get transmitted through contaminated objects or insects such as cockroach.

Clinical Features

The presenting symptoms are cough, shortness of breath, hypoxia and fever greater than 100.5 $^\circ$F. Radiographic examination reveals findings of pneumonia. The incubation period for SARS is 2 to 7 days.

Identifying SARS Patient in Dental Clinic

If the dental surgeon encounters a patient who presents with above mentioned symptoms of respiratory illness that is of unknown etiology and radiographic findings of pneumonia, he may suspect of having SARS in his/her patient. The dental surgeon should immediately send the patient to a hospital for diagnosis and proper care.

Preventive Measures

The preventive measures for SARS in dental clinic should include the following:
a. Dental staff should be educated about SARS specific infection control and identifying the case of SARS.
b. Strict infection control measures should be taken. Dental clinic should be disinfected by hospital grade disinfectant or 1:100 dilution of household bleach.
c. Dental clinic should have good ventilation.
d. Dental surgeon and auxiliaries should adopt barrier techniques which should include chin length plastic face shields, disposable gloves, surgical masks and gowns.
e. While taking patient's medical history, dental surgeon should ask about fever or recent onset of respiratory problem.

BIBLIOGRAPHY

1. Bryan CS. Blood cultures for community-acquired pneumonia. No place to skimp. Chest 1999;116:1153.
2. Cross JT Jr, Campbell GD Jr. Drug-resistant pathogens in community- and hospital—acquired pneumonia. Clin Chest Med 1999;20:499.
3. Ewig S. Community-acquired pneumonia. Definition, epidemiology, and outcome. Semin Respir Infect 1999;14:94.
4. Macfarlane J. Lower respiratory tract infection and pneumonia in the community. Semin Respir Infect 1999;14:151.
5. Mygind N, Gwaltney JM Jr. Winther B, Hendley JO. The common cold and asthma. Allergy 1999;54 Suppl, 57:146.
6. Peebles RS Jr. Hartert TV. Respiratory viruses and asthma Curr Opin Pulm Med 2000;6:10.
7. Pozzi E. Community-acquired pneumonia. The ORIONE Board. Monaldi Arch Chest Dis 1999;54:337.
8. Ramilo O. Role of respiratory viruses in acute otitis media. Implications for management. Pediatr Infect Dis J 1999;18;1125.
9. Scannapieco FA. Role of oral bacteria in respiratory infection. J Periodontal 1999;70:793.
10. Schneider LC, Lester RM. Atopic diseases and upper respiratory infections. Curr Opin Pediatr 1999;11:475.
11. Shanker S, Vig KWL, Beck FM, et al. Dentofacial morphology amd upper respiratory function in 8-10 year-old children. Clin Orthod Res 1999;2:19.
12. Temte JL, Shult PA, Kirk CJ, Amspaugh J. Effects of viral respiratory disease education and surveillance on antibiotic prescribing. Fam Med 1999;31:101.
13. Van Kempen M, Bachert C, Van Gauwenberge P. An update on the pathophysiology of rhinovirus upper respiratory tract infections Rhinology 1999;37:97.

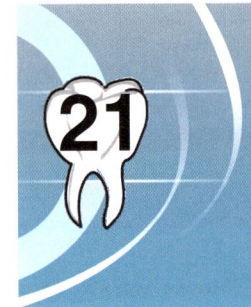

Gastrointestinal Diseases Related to Oral Medicine

Dental surgeons are responsible for diagnosis of oral manifestations of gastrointestinal (GI) diseases, risk of infection, homeostasis, actions and interactions of the drugs and when required proper medical referral. A comprehensive knowledge of working of GI system is essential. Digestive system consists of esophagus, stomach, small intestine and large intestine. Each of these parts perform specific functions. Besides these exocrine functions of the liver, pancreas and gallbladder complete the assimilation of dietary calories and nutrients.

ESOPHAGEAL DISEASES

Dysphagia

Dysphagia or difficulty in swallowing may occur either due to mechanical obstruction in the esophagus or due to disorders of the nervous system. Mechanical obstruction of the esophagus can be seen in obstructing tumors, enlargement of paraesophageal lymph nodes and obstruction by a foreign body.

In neurologic disorders, coordinated reflex contraction of muscles necessary for normal swallowing fails to take place due to which patient is unable to swallow liquids and solids. Diseases associated with neurologic disorders are myasthenia gravis, sarcoidosis, poliomyelitis, myotonic dystrophy, multiple sclerosis and scleroderma.

Esophageal Ulcers

Esophageal ulcers may occur due to swallowing of the tablet or capsules without adequate amount of liquid, especially at bed time. These ulcers are also associated with tetracycline and other antibiotic therapy. The patient manifests severe retrosternal burning pain.

Dental Considerations

The patient with above esophageal diseases may seek help from the dental surgeon for the problem of dysphagia. Dental surgeon should take precautions to prevent the patient's aspirating material during dental procedure. Patients on tetracycline therapy complaining of retrosternal burning should substitute another antibiotic. Patient should be instructed to swallow tablets or capsules with adequate amount of liquid.

PEPTIC ULCERS

The peptic ulcers in the gastrointestinal tract are most frequently caused by infections with *Helicobacter pylori* and use of non-steroidal anti-inflammatory drugs. Stress, smoking, hypoglycemia, foods such as coffee and alcohol are the contributing factors for peptic ulcerations in the presence of gastric *H. pylori* infection or use of NSAID. Peptic ulcers involve lower part of esophagus, stomach and duodenum.

Duodenal Ulcers

Duodenal ulcers account for 80 to 85% of all peptic ulcers and are most commonly seen in males. The primary cause for duodenal ulcer is *Helicobacter pylori* infection. Other factors responsible for duodenal ulcers are stress, parathyroid disease, cirrhosis, gastrinoma of the pancreas, polycythemia vera and steroid therapy. Ulcers are usually seen in the first part of the duodenum.

Clinical Features

The presenting symptom is epigastric pain that occurs either before eating or few hours after eating. The pain is described as burning and is sometimes associated with nausea and vomiting. The pain is generally relieved by food intake. Large ulcers may erode an artery leading to gastrointestinal bleeding which is manifested by black-colored stools.

Treatment

Treatment of duodenal ulcers includes the following:
a. Avoidance of food that causes discomfort to the patient.

b. Use of alcohol, tobacco and drugs such as aspirin should be stopped.
c. Administration of metronidazole with amoxycillin or tetracycline to eliminate *H. Pylori* infection
d. Other drugs prescribed are sedatives to reduce stress, anticholinergic drugs, H$_2$ histamine receptor blockers and omeprazole to decrease acid production, and antacids to neutralize the excess acid present in the stomach.

Dental Considerations

Patients with gastric reflex disease complain of dysgeusia (foul taste), dental sensitivity, erosion with or without pulpal involvement.

Dental sensitivity is usually due to erosion of enamel by gastric acid.
a. Dental surgeon should avoid administration of non-steroidal anti-inflammatory drugs in patients with the history of peptic ulcerations, as these drugs may aggravate ulcerations.
b. Anticholinergic drugs used to decrease acid production may cause xerostomia which may lead to increased incidence of caries and discomfort in wearing complete dentures.
c. Antacids containing calcium, magnesium and aluminium salts may interfere with absorption of antibiotics, such as erythromycin and tetracycline. So these drugs should be administered one or two hours after antacid therapy.
d. Chronic gastrointestinal bleeding in peptic ulcers may lead to anemia. So patient's hemoglobin concentration should be determined before starting any oral surgical or periodontal procedure in which blood loss takes place.
e. Patients who are in stress and nervous for dental procedure should be sedated before dental treatment, as mental stress is an etiological factor for peptic ulcers.
f. Nausea causing medicaments should be avoided as far as possible because of the increased chances of regurgitation and possible aspiration. Mouth rinses with baking soda (half teaspoon of sodium bicarbonate in ¼ litre water) are helpful in dysgeusia.
g. Atropine used to treat peptic ulcer may lead to xerostomia.

Gastric Ulcers

Gastric ulcers or ulcers of the stomach are mostly seen in males usually above the age of 50 years. Factors responsible for gastric ulcers are same as duodenal ulcers. Peptic ulcerations of the stomach may require surgical treatment if they do not respond to drug therapy. Dental considerations are also same for both patients with gastric ulcers and duodenal ulcers.

DISEASES OF LIVER

Jaundice (Icterus)

Jaundice results from excess of bilirubin in the circulation. Jaundice manifests as yellow discoloration of skin, oral mucous membrane and sclera when the serum bilirubin exceeds 2 to 3 mg/dl. Jaundice may be caused by destruction of red blood cells (Hemolytic jaundice), obstruction of bile duct (obstructive jaundice) or due to hepatic diseases (hepatocellular jaundice).

Jaundice is of dental consideration as it may indicate presence of hepatitis which may be hazardous to dental surgeon and other patients. Presence of liver dysfunction may decrease tolerance to anesthetics and other medications and may also cause severe bleeding after oral surgical or periodontal procedures.

Hepatitis

Etiology

Hepatitis may be caused by following etiological agents.
a. Chemical agents: Phosphorus or carbon tetrachloride and Isoniazid hydrochloride.
b. Collagen disease: Lupus erythematosus
c. Bacterial Infections: Syphilis
d. Viral Infections: Infectious mononucleosis and cytomegalovirus.

Viral hepatitis is caused by the hepatitis A, B, C, D, E and F or Non A, non B viruses.

Clinical Features

The clinical course of disease is characterized by the following three phases.

Prodromal phase: Prodromal symptoms of hepatitis are arthralgia, myalgia, upper respiratory tract infection and general malaise. Some patients may experience nausea, anorexia and high fever.

Icteric phase: In this phase there is appearance of jaundice after which the fever subsides. Splenomegaly, hepatomegaly and lymphadenopathy are also present.

Recovery phase: The initial feature of this phase is disappearance of jaundice. Complete recovery occurs within four months after the onset of jaundice.

Oral Manifestations

Hepatitis manifests itself in oral cavity as icterus of oral mucosa, which is mostly seen on the palate and in sublingual area. Hepatic dysfunction or severe jaundice may lead to severe bleeding after periodontal operation and spontaneous bleeding in oral cavity.

Types of Viral Hepatitis

Hepatitis A: Hepatitis A is an infectious disease, caused by Hepatitis A virus, an enterovirus. It spreads by fecal-oral route, most often through ingestion of contaminated food or water. The incubation period is of 2 to 6 weeks. The disease occurs most frequently before 35 years of age and has an acute onset with high fever.

Treatment: Treatment of hepatitis is usually symptomatic which includes complete bed rest during early weeks of disease. High protein and high carbohydrate diet is recommended. The fatality rate is very low and recovery is complete which takes place in 6 to 8 weeks.

Prevention: People who accidentally had contact with a hepatitis A patient either through fecal-oral route or by infected blood should be given prophylactic gammaglobulin injections.

Hepatitis B: Hepatitis B is a viral disease caused by hepatitis B virus, a DNA virus. It has a long incubation period that varies from two to six months. It is transmitted by percutaneous and non-percutaneous modes. In non-percutaneous modes, virus gets transmitted through body secretions such as saliva, blood and semen.

Percutaneous mode of transmission occurs by small amount of blood through skin with minor-cuts. Hepatitis-B virus infection may lead to cirrhosis, hepatic failure and hepatocellular carcinoma in chronic carriers.

Treatment: Treatment of acute hepatitis B is symptomatic as that for hepatitis A. Chronic hepatitis B is treated by interferon alpha-2b.

Prevention: Individuals exposed to Hepatitis B virus are protected by passive immunity being provided by Hepatitis-B immunoglobulin (HBIG). Vaccination for hepatitis-B is now available which is given in three doses over a period of six months (0,1, 6 months). Vaccination is necessary for all high-risk groups, such as dental surgeons, surgeons, physicians and nurses. Immersion in solution of isopropyl alcohol for 15 minutes is not effective in inactivating Hepatitis B virus.

Hepatitis non-A, non-B (NANB hepatitis): It is caused by hepatitis NANB virus. This type of hepatitis is predominantly seen in transfusion recipients and intravenous drug abusers. It has an incubation period of 60 to 150 days. Hepatitis NANB is less severe and has a shorter clinical course than Hepatitis B. Some patients may develop chronic liver diseases. Treatment is same as for hepatitis A and hepatitis B.

Hepatitis C: Hepatitis C virus is the principal cause of non-A, non-B post transfusion hepatitis. The incubation period is of 6 to 8 weeks. About one-third of the cases of Hepatitis C are associated with intravenous drug abuse. More than half of the cases of Hepatitis C lead to chronic hepatitis, and 20% of these chronic carriers develop cirrhosis and hepatic carcinoma.

Hepatitis D: Hepatitis D is caused by the hepatitis delta virus, a defective RNA virus that requires HBsAg to replicate. The acute Hepatitis D occurs in two following forms:

i. As a coinfection with acute Hepatitis B, which is usually self-limiting.
ii. As a superinfection in chronic hepatitis B carrier.

The infection is primarily transmitted by the parenteral route. The clinical manifestations in hepatitis D are of severe type and occur suddenly. The possibility of chronic liver disease in hepatitis B patient co-infected with hepatitis D is increased by four times. Treatment of hepatitis D is supportive.

Dental considerations: Hepatitis B, C, D, E and F and some types of NANB can be transmitted to dental surgeons and auxiliaries by a blood contaminated needle or instrument from an infected patients. The HBsAg may be present in saliva of patients with acute type-B hepatitis.

Dental surgeon should be able to identify the patients that may transmit the disease. Multiple blood transfusion recipients, percutaneous drug abusers, hemodialysis patients and immuno-suppressed patients have much higher carrier state than the general population.

Universal infection control practice is very important to protect dental surgeons and auxiliaries and patients from hepatitis. Dental instruments should be sterilized by any one of the following suitable method (a) by immersing them in 100°C boiling water for 30 minutes, (b) dry heat at 106°C for one hour (c) by autoclaving by exposure to saturated steam at 121°C and 15 psi pressure for 30 minutes autoclaving is best.

Preventive measures while treating patient with hepatitis: The least amount of infected blood capable of transmitting hepatitis virus is 0.004 ml. Therefore following precautions must be observed.

a. The patient should be treated at the end of the session or day
b. Disposable gloves, masks, gowns and eye glasses should be used.
c. Ultrasonic scalers should not be used.
d. Sharp instruments and needles should be handled properly to prevent minor-cuts.
e. Cavity preparation should be carried out with rubber dam isolation.
f. Dental impressions should be taken with silicon-based impression material. The impression should be immersed in 2% glutaraldehyde or iodophor or 0.5 % Sodium hypochlorite for one hour, washed, and then again soaked in 2% glutaraldehyde for 3 hours before pouring the cast.
g. Non-disposable instruments should be cleaned with detergent before sterilization.
h. External surfaces of the equipment in the dental clinic should be cleaned with sodium hypochlorite solution.

INFLAMMATORY DISEASES OF THE INTESTINE

Chronic inflammatory disease of the intestine occurs in two major forms.

Ulcerative Colitis

It is a chronic inflammatory disease of mucosa and submucosa of the colon. It is characterized by abdominal pain, rectal bleeding and diarrhea. It frequently causes anemia, hypoproteinemia and electrolyte imbalance.

Crohn's Disease

It is an inflammatory disease involving the entire thickness of intestinal wall. It is characterized by patchy deep aphthous like ulcers that may cause fistulas, and narrowing and thickening of the bowel. Symptoms include cramping abdominal pain, fever, diarrhea and weight loss. Crohn's disease usually involves the small intestine.

Treatment

The treatment of chronic inflammatory diseases of intestine includes the following:
a. Drugs such as sulfasalazine, and 5-aminosalicylic acid
b. Corticosteroid therapy (both corticosteroids and ACTH are used).
c. Immunosuppressive therapy (cyclosporine, azathioprine, methotrexate and mercaptopurine)
d. Surgery is required in 15 to 20% of patients with ulcerative colitis and in approximately 40 to 50% of patient's with Crohn's disease.

Oral Manifestations

Crohn's disease of the colon may produce lesions in certain areas of the oral cavity. The appearance of these lesions depends on their location. The lesions may be described as follows:
a. Nodular mass on the buccal mucosa showing cobblestone pattern.
b. Ulcers on the vestibule or palate
c. Lesions on the lips which appear swollen and hardened.
d. Granular erythematous lesions on the gingiva and alveolar mucosa.
e. Aphthous like ulcerations may be present in few patients with Crohn's disease.

Dental Considerations

Medications taken by the patients for the treatment of inflammatory bowel disease may necessitate alteration in the course of dental therapy. Immunosuppressive drugs may produce changes in white and red blood cell counts. Inflammatory bowel diseases may cause anemia due to gastrointestinal bleeding.

Therefore, total and differential white blood cell counts and hemoglobin concentration should be taken before starting any oral surgical procedure. Corticosteroids may lead to hyperglycemia and osteoporosis, which have adverse effects on dental therapy.

BIBLIOGRAPHY

1. Chatoor I. Feeding and eating disorders of infancy and early childhood. In: Kaplan HI, Sadock BJ, (Ed.). Comprehensive textbook of psychiatry. 7th ed. Baltimore (MD): Willimas & Wilkins 2000;2740-10.
2. Fenoglio-Preiser CM, Noffsinger AE, Lantz PE, et al. Gastrointestinal pathology. 2nd ed. Philadelphia: Lippincott-Raven 1999.
3. Ming SC, Goldman H, (Ed.). Pathology of the gastrointestinal tract 2nd ed. Baltimore: Williams and Wilkins 1998.
4. Siegel MA, Jacobson JJ. Inflammatory bowel diseases and the oral cavity. Oral Surg Oral Med Oral Pathol Oral Radiol Endod 1999;87:2-4.
5. Spivak H, Farrell TM, Trus TL, et al. Laparoscopic fundoplication for dysphagia and peptic esophageal stricture. J Gastrointest Surg 1998;2(6):555-60.
6. Yagiela JA, Neidle EA, Dowd FJ. Pharmacology and therapeutics for dentistry. 4th ed. St Louis (MO): Mosby 1998;449-52.

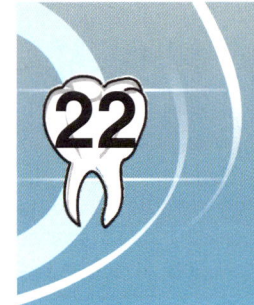

Renal Diseases and Oral Medicine

Renal diseases are one of the major causes of morbidity and mortality in the developed countries. The kidneys are vital organs and maintain a stable internal environment (homeostasis). The important functions of the kidneys are (a) Filtering the blood to regulate the acid-base and fluid electrolytes balances of the body (b) Selective resorption of water and electrolytes (c) Excreting urine (d) Excretion of metabolic waste products including urea, creatinine, uric acid and foreign chemicals.

Important disorders of the kidneys are as follows:

CHRONIC RENAL FAILURE

Chronic renal failure can be caused by number of diseases such as glomerulonephritis, pyelonephritis, diabetes, nephrosclerosis, collagen vascular diseases and polycystic renal diseases.

Glomerulonephritis

Glomerulonephritis is characterized by diffused inflammatory changes in glomeruli, that produce irreversible impairment of function. It may occur as acute glomerulonephritis which is of either streptococcal or non-streptococcal origin.

Chronic glomerulonephritis is of insidious onset or a late sequelae of acute glomerulonephritis. Typical examples are idiopathic membranous glomerulonephritis and membrano-proliferative glomerulonephritis. Glomerulonephritis accounts for 55% of cases of renal failure.

Pyelonephritis

Pyelonephritis is the second most common cause for renal failure. Pyelonephritis refers to inflammation of renal parenchyma and pelvis due to bacterial infection. The most frequent cause of infection is *Escherichia coli*. The disease may occur in acute or chronic form. The clinical features of pyelonephritis are sudden increase in body temperature, pain in costovertebral areas, chills and symptoms of bladder inflammation.

MANIFESTATIONS OF RENAL DISEASES (UREMIC SYNDROME)

In chronic renal failure, number of signs and symptoms appear related to dysfunction of every organ system of the body. In end stage of renal failure oliguria develops, sodium retention takes place resulting in edema, hypertension, and congestive heart failure.

Gastrointestinal

The common symptoms include vomiting, nausea and anorexia. In late renal failure there may be inflammation of gastrointestinal tract, such as esophagitis, gastritis and duodenitis. Gastrointestinal bleeding may also be present.

Hematologic

Anemia and bleeding are the common hematological problems associated with chronic renal dysfunction The anemia is usually normocytic-normochromic. The factor responsible for anemia is inability of the diseased kidney to produce erythropoietin which helps in production of red blood cells. Bleeding is caused due to intrinsic coagulation defect or administration of anticoagulants with dialysis and access-site maintenance.

Cardiovascular

Renal diseases may lead to hypertension, pericarditis, arrhythmias, cardiomyopathy and congestive heart failure. Retinopathy and encephalopathy may result due to severe hypertension.

Neuromuscular

Early signs and symptoms of renal dysfunction are related to neuromuscular system which are characterized by headache, seizures, myoclonic jerks, muscle weakness, paralysis and peripheral neuropathy.

Metabolic-endocrine

Metabolic and endocrinal changes resulting from chronic renal failure are impaired growth and development, renal osteodystrophy (osteomalacia, osteosclerosis and osteoporosis), secondary hyperparathyroidism, amenorrhea and loss of sexual function.

Dermatologic

Dermatologic manifestations in renal diseases are characterized by hyperpigmentation, pruritus, pallor, ecchymosis and uremic frost.

Immunologic

Chronic renal failure may lead to granulocyte dysfunction and suppressed cell—mediated immunity. This increases risk of infection in uremic patients and may be the cause of their disability and death.

Oral Manifestations

Oral cavity also shows variety of changes in chronic renal failure which are as follows:

Bad taste and odor: Patients with renal failure may complain of ammoniacal taste and smell particularly in the morning. This is due to high concentration of urea in the saliva and its breakdown to ammonia.

Stomatitis: In kidney failure, blood urea level increases which results in uremic stomatitis. Uremic stomatitis occurs in the following two forms:
a. Erythemopultaceous form characterized by red mucosa covered with thick exudates and pseudomembrane.
b. Ulcerative form is characterized by ulcerations with redness and pultaceous (pulpy) coating.

Xerostomia: Xerostomia is caused by involvement of salivary glands, dehydration and mouth breathing.

Bony changes: Defective kidney function may lead to compensatory hyperactivity of the parathyroid glands. This compensatory hyperparathyroidism generally involves skeletal system. The oral manifestations of hyperparathyroidism appear frequently in the mandibular molar region these changes are as follows. (a) Total or partial loss of lamina dura, (b) Bone demineralization (c) Loss of trabeculation, (d) Giant cell tumors (e) Tooth mobility (f) Malocclusion (g) Metastatic soft tissue calcifications (h) The teeth may be painful on percussion and mastication. Malocclusion is due to increased mobility and drifting of teeth and demineralization of temporomandibular and paratemporomandibular bones.

Young patients with renal diseases may exhibit enamel hypoplasia with brownish discoloration.

MANAGEMENT OF CHRONIC RENAL FAILURE (CRF)

Management of CRF is divided into (1) Conservative therapy (2) Replacement therapy. Replacement therapy is done when conservative therapy is unable to sustain life.

Conservative Therapy-Medical Management of Chronic Renal Failure

When the patient becomes azotemic conservative therapy is started. Dietary modification is done. Blood pressure should be maintained lower than 130/85 mmHg. Hemoglobin level is maintained at 10 to12 g/dl with Erythropoietin. When the serum creatinine reaches > 4.0 mg/dl or the GFR falls to < 20 ml/minute, access for dialysis should be created. Nutritional status should be closely monitored to (a) avoid protein deficiency (b) correct metabolic acidosis (c) prevent hyperphosphatemia (d) prevent vitamin deficiency and (e) guide the initiation of dialysis. Special evaluation by a nephrologist must be done when serum creatinine is > 3.0 mg/dl.

DIALYSIS

Life span in patients with irreversible kidney disease can be increased by dialysis therapy. Dialysis is of two types, hemodialysis and peritoneal dialysis.

Hemodialysis

In hemodialysis, nitrogenous and toxic products of metabolism are removed from blood by a dialysis system. Exchange of toxic products occurs between the patient's plasma and dialysate across a semi-permeable membrane, that allows toxins to diffuse out of the plasma and retain formed elements and protein composition of blood. Anticoagulants are administered during and after the dialysis to prevent clotting in dialyser, tubing and access site.

Peritoneal Dialysis

In peritoneal dialysis, 1 to 2 litres of dialysate is instilled into peritoneal cavity and left inside for varying intervals of time. Toxic products diffuse across the semi-permeable peritoneal membrane into the dialysate. The dialysate is then drained out. Peritoneal dialysis is more beneficial and safe for patients than hemodialysis.

Orodental Considerations

Preoperative considerations in the dental management of the dialysis patient are as follows:

A. Extractions and other oral surgical procedures should be carried out early in the dialysis cycle, (within 24 hours after the dialysis) much before next dialysis because at this time patient's blood is free from anticoagulant and sufficient time is available for clotting to occur before the next dialysis.
B. The arm from which vascular access is created should not be used for (a) injection of medication, either intravenously or intramuscularly and (b) taking blood pressure.
C. The presence of vascular access site increases the susceptibility to infective endocarditis and endarteritis. So, antibiotic prophylaxis is necessary, which includes administration of streptomycin and penicillin or broad-spectrum antibiotics such as amoxycillin or any other suitable antibiotic.
D. Infection with hepatitis B and C and HIV are of major consideration in the dialysis patients because of large number of transfusions and increased exposure of dialysis patients. All available precautions and preventive measures should be taken to avoid transmission of Hepatitis B and HIV during dental treatment.
E. Patients on dialysis may present with reduced platelet count, decreased platelet adhesiveness and prolonged bleeding and clotting time which may lead to ulcerations and petechial lesions on the oral mucosa, hemorrhage from gingiva and hematoma formation after alveolectomy or periodontal surgery.
F. Medications recommended during the dialysis therapy are also of major consideration. Some drugs may lead to further renal damage. Nonsteroidal antiinflammatory drugs may cause sodium retention, prevent aldosterone production and cause acidosis. Phenacetin is nephrotoxic and puts strain on an already damaged kidney. Tetracyclines and steroids are antianabolic and increases urea nitrogen.
Such drugs should be avoided or limited when treating dialysis patients.
G. If fluoridated community water is used to mix the dialysates, it may lead to fluoride toxicity, fluorosis and renal osteodystrophy. So, dialysis patients should receive dialysates that are mixed with purified and de-ionized water.

KIDNEY TRANSPLANTATION

Patients with last stage renal failure may require renal transplantation for survival. In kidney transplantation, healthy kidney is surgically removed from the donor and implanted into the recipient. The kidney is usually taken from a blood relative or from someone who has recently died in an accident. In most of the cases of transplantation, except between monozygotic twins, transplantation rejection occurs which is mediated through the lymphocytic system.

Kidney transplantation patients require continuous immunosuppressive therapy for graft survival. The immunosuppressive therapy involves the combination of following drugs.

a. Immunosuppressive medications such as azathioprine or cyclosporin.
b. Corticosteroids such as prednisone. Recommended dose of prednisone is 10 to 40 mg/day.
c. Alkylating agents such as cyclophosphamide
d. Local graft irradiation
e. Antilymphocyte globulin.

Clinical Manifestations

Most of the clinical manifestations occurring in the transplant patients are due to immunosuppressive drugs.

A. Immunosuppressive drugs may cause increased susceptibility to gram-negative, viral and fungal infections in patients, due to reduction in T-lymphocyte competence.
B. Steroid therapy may lead to cushingoid effect that is characterized by deposition of fat around the upper portion of the body.
C. Patients on corticosteroid are also more susceptible to fungal infections due to decreased migration and phagocytic function of leucocytes and macrophages.
D. Corticosteroids also affect the healing potential
E. Excessive administration of cortisone inhibits new capillary formation, fibroblast proliferation and synthesis of mucopolysaccharides.
F. Cyclosporine may some times lead to renal and hepatic dysfunction.

Orodental Considerations

A. After transplantation only routine minor conservative dental treatment should be carried out until the maintenance dose of immunosuppressive drugs is reached. Emergency treatment should be carried out in consultation with nephrologist of the patient.
B. Immunosuppressive drugs used to reduce transplant rejection increase the risk of infection. Oral microbial flora can cause many of these infections. Oral ulcers, pulpal infection and periodontal disease may contribute in spreading oral microorganisms into the blood stream or their aspiration may spread them to respiratory tract.
C. Corticosteroid therapy at adrenal suppressive level increases susceptibility to shock because the body is unable to cope with the added stress of a dental procedure or the emotional stress associated with it. To avoid this condition following steps should be taken.
   a. Long acting anesthetic should be used.
   b. Mild sedatives should be administered to patients before dental procedure.
D. Elective procedures should be carried out in morning.
E. Postoperative analgesics should be prescribed.
F. For proper management of renal transplant patients, following steps should be considered.
   i. Dental treatment should be carried out in consultation with patient's physician or nephrologist.
   ii. Broad-spectrum antibiotic should be given prophylactically before dental treatment because of decreased immune response, e.g. amoxicillin 3 gm 1 hour before treatment, then 500 mg every 8 hours.
   iii. Vital signs should be monitored during dental procedure.
   iv. A complete blood count with differential and platelet count should be obtained before any surgical procedure.
   v. Culture and sensitivity testing of the area where surgery is planned, should be obtained.
   vi. A supplemental dose of steroids should be available for administration during hypoadrenal crisis.

ORAL MANIFESTATIONS

The orofacial manifestations of renal disease, indications of dialysis and renal transplantation are as follows:

1. Metallic taste
2. Smell of urea in breath
3. Enlarged salivary glands
4. Decreased salivary flow
5. Xerostomia
6. Enamel hypoplasia
7. Brownish discoloration of crowns of teeth
8. Low caries rate
9. Increased calculus formation
10. Low grade gingival inflammation
11. Cyclosporine induced gingival hyperplasia
12. Candidal infections of oral mucosa
13. Burning, tenderness and dryness of mucosa
14. White plaque like lesions of oral mucosa in immunosuppressed renal transplant patients.
15. Petechia and ecchymosis on the oral mucosa
16. Prolonged bleeding
17. Hemorrhage from gingiva
18. Dehiscence of wounds
19. Demineralization of bone
20. Loss of lamina dura specially in mandibular posterior teeth
21. Pulpal narrowing and calcifications
22. Tooth mobility
23. Socket sclerosis and abnormal bone repair after extraction
24. Erosion of teeth due to regurgitation associated with dialysis
25. Arterial and oral calcifications
26. Peri-oral dermatitis characterized by red papules and scaling on upper lip and nasolabial fold is seen in transplant patients.

BIBLIOGRAPHY

1. Dishart MK, Kellum JA. An evaluation of pharmacological strategies for the prevention and treatment of acute renal failure. Drugs 2000;59(1):79-91.
2. Levy NB. Psychiatric considerations in the primary medical care of the patient with renal failure. Adv Ren Repalce Ther 2000;7(3):231-8.
3. Lieberthal W, Nigam SK. Acute renal failure. II. Experimental models of acute renal failure: Imperfect but indispensible. Am J Physiol Renal Physiol 2000;278(1)F1-12.
4. O' Neill WC. Sonographic evaluation of renal failure. Am J Kidney Dis 2000;35(6):1021-38.
5. Orth SR. Smoking-a renal risk factor. Nephron 2000;86(1):12-26.

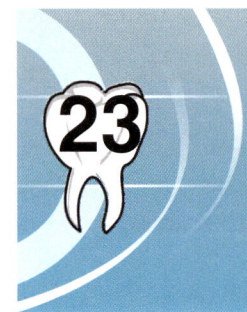

Relation of Immunologic Diseases with Oral Medicine

INTRODUCTION

Immunity refers to ability of the body to resist infections. In recent years scope of immunology has increased to many fold. It has explained many disease processes. It also provide methods to investigate a continually growing number of clinical conditions. Due to the everincreasing information added by immunologic research the concepts of diseases are very rapidly changing. The function of the immune system is to eliminate destructive foreign substances from the body. Lymphocytes are responsible for the immune response that form two components of immune system- thymus-dependent or the T-cell system and B-cell system. X-linked gammaglobulinemia is caused by defect in B-cell function.

T-cell system or T-lymphocytes provide cell-mediated immunity, which is responsible for body's primary defense against viruses and fungi and also takes part in delayed hypersensitivity reactions. B-lymphocytes carry immunoglobulin receptors on their surface. These receptors combine with antigen and produce antibody, which is necessary for the body's defense against bacterial infections and other toxic foreign substances.

Major classes of immunoglobulins (Ig) or antibodies are IgM, IgG, IgA, IgD and IgE. Macrophages also play major role in immune response. They secrete interleukins which activate T-lymphocytes. The immune response essential for protection against disease, can also cause disease when it reacts against host tissue.

PRIMARY IMMUNODEFICIENCIES

Primary immunodeficiencies are essentially by hereditary abnormalities characterized by an inborn defect in the immune system. There may be involvement of either B-cell system with deficiency of humoral antibodies or T-cell system with deficiency of cellular immunity. There may be combined deficiencies of both B- and T-cell systems.

Selective Immunoglobulin Deficiencies

In selective immunoglobulin deficiency there is a group of abnormality of B-cell or humoral antibody system. Usually only one or two immunoglobulins classes are deficient. The disease is usually asymptomatic throughout the childhood and becomes apparent after third decade of life. The common symptoms of selective immunoglobulin deficiencies are recurrent gram positive bacterial infections of upper and lower respiratory tract.

The most common deficient immunoglobulin is IgA. Abnormalities particularly associated with IgA deficiency are chronic pulmonary infection, chronic sinusitis and malabsorption syndrome. There is increased incidence of collagen vascular diseases such as rheumatoid arthritis and systemic lupus erythematosus in B-cell deficiencies.

Thymic Hypoplasia

Thymic hypoplasia is seen in DiGeorge's syndrome and Nezelof's syndrome. Hypoplasia of the thymus leads to deficiency of T-lymphocytes. Patients with these syndromes have normal levels of serum immunoglobulin but impairment of cell-mediated immunity. T-lymphocyte deficiency increases susceptibility to infections with viruses and fungi. Infections with Candida albicans are most common.

Combined Immunodeficiency

Combined immunodeficiency is a genetic disease characterised by low peripheral lymphocyte counts, lack of cellular immunity and severe deficiency of immunoglobulins. The clinical manifestations of this disease appear in the first few weeks of life which include the following:

a. Bacterial, viral and fungal infections
b. Localized or systemic candidiasis
c. Cutaneous granulomas.

X-linked Agammaglobulinemia

In this there is absence of, or extremely low levels of, the gamma fraction of serum globulin. It is a hereditary disease of male children, X-linked agammaglobulinemia (XLA). The disease is caused by abnormality in B-cell function due to which synthesis of all classes of antibodies or immunoglobulins does not take place. The symptoms begin at six months of age, characterized by severe recurrent bacterial infections of lungs, skin, meninges and sinuses. There is also increased incidence of rheumatoid arthritis, lymphoma and leukemia. Treatment consists of intravenous administration of gammaglobulin at doses from 100 to 400 mg/kg body weight once in a month and broad-spectrum antibiotics.

Partial Combined Immunodeficiency with Ataxia Telangiectasia (PCIAT)

This immune disorder is characterized by combined T-cell and B-cell deficiency leading to abnormal cellular response and deficiency of immunoglobulins. The clinical features of the disease are as follows.
a. Telangiectasias of skin and eyes
b. Cerebellar ataxia
c. Severe pulmonary infections
d. Gonadal dysgenesis
e. Endocrinal disorders.
Treatment is limited to supportive care as no direct cure is recommended.

Oral Manifestations of Primary Immunodeficiencies

a. Abnormalities of T-lymphocytes lead to chronic fungal and viral infections of the oral mucosa, whereas deficiency of B-lymphocytes leads to recurrent bacterial infections.
b. Chronic oral candidiasis is seen in patients with T-cell deficiency.
c. Patients with B-cell abnormality may exhibit chronic maxillary sinusitis.
d. Skin and mucosal telangiectasias
e. Congenital defects such as micrognathia, cleft palate, bifid uvula, and short philtrum of upper lip are seen in patients with thymic hypoplasia.
f. Herpes simplex virus infections localised to mouth are also common in patients with T-cell disease.
g. Oral ulcerations may also occur occasionally in few patients.
Treatment—Antiviral medication.

Orodental Management

The chances of infection must be reduced in patient with primary immunodeficiency. The following additional precautions must be taken.
A. Patients with oral candidiasis and T-cell deficiency should be given prophylactic antifungal therapy before dental treatment to reduce risk of systemic fungal infections.
B. Patients with B-cell abnormalities are given monthly therapy with gammaglobulin. Before starting a dental treatment, the gammaglobulin level should be checked to make sure that it is atleast 200 mg/dl. An extra dose of 100 to 200 mg/kg body weight, should be administered a day before carrying out any oral surgical procedure.
C. Dental infections in patients with primary immunodeficiencies should be managed carefully and vigorously. Before prescribing an antibiotic, a culture sensitivity for bacteria and fungi should be taken because usually these patients get unusual infections with fungi and gram-negative bacteria.

SECONDARY IMMUNODEFICIENCY

Secondary immunodeficiencies are caused by HIV infections, immunosuppressive therapy, malignancies, protein-depleting diseases and granulomatous diseases of lymphoid system. Specific diseases such as Hodgkin's disease, non-Hodgkin's disease, non-Hodgkin's lymphoma, leukemia, multiple myeloma, sarcoidosis, nephrotic syndrome and AIDS result in secondary immunodeficiency.

Hodgkin's Disease

In Hodgkin's disease there is loss of T-lymphocyte function. Lymphocytes in patients with Hodgkin's disease show an abnormal response to antigens. The major clinical infections seen in Hodgkin's disease are fungal, viral and protozoal. As the disease progresses the condition become bad to worse.

Chemotherapy and radiotherapy used for the treatment of disease also suppress neutrophil and antibody function, which increases the patient's susceptibility to bacterial infections.

Non-Hodgkin's Lymphoma

There is deficiency of the B-cell or T-cell system. Lymphoma patients have increased infections with bacteria, virus and fungi. Non-Hodgkin's lymphoma is the second most common tumor in AIDS patients.

Leukemia

The major clinical manifestation in patients with leukemia is infection by microorganisms that rarely cause illness in normal individuals such as gram-negative bacilli, fungi and herpes viruses. Such infections are caused by decrease in mature, functioning granulocytes due to cytotoxic chemotherapy used for treatment of leukemia.

In acute leukemia there is impaired ability of neutrophils to migrate and reduced bactericidal and chemotactic functions. Chronic lymphatic leukemia affects humoral antibody response resulting in secondary bacterial infections.

Multiple Myeloma

Multiple myeloma is a malignant disease of plasma cells which are required for the humoral antibody response. These abnormal plasma cells produce myeloma protein instead of normal immunoglobulins.

Deficiency of immunoglobulin leads to repeated episodes of bacterial infections, especially pneumococcal pneumonia. Chemotherapy used for treatment of malignancy also increases patient's susceptibility to infections. *Varicella-zoster* virus infection is also common in multiple myeloma patients.

Nephrotic Syndrome

In nephrotic syndrome, damaged glomeruli lose large amount of serum protein that causes secondary hypogammaglobulinemia. Hypogammaglobulinemia leads to bacterial infections involving skin, lungs and oropharynx and may result in death in children with nephrotic syndrome. The incidence of infection is dramatically reduced by prophylactic use of gammaglobulin and antibiotics.

ACQUIRED IMMUNODEFICIENCY SYNDROME (AIDS)

Acquired immunodeficiency syndrome is caused by human immunodeficiency virus (HIV). HIV is a retrovirus belonging to subfamily of Lentivirinae, that causes slow infection in which signs and symptoms appear many months or years after infection.

Immunopathogenesis

A. Human immunodeficiency virus has ability to suppress cell-mediated immunity by infecting T_4 cells, the helper lymphocytes. These lymphocytes contain CD_4 surface molecule which bind the virus to the cell.
B. HIV decreases T_4 lymphocyte count below 200 mm^3, at which the patient becomes susceptible to infections and tumors.
C. Infection with HIV causes abnormalities of monocytes and natural killer cells (macrophages).

Clinical Manifestations

The clinical manifestations in AIDS patients can be divided into following groups:

Acute Infections

Acute infections occur 3 to 6 weeks after initial contact with HIV, which are mostly asymptomatic. Some patients may develop fever, gastrointestinal symptoms, joint pain and maculopapular rash. These are self-limiting symptoms which remain for 2 to 3 weeks.

Asymptomatic Phase

a. Asymptomatic phase of the disease is a period between the initial contact with HIV and development of clinical manifestations. The average time is 8 to 10 years.
b. During this phase, the number of T_4 lymphocytes gradually decrease from the normal levels of 700 mm^3 to 1200 mm^3 (above 600 mm^3) to below 200 mm^3.
c. Persistent generalized lymphadenopathy occurs during asymptomatic phase characterized by enlarged lymph nodes of more than 1 cm in diameter at extra-inguinal sites for more than 3 months.

Clinical Signs and Symptoms

Clinical signs of AIDS can be divided into following subgroups.

Constitutional symptoms: Constitutional symptoms related to AIDS include fever, weight loss more than 10% without any effort for it or diarrhea persisting for more than one month.

Neurologic diseases: Neurologic diseases occur more frequently and severely in last stages of AIDS. The common AIDS related neurologic complications are B-cell lymphoma, AIDS dementia complex, neuropathies and myelopathies. AIDS related CNS infections result from cryptococcus, cytomegalovirus and toxoplasmosis.

Secondary Infections (Opportunistic Infections)

The main clinical manifestations in an AIDS patient are opportunistic infections. Some of the opportunistic infections associated with AIDS are as follows:
  i. The major opportunistic infection that is an initial infection in 60% of the patients and infects 80% of the AIDS patients during course of disease, is Pneumocystis carinii pneumonia (PCP).
  ii. Candida albicans also cause infection in AIDS patients leading to esophagitis.
  iii. Herpes simplex and herpes zoster cause extensive mucocutaneous disease.
  iv. Cytomegalovirus causes gastrointestinal ulcers, pneumonia and retinitis.
  v. Pulmonary Mycobacterium tuberculosis is also common in AIDS patients.

Neoplasms

The most common neoplasm among AIDS patients is Kaposi's sarcoma. Kaposi's sarcoma clinically presents as macule, papule or nodule on the skin or mucosa (Fig. 14.10). The second most common tumor associated with AIDS is non-hodgkin's lymphoma, particularly B-cell lymphoma.

Oral Lesions Associated with HIV Infection

Oral lesions are prominent in AIDS patients. They may be the first sign of HIV disease. They have prognostic value and their proper treatment increases the life of HIV patients.

Viral Infections

Hairy leukoplakia: Hairy leukoplakia is caused by Epstein-Barr virus infection. It appears as corrugated white patch which occurs most frequently on lateral borders of tongue.

Cytomegalovirus: Cytomegalovirus is responsible for large painful ulcers in the oral cavity. Other large oral ulcers of unknown etiology, which resemble major aphthous ulcers also occur in HIV patients.

Herpes virus infection: Recurrent herpes simplex virus infection in HIV patients causes large, chronic oral lesion involving lips and intraoral mucosa. The lesions are surrounded by raised white border comprising small vesicles.

Human papilloma virus: Oral human papilloma virus lesion clinically presents as single wart, large cauliflower like masses or flat lesions.

HIV related gingivitis: HIV related gingivitis is characterized by generalized erythema of the marginal gingiva that does not respond to routine periodontal therapy and debridement.

HIV-associated periodontal disease: In HIV-associated periodontitis there is painful rapid destruction of the gingiva, periodontal ligaments and alveolar bone, localized in one or two teeth or generalized over the entire gingiva. Lesions if not treated lead to destruction of tissue, bone exposure and bone sequestration.

Treatment

The management of AIDS includes recommendation of following drugs.
A. The main drug used for treating AIDS is azidothymidine (AZT). The recommended dose is 200 mg every 4 hrs.
B. Didanosine is also effective in treating HIV infection.
C. Aerosolized pentamidine or trimethoprim/sulphamethoxazole is used to manage Pneumocystis carinii pneumonia
D. Fungal infections are treated by ketoconazole (KTZ), fluconazole or amphotericin B (AMB).
E. Herpes or cytomegalovirus infections are managed by acyclovir, ganciclovir or foscarnet.

Fungal Infection-candidiasis

Oral candidiasis occurs in about 1/3rd of HIV-infected patients. Both erythematous and pseudomembranous form of candidiasis occur frequently in AIDS patients. Denture wearing and use of corticosteroids and antibiotics increase severity of candidiasis.

Oral Neoplasms

The most common oral neoplasm in AIDS is Kaposi's sarcoma. Early lesions of Kaposi's sarcoma appear as multifocal vascular nodule on the mucosa. As the lesion progresses, it may ulcerate and cause pain and bleeding. On further progression, lesion covers large portion of anterior mucosa or gingiva, which causes difficulty in speech and eating (Fig. 14.10).

DISEASES OF THE CONNECTIVE TISSUE

They are also called as collagen diseases, collagen vascular diseases, autoimmune diseases or hyperimmune diseases. They are called 'autoimmune' diseases because autoantibodies which react with normal tissues in vitro have been observed in sufficient quantities in patients with these diseases.

Systemic Lupus Erythematosus (SLE)

Systemic lupus erythematosus is a disease that shows presence of abnormal serum antibodies and immune complexes. The disease affects young females between 20 to 40 years of age. The disease is characterized by multiorgan involvement because autoantibodies of SLE are directed against erythrocytes, leukocytes, platelets, nucleoproteins and liver, kidney or heart tissue.

Clinical Manifestations

SLE has a variety of clinical manifestations.
a. Skin lesions in SLE begin as erythematosus scaling with sharp borders, which progress to form depigmented scars.
b. Glomerular destruction is seen in about 50% of patients leading to nephrotic syndrome
c. Pericarditis, muscle atrophy, pulmonary infiltration may also occur.
d. Central nervous system involvement is characterized by seizures, neuropathies and psychiatric abnormalities.

Common Problems

The more common problems with SLE are as follows:

Adrenal suppression: High doses of corticosteroid taken for SLE may suppress adrenal function and makes these patients susceptible to shock. Patients physician should be consulted before any dental treatment is done.

Infection: Cytotoxic and immunosuppressive drugs cause increased risk of infection. Preoperative prophylactic antibiotics should be used.

Hematologic abnormalities: SLE patients develop normochromic normocytic anemia, hemolytic anemia, leukopenia and thrombocytopenia.

Cardiac diseases: SLE patients may develop bacterial endocarditis. Such patients with SLE and heart murmurs must be given antibiotics before dental treatment.

Renal disease: In SLE patients renal disease is common. Patients who are undergoing hemodialysis must receive dental treatment on nondialysis days.

Exacerbation by drugs: Penicillin, sulfonamide and nonsteroidal anti-inflammatory drugs (NSAIDS) cause lupus flares, hence these should be used carefully.

Exacerbation by surgery: In patients with history of lupus flares following surgery, the clinician should be careful.

Oral Manifestations

a. The most common site for oral lesions and ulcerations are buccal mucosa, lips and palate.
b. About 75% of patients with SLE complain of xerostomia, burning mouth or soreness.
c. The lesions of lips appear as central atrophic area with small white dots surrounded by keratinized border.
d. Intra-oral lesions occur as a central, depressed, red atrophic area surrounded by elevated keratotic zone.
e. Salivary gland disease and TMJ disorders usually occur.

Dental Considerations

a. SLE is a widespread disease affecting many organ systems hence the dental management of a SLE patient requires a good understanding of general medicine.
b. Patients with SLE should have antibiotic prophylaxis before dental treatment to prevent bacterial endocarditis.
c. Surgery can aggravate SLE, so all the elective dental procedures should be avoided.
d. There may be severe thrombocytopenia, so platelet count should be determined before carrying out oral surgical procedures.

Treatment

Oral ulcers of SLE are transient, occur with acute lupus flares.

Treatment includes bed rest with high doses of systemic corticosteroids. Immunosuppressive drugs such as azothioprine or methotrexate can be prescribed in resistant case. Symptomatic lesions can be treated by high-potency topical corticosteroids or intralesional steroid injections.

Dermatomyositis (DM)

It is an inflammatory disease characterized by skin lesions and muscle atrophy. The onset of disease is associated with infection, cancer or drug therapy. Diseases occur most frequently in childhood and between fourth and sixth decades of life.

Clinical Features

a. Painless muscle weakness of arms, legs and trunk.
b. Weakness may spread to face, neck, pharynx, larynx and heart.

c. Typical skin lesions occur around face and fingers.
d. There may also be arthritis, renal damage and cardiac failure.
e. Fever and leukocytosis.

Oral Manifestations

Oral involvement is rare.
a. Diffuse stomatitis and pharyngitis.
b. Weakness of pharyngeal and palatal muscles may lead to difficulty in swallowing and nasal speech.
c. Lesions present on oral mucosa are characterized by shallow ulcers, erythematous patches and telangiectasis.
d. There may be swelling of face, eyelids and lips.
e. There may be weakness of muscles of mastication and phonation leading to difficulty in chewing and speech.

Treatment

Symptomatic treatment is provided as there is no specific treatment. It may be fatal in very severe cases. In mild and moderate cases there may be recovery. Occasionally with a residual disability.

Scleroderma (Systemic Sclerosis, Dermatosis, Hidebound Disease)

Scleroderma is a multi system disease characterized by fibrosis of connective tissue and blood vessels. The most typical feature of disease is hardening and tightening of skin and mucosa. Disease may occur as localized scleroderma or progressive systemic sclerosis. Women are more affected than men.

The disease starts with pitting edema of extremities and face which is replaced by tightening and hardening of skin leading to restricted movement of affected part.

Oral Manifestations

a. Lips become rigid with narrowing of oral aperture
b. Tongue also becomes hard and rigid leading to difficulty in speech and swallowing
c. Thickening of periodontal membrane, especially in posterior teeth
d. There may be resorption of mandible at body and angle due to severe tightening of face
e. Skin folds are lost around the mouth giving a mask like look to the face
f. If the soft tissues around the TMJ are affected, the movement of the TMJ will be restricted resulting into pseudoankylosis.
g. Due to rigidity of the muscles forceful movement may cause resorption of the mandible which may lead to pathological fracture.

Treatment

There is no adequate treatment. Partial remission may be obtained with cortisone therapy.

Dental Management

a. Dental procedures in scleroderma patients are difficult because of narrowing of oral aperture and rigidity of tongue, making speaking and swallowing difficult.
b. Extensive resorption of the angle of mandible may lead to pathologic fracture from minor trauma or dental extraction.
c. The mouth opening can be increased by use of stretching exercises by about 5 mm.
d. Daily topical application of fluoride and fluoride tooth paste.
e. Monthly or bimonthly dental checkup and oral prophylaxis.
f. If necessary a bilateral commissurotomy may be done.

Rheumatoid Arthritis (RA)

RA is characterized by inflammation of the synovial membrane. Females are about 3 times more affected usually between the age group of 35 to 50 years. Weakness and fatique followed by stiffness of joints occur.

Oral Manifestations

The treatment of RA may give rise to oral manifestations like stomatitis, gingival over growth, periodontal disease, loss of alveolar bone and teeth. RA of TMJ can also occur.

Dental Management

1. Precautions against bleeding be taken if the patient is taking about 5 gm per day of aspirin or NSAIDS.
2. IM dose of gold salts may produce stomatitis, blood dyscrasias and nephrotic syndrome.
3. If patient is taking corticosteroids and immunosuppressive drugs, proper precautions must be taken before surgery.

Mixed Connective Tissue Disease (MCTD)

The mixed connective tissue disease (MCTD) has the combined clinical features of SLE, Progressive systemic sclerosis (PSS) and Dermatomyositis (DM). The oral manifestations are xerostomia and decreased mandibular movements.

ALLERGY

Allergy refers to hypersensitivity reaction caused by exposure to a particular antigen (drug, spice, food or air borne substance) resulting in marked increase in reactivity to that antigen upon subsequent exposure. Acute allergic reactions are caused by an immediate type hypersensitivity reaction. This include vasodilation and increased permeability. The fluid and leukocytes leave the blood vessels and accumulate in the tissues resulting in the edema in the areas where histamine is released. Urticaria of lips and oral mucosa are commonly seen.

Localized Anaphylactic Reactions

Anaphylactic reactions refers to immediate, transient kind of allergic reactions characterized by contraction of smooth muscles and dilatation of capillaries. Localized anaphylactic reactions are of two types:

Urticaria

When superficial blood vessels are involved in localized anaphylactic reaction, it results in urticaria. Urticaria of lips and oral mucosa occurs after ingestion of particular food or spice to which individual is allergic. Drugs such as penicillin and aspirin may cause urticaria. Urticaria starts with pruritus in the areas where histamine is released. Urticaria of lips and oral mucosa are commonly seen. Drugs like penicillin and aspirin and some edibles may also cause urticaria.

Angioneurotic Edema (Angioedema)

When blood vessels deeper in the subcutaneous tissues are affected, angioneurotic edema results. It is characterized by large diffuse area of subcutaneous swelling under normal overlying skin. Angioedema mostly occurs on lips, tongue and around the eyes. If posterior portion of tongue or larynx is involved it may lead to respiratory distress.

The treatment for respiratory distress includes administration of 0.5 ml (1:1000) epinephrine subcutaneously or 0.2 ml epinephrine slowly intravenously.

Generalized Anaphylactic Reactions

Generalized anaphylaxis is an immediate response to allergen, involving smooth muscles of respiratory and intestinal tract and capillaries.

Factors that may increase risk of anaphylaxis are as follows:
a. History of asthma
b. Family history of allergy
c. Intravenous administration of drugs
d. Administration of drugs such as penicillin.

The generalized anaphylactic reaction affects the following four systems.
a. *Skin:* Initial symptoms occur on skin characterised by angioedema, urticaria, pruritus and erythema.
b. *Intestinal:* Gastro-intestinal tract symptoms are vomiting, cramps and diarrhea.
c. *Respiratory:* Respiratory symptoms include dyspnea, asthma and wheezing.
d. *Cardiovascular:* Cardiovascular symptom is hypotension due to loss of intravascular fluid.

Treatment

a. Emergency allergy drugs should be at hand.
b. Intramuscular or subcutaneous administration of 0.5 ml of epinephrine (1:1000 dilution) in an adult and 0.1 ml to 0.3 ml in children.
c. Bronchospasm can be managed by intravenous injection of aminophylline 250 mg over a period of 10 minutes.
d. IV injection of hydrocortisone.
e. IM injection of antiallergic drug.

Latex Allergy

The latex gloves sometimes produce cutaneous and mucosal reactions. The allergy can be the patients, clinicians and auxiliary staff. Nonlatex gloves and products should be used. Emergency allergy drugs must be available at hand.

Clinicians and auxiliary staff allergic to latex should change the (a) type of the gloves used (b) soap for scrubbing hands.

All patients allergic to latex should carry an epinephrine autoinjection kit and wear Medic Alert identification.

The treatment for all allergies is almost same which is as follows.
a. Maintenance of proper airway and circulation
b. Administration of epinephrine
c. IV administration of steroids as required
d. Administration of oxygen
e. Administration of antiallergic injections.

BIBLIOGRAPHY

1. Alam R. A brief review of the immune system. Primary Care 1998;25:727-38.
2. Arkachaisri T, Lehman TJ. Systemic lupus erythematosus and related disorders of childhood. Curr Opin Rheumatol 1999;11:384-92.
3. Froland SS. Antimicrobial chemoprophylaxis in immunocompromised patients. Scand J Infect Dis 1990;70:130-4.
4. Hillebrand G, Siebert R, Simeoni E, Santer R. DiGeorge syndrome with discordant phenotype in monozygotic twins. J Med Genet 37; E23.
5. Hong R. The DiGeorge anomaly. Clin Rev Allergy Immunol 2001;20:43-60.
6. Johnson KJ, Chensue SW, Ward PA. Immunopathology. In: Rubin E, Farber JR, (Ed). Pathology. 3rd ed. Philadelphia: Lippincott-Raven Publishers 1999.
7. Jones RE, Chatham WW. Update on sarcoidosis. Curr Opin Rheumatol 1999;11:83-7.
8. Kujala V. A review of current literature on epidemiology of immediate glove irritation and latex allergy. Occup Med 1999;49:3-9.
9. Mohamed AJ, Nore BF, Christensson B, Smith CI. Signalling of Bruton's tyrosine kinase Btk. Scand J Immunol 1999;49:113-8.
10. Nononyama S. Recent advances in the diagnosis of X-linked agammaglobulinemia. Intern Med 1999;38:687.
11. Pizzo PA. Fever in immunocompromised patients. N Engl J Med 1999;341:893-900.
12. Rogers MH, Lwin R, Fairbanks L, et al. Cognitive and behavioral abnormalities in adenosine deaminase deficient severe combined immunodeficiency. J Pediatr 2001;139:44-50.
13. Roitt IM. Primary immunodeficiency. In. Roitt IM, Brostoff J, Male D (Ed). Clinical immunology. 5th ed. London: Mosby 1998;285-92.
14. Rubin RL. Etiology and mechanisms of drug-induced lupus Curr Opin Rheumatol 1999;11:357-63.
15. Secondary immunodeficiency. In: Roitt IM, Brostoff J, Male D (Ed). Clinical immunology. 5th ed. London: Mosb 1998;293.
16. Treister N, Glick M. Rheumatoid arthritis: A review and suggested dental care considerations. J Am Dent Assoc 1999;130:689-98.

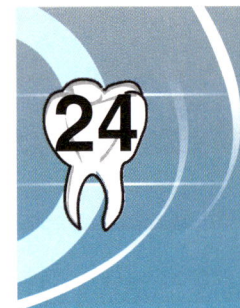

Neuromuscular Diseases Affecting the Orofacial Region

There are many diseases of nerve and muscle tissues of orofacial region which are important for the management of dental patients. Neuromuscular disease affecting the orofacial region can be classified as follows:

MOVEMENT DISORDERS

Cerebral Palsy (CP)

Cerebral palsy refers to various types of non-progressive motor dysfunctions usually present at birth or beginning in early childhood. Congenital infections, anoxia and ischemia during labor or at birth are the causes of cerebral palsy. The incidence of CP is 2 to 6 in every 1000 live birth.

Clinical Features

a. Spasm of muscles used for speaking, results in disturbance of speech
b. Difficulty in chewing and swallowing
c. Seizures associated with mental retardation
d. Athetotic purposeless movement of fingers and hands.

Treatment

Treatment includes the following:
a. Physiotherapy to prevent contractures
b. Seizures are treated by administration of drugs such as diazepam and L-dopa
c. Systemic corticosteroids with acyclovir medicine.

Orodental Considerations

a. Children suffering from cerebral palsy exhibit increased incidence of enamel defects
b. Sialorrhea and drooling are also seen in patients with cerebral palsy.

Parkinson's Disease (Parkinsonism, Paralysis Agitans)

It is a neurologic disease resulting from deficiency of neurotransmitter dopamine due to degenerative, vascular or inflammatory changes in the basal ganglia, characterized by rigidity, tremors, bradykinesia and impaired postural reflexes, mainly affects adults in middle or late life.

Clinical Features

a. Tremors of the hand and muscular rigidity of extremities are the early signs of the disease
b. Mask-like expression due to rigidity of the facial muscles
c. Difficulty in speech due to lack of muscle control
d. Rigidity of facial muscles causes difficulty in swallowing, resulting in drooling
e. Mandibular tremors create difficulty in patients with removable partial denture.

Treatment

The drug of choice for treatment of parkinsonism is Levodopa, a dopamine precursor. Mild form of disease can be managed by anticholinergic drug (trihexyphenidyl).

Dental Considerations

a. Due to dysplasia and an altered gag reflex, care must be taken to avoid the aspiration of water or materials used during dental procedures. Antiparkinsonism drugs cause xerostomia resulting in root caries and recurrent caries.
b. More frequent dental checkup should be done
c. More frequent—topical fluoride application should be done
d. Abnormal oral behavior such as purposeless chewing and grinding movement makes dental procedure difficult
e. Pretreatment sedation is necessary as anxiety increases both tremors and muscle rigidity.

Bell's Palsy

Bell's palsy is described as unilateral paralysis of the facial muscles due to dysfunction of the facial nerve. Inflammation of nerve, trauma and herpes simplex infection are the etiological factors.

Clinical Features

a. The disease starts with slight pain around the ear, followed by paralysis of the facial muscles of that side. The eye of that side stays open
b. The corner of the mouth on affected side drops, and there is drooling
c. Food is retained in upper and lower buccal and labial fold due to weakness of buccinator muscle
d. Loss of taste on anterior two third of the tongue and reduced salivary secretion
e. Corneal ulcerations may result from foreign body as the eye stays open on affected side.

Treatment

Steroids with antiherpetic drugs such as acyclovir may decrease the severity and duration of paralysis.

Guillain-Barré Syndrome (Acute Idiopathic Polyneuropathy)

Guillain-Barre Syndrome is an autoimmune disease caused by progressive demyelinating neuropathy. It often occur 1 to 3 weeks after an acute infection. This syndrome often follows a non specific respiratory or gastrointestinal illness.

Clinical Features

a. Early signs of disease are difficulty in swallowing and paresthesia of mouth due to weakness of pharyngeal and facial musculature and myalgia or paresthesia of the lower limbs
b. Anesthesia and paralysis of legs and trunk due to weakness of associated muscles
c. There may be changes in blood pressure and pulse rate
d. Respiration is compromised
e. The seventh cranial nerve is frequently involved.

Treatment and Prognosis

The paralysis may progress for 10 days and remain constant for 2 weeks. Recovery is very slow and may take 6 months to 24 months.

Huntington's Chorea [Huntington's Disease (HC)]

Huntington's chorea is a hereditary neurodegenerative disease characterized by involuntary movements of limbs and facial muscles and dementia. The disease occurs mainly in adults in third to fifth decades of life.

The main clinical feature is spasmodic or excessive muscular activity of tongue, face and head. This muscular activity progressively becomes worse, resulting in violent movements and difficulty in speech. Pretreatment sedation with diazepam is recommended before carrying out dental procedure.

Clinical Manifestation

Progressively worsening choreic movements in the face, tongue and head. Gradually hyperkinesia becomes aggravated, movements become violent with difficulty in speech and swallowing.

Treatment

Symptomatic

Orodental Considerations

Before treatment sedation with diazepam is helpful. Removable appliances like RPD or RCD must be avoided.

MULTIPLE SCLEROSIS (MS)

Multiple sclerosis is a chronic neurologic disease characterized by demyelination of axons within the central nervous system. It occurs primarily in adult woman, usually starting from fourth decade of life. There is prevalence increase with increase in distance from equator, hence more in countries away from equator like New Zealand, Canada and Norway etc.

Clinical Features

a. Intermittent loss of vision for several days with partial recovery within one month and complete in few months, to be followed again after years
b. Color blindness and diplopia due to involvement of third, fourth and sixth cranial nerves
c. Weakness and paresthesia of the extremities
d. Other signs of disease are bladder dysfunction, ataxia and generalized incoordination
e. Uthoff's sign and Marcus Gunn's pupillary sign are found in multiple sclerosis.

Orodental Considerations

a. There may be involvement of trigeminal nerve, leading to paresthesia and anesthesia of its divisions leading to facial palsy.
b. Few patients may develop either trigeminal or glossopharyngeal neuralgia. Pain is severe and lancinating with no trigger zones.
c. In later course of the disease facial paralysis takes place which is difficult to differentiate with Bell's palsy.

Treatment

Carbamazepine, baclofen, gabapentin and phenytoin supplemented by alcohol injection and surgical cutting and removing part of the nerve.

CEREBRAL ABSCESS

Cerebral abscess is caused by spread of pyogenic bacteria from infections of the middle ear, paranasal sinuses and lungs. The bacteria isolated from abscesses include Staphylococci, Enterococci, Bacteroids and Pepto-streptococcus found in dental plaque; and *Streptococcus milleri* (common oral commensals of streptococcus group).

The clinical features are same as those of general systemic infections such as fever and malaise. Treatment includes antibiotic therapy towards the causative organism.

AMYOTROPHIC LATERAL SCLEROSIS (ALS)

ALS is also called as Lou Gehrig disease and motor neuron disease. Amyotrophic lateral sclerosis is a fatal degenerative disease affecting upper and lower motor neurons of the central nervous system. The disease occurs between fourth and sixth decades of life and is caused by slow viral infections.

Clinical Features

a. Fatigue and weakness of muscles of mastication and tongue resulting in difficulty in mastication and speech and also of upper limbs
b. Dysfunction of temporomandibular joint
c. Development of malocclusion may occur as the disease progresses
d. Aspiration pneumonia may also occur in patients with amyotrophic lateral sclerosis due to reduced functions of the muscles of breathing
e. Aspiration pneumonia is usually the cause of death in ALS patients.

Treatment

1. No effective treatment. Usually survival is for 3 years.
2. Ceftriaxone, guanidine, hydrochloride, gabapentin, gangliosides, interferons may be tried but have not proved effective.
3. Supportive measures and medicaments may be used.

Orodental Considerations

1. Orofacial muscles become weak.
2. Patient may not be able to cough or clear the throat hence a reclining position for dental treatment is contraindicated due to risk of aspiration.
3. Any type of nerve stimulation induce gagging or vomiting hence must be avoided.
4. Topical anesthetics must be avoided.
5. Patient should be nil per os (NPO or nil per os) for 12 hours before treatment.
6. During treatment dentist should avoid touch of soft tissue areas to avoid gagging.
7. Avoid topical strong fluoride as they induce nausea.
8. Mild mechanical toothbrushing, mild fluoride oral rinses and more frequent dental checkup should be done.

MUSCULAR DYSTROPHY (MD)

Muscular dystrophy is a hereditary progressive degenerative disorder characterized by muscle atrophy leading to weakness.

Clinical Features

Muscular dystrophy can be classified into four major types according to clinical manifestation.

Duchenne's Pseudohypertrophic Dystrophy

a. Onset of clinical manifestation is during first three years of life
b. Disease is seen only in males
c. Early signs are frequent falling, difficulty in walking and inability to run
d. Patient is unable to walk at the end of first decade of life due to atrophy of muscles.

Facioscapulohumeral Dystrophy

a. Muscles of pectoral girdle are most frequently involved
b. Patient exhibits weakness of arms and winging of scapulae
c. There is also weakness of muscles of eyes and mouth.

Limb Girdle Dystrophy of ERB (A Type of Paralysis)

a. The disease begins in second and third decades of life.
b. Patient experiences weakness in shoulders and pelvis.

Myotonic Dystrophy

a. It is most common muscular dystrophy in adults.
b. There is involvement of muscles of head, neck and distal extremities.
c. Patient is unable to relax his muscles after contraction.
d. There is wasting and subsequent weakness of cranial innervated muscles.

Oral Manifestations

a. There is severe atrophy of sternomastoid muscles resulting in inability to turn the head.
b. Muscles of mastication are commonly affected that causes difficulty in chewing.
c. There may be enlargement of the tongue and weakness of facial muscles due to fat deposition.

Dental Considerations

a. Lack of proper muscle tension to keep teeth in proper alignment in the dental arch results in occlusal abnormalities.
b. Severe open bite and diastema may result from enlarged tongue and weak facial muscles.
c. Temporomandibular joint dysfunction characterized by inability to chew, frequent dislocation and clicking of jaws is also observed in patients of muscular dystrophy.

MYASTHENIA GRAVIS

In myasthenia gravis, striated muscles get fatigued due to disorder at a neuromuscular junction. The disease is most prominent in women during third and fourth decades of life.

Clinical Features

a. Muscular weakness after exercise is the chief complaint in patients with myasthenia gravis.
b. Diplopia due to weakness of extraocular muscles and ptosis due to weakness of lid are the early signs of the disease.
c. The disease may also affect limbs and shoulders.
d. In severe cases, respiratory difficulty may arise.

Oral Manifestations

a. Patient exhibits mask-like, expressionless appearance due to involvement of facial muscles.
b. Difficulty in chewing due to involvement of muscles of mastication.
c. Weakness of tongue and palatal muscles may also occur.

Dental Considerations

1. Dental treatment should be done in a hospital where endotracheal tube if required can be inserted
2. Airway must be kept clear
3. Adequate suction and use of rubber dam are helpful
4. Avoid prescribing drugs like narcotics, tranquilizers and barbiturates which may affect the neuromuscular junction.
5. Certain antibiotics which reduce neuromuscular activity must be avoided like tetracycline, streptomycin, sulfonamides and clindamycin.

CEREBROVASCULAR DISEASE

Cerebrovascular disease is a general term used for a brain dysfunction caused by damage to or an abnormality in cerebral blood supply causing severe interruption in the blood flow to the brain.

Complete stoppage of blood for 3 to 4 minutes may render cerebral infarct. General symptoms include sensory loss, motor paralysis, visual difficulty and difficulty in speech.

Stroke

Stroke refers to acute neurologic deficit or injury caused by impairment in the blood flow to the brain.

Etiology

Transient cerebral ischemia due to embolism. Ischemia may be caused by (a) Rheumatic heart disease (b) Mitral value disease (c) Infective endocarditis (d) Cardiac arrhythmia and (e) Neural thrombi complicating myocardial infarction.

Clinical Manifestation

The onset is abrupt without warning and recovery occurs rapidly within few minutes. Depending on the site of the brain involved in ischemia, a wide variety of neurologic signs and symptoms can be observed. When the vertebrobasilar arterial system is involved short episodes of dizziness, diplopia, dysarthria, facial paresthesia and headache are observed.

Stroke may be clinically categorized as follows:

Transient ischemic attack:
  i. It is a reversible neurologic deficit lasting for few minutes to twenty-four hours
  ii. Dizziness, diplopia, facial paresthesia, disturbance in speech and headache are symptoms when vertebrobasilar arterial system is involved
  iii. Ischemia in contralateral frontal lobe leads to short episodes of arms and hand weaknesses.

Stroke in evolution:
Stroke in evolution refers to a condition in which symptoms of cerebral ischemia become worse while the patient is under observation. It may be due to propagation of a thrombus in the carotid artery.

Completed stroke:
Completed stroke develops when clot blocks a cerebral vessel. The symptoms include aphasia, hemiplegia and defects involving cranial nerves V, VII, IX, and X.

Management

a. Correction of etiological and immediate pathological problem like embolism
b. Good results are obtained by use of aspirin
c. Control of hypertension and coagulopathy
d. Anticoagulant therapy with heparin or coumadin is often used
e. Vascular surgical endarterectomy if transient ischemic attack (TIA) is caused by carotid stenosis.

Orodental Considerations

In patients prone to stroke following precautions should be taken:
a. A complete medical history
b. Complete blood examination specially BT and CT, as patient may be taking anticoagulants and may excessively bleed during procedures
c. Consult patient's treating physician
d. Xerostomia may be a side effect of the medicines, hence proper oral hygiene, frequent topical fluoride application and dental checkup are important
e. Poor oral hygiene is a significant problem in poststroke patients. Due to paralysis, patients are physically unable to brush their teeth. Dental surgeon should help in maintaining proper oral hygiene
f. Patients with removable dental prostheses face difficulty after stroke if V, VII and IX cranial nerves are involved. Cheek-biting and accumulation of food in buccal sulci can be reduced by adding large buccal flange to the lower denture
g. Lengthy appointments should be avoided
h. Careful history taking and checking of blood pressure prior to dental treatment is necessary.

EPILEPSY

Epilepsy refers to neurologic disorder characterized by brain dysfunction due to abnormal, recurrent excessive neuronal discharges. This results in sensory and motor abnormalities and loss of consciousness.

Clinical Features

Men and women are equally affected. The clinical manifestations of epilepsy can be classified into following phases.

Tonic Phase

Tonic phase begins with aura. Aura is characterized by epigastric discomfort, hallucination of vision, smell or hearing. The aura is followed by unconsciousness and spasm of tonic muscles. Patient is unable to breathe due to spasm of respiratory muscles and becomes cyanotic.

Clonic Phase

Clonic phase consists of tongue biting, convulsive jerky movements and incontinence.

Postictal Phase

This phase is characterized by headache, lethargy, confusion and deep sleep.

Status Epilepticus

Status epilepticus is a severe form of epilepsy characterized by series of seizures that follow each other before the patient gains consciousness.

Petit Mal Seizure

This type of epileptic seizures occur in children and disappear during the second decade of life. The seizures lasts for seconds and occur without aura and little clonic or tonic phase.

Treatment

The treatment includes administration of anticonvulsant drugs such as phenytoin, carbamazepine, benzodiazepines, phenobarbital and valproic acid.

Dental Considerations

a. Proper medical history will indicate the type of seizures and their management.
b. Patients with epilepsy must be treated in the room where other patients are not observing.
c. If the patient has seizures change the line of treatment.
d. Never use removable appliances, always use fixed appliances.
e. Gingival overgrowth may be seen in patients taking phenytoin (anticonvulsant). First interdental papillae are affected. The papillae are firm, pink, and covered with normal mucosa. Careful proper oral hygiene can prevent gingival overgrowth upto some extent. Proper oral hygiene and gingival curettage of each patient taking anticonvulsant therapy should be done.
f. If oral hygiene is neglected gingivectomy may be required. After gingivectomy proper oral hygiene must be observed otherwise gingival overgrowth may recover.
g. Before dental treatment there is no need for increasing the dose of anticonvulsant drug.
h. Routine sedation is contraindicated in epilepsy patients.
i. Patient on anticonvulsant drug such as phenytoin are subjected to gingival hyperplasia. Such patients should be referred for oral hygiene instruction and gingival curettage.
j. Patients with gross gingival enlargement may require gingivectomy.
k. Routine dental treatment can be carried out in controlled epileptic patients without any change in normal treatment.
l. There is no requirement for increasing the dose of anticonvulsant drug and sedation prior to dental treatment.

Cavernous Sinus Thrombosis (CST)

CST is mostly secondary to dental, nasal or ocular infections. It is rare but usually fatal. Infections from maxillary teeth may spread to cavernous sinus.

Clinical Manifestations

Exophthalmos, periorbital edema, retinal vein thrombosis, involvement of ophthalmic nerve leading to ptosis, dilated pupils and lack to corneal reflexes.

Treatment

Immediate heavy antibiotics and removal of etiology.

BIBLIOGRAPHY

1. Arahata K. Muscular dystrophy. Neuropathology Sep; 20 Suppl 2000;S34-41.
2. Browne TR, Holmes GL. Epilepsy. N Engl J Med 2001; 344(15):1145-51.
3. Gilroy J. Basic neurology. 3rd ed. New York. McGraw-Hill 2000.
4. Urtizberea JA. Therapies in muscular dystrophy. Current concepts and future prospects. Eur Neurol 2000;43(3):127-32.
5. Van der Meche FG, Aan Doorn PA, Meulstee J, et al. Diagnostic and classification criteria for the Guillain-Barre syndrome. Eur Neurol 2001;45(3):133-9.
6. Victor M, Ropper AH. Adams and Victor's principles of neurology. 7th ed. New York. McGraw-Hill 2001.
7. Wolf PA, Clagett GP, Easton JD, et al. Preventing ischemic stroke in patients with prior stroke and TIA. A statement for healthcare professionals from the stroke council of the American Heart Association. Stroke 1999;30:1991-4.

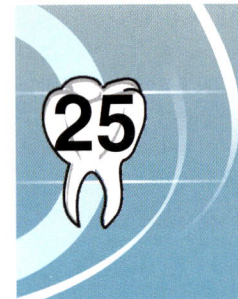

Diabetes Mellitus and Its Oral Manifestations

INTRODUCTION

Diabetes mellitus is a metabolic condition which affect multiple organs. In this oral cavity is also frequently affected. Diabetes mellitus is a chronic metabolic disorder in which metabolism of carbohydrates, proteins and lipids is disregulated. It is caused by an absolute or relative deficiency of insulin and the primary feature of this disorder is elevation of blood glucose levels (hyperglycemia). It results from either a defect in insulin secretion from the pancreas, a change in insulin action or both. It is characterized by hyperglycemia, glycosuria, ketoacidosis and water and electrolyte loss. Long-term complications of disease involve eyes, kidneys, blood vessels and nerves. The complications are responsible for the high degree of morbidity and mortality of the diabetic population.

ETIOLOGICAL CLASSIFICATION OF DIABETES

Primary Diabetes

A. Type I or insulin-dependent diabetes mellitus, juvenile diabetes (IDDM)
B. Type II or Non-insulin dependent diabetes mellitus (NIDDM), adult onset diabetes.
   a. Non-obese NIDDM
   b. Obese NIDDM
   c. Maturity onset diabetes of youth
C. Gestational diabetes (pregnancy diabetes)

Secondary Diabetes or Other Types of Diabetes

A. Pancreatic Disease or Injuries

a. After total or partial pancreatectomy
b. Pancreatitis, hemochromatosis
c. Tumor or wound
d. Cystic fibrosis
e. Pancreatic ulcer

B. Endocrine Disease

a. Hypersomatotropism (acromegaly)
b. Hyperthyroidism
c. Hyperadrenalism (Cushing's syndrome, Conn's syndrome, pheochromocytoma)
d. Glucagonoma

C. Genetic Defects Affecting Beta Cell Function or Insulin Action

D. Drug-induced Diabetes

a. Corticosteroids
b. Thiazides
c. Phenytoin

E. Other Genetic Syndromes (With Associated Diabetes)

F. Infectious (Congenital Rubella, Cytomegalovirus Infection)

Impaired Glucose Tolerance (IGT) and Impaired Fasting Glucose (IFG)

IGT and IFG are not clinical entities, but are risk factors for future diabetes. They represent metabolic states lying between diabetes and normoglycemia. Persons with increased IFG have increased fasting blood glucose levels but have normal levels after taking food. Persons with IGT are normoglycemic but become hyperglycemic after heavy dose of glucose.

ETIOLOGY OF DIABETES

Type 1 Diabetes (IDDM)

Etiological factors are as follows:

Genetic

Histocompatibility Leukocyte Antigen (HLA) present on short arm of chromosome 6 is associated with Type 1 diabetes.

Viruses

Viruses related to onset of IDDM are mumps, rubella, coxsackie B_4 and cytomegalovirus.

Stress

Stress may progress development of Type 1 Diabetes.

Type 2 Diabetes (NIDDM)

Diet

Overeating when combined with obesity and under activity is associated with development of Type 2 diabetes.

Age

Age is an important risk factor for type 2 diabetes. NIDDM affects older age group, i.e. usually above 35 years of age.

CLINICAL FEATURES

Type 1 Diabetes Mellitus

a. Classical symptoms of diabetes mellitus are polydipsia (increased thirst), polyuria (increased urination) and polyphagia (increased appetite).
b. Rapid weight loss
c. Salt and water depletion
d. Loss of skin turgor,
e. Tachycardia and hypotension
f. Increased susceptibility to infection
g. Severe hyperglycemia and ketoacidosis

Type 2 Diabetes Mellitus

a. Most of the patients are asymptomatic but may complain of chronic fatigue and malaise.
b. Patients are overweight with abdominal obesity.
c. Paresthesia, pain and muscle weakness in legs.
d. Hypertension is present in 50% of the patient
e. Hyperlipidemia
f. Diminished or inpalpable pulse in the feet.
g. Trophic brownish scars on the shins.

COMPLICATIONS OF DIABETES

(A) Diabetic Retinopathy

There may be progressive color blindness to total blindness due to involvement of retina in diabetes. The clinical features of diabetic retinopathy are as follows:
a. Retinal hemorrhages
b. Vitreous hemorrhages
c. Hard and soft exudates
d. Microaneurysms
e. Intraretinal microvascular abnormalities

(B) Diabetic Neuropathy

Sensory: Loss of sensation in extremities, impotence, other sensory dysfunction.

Peripheral neuropathy is the most common complication in diabetes. Symptoms include paresthesia in the feet, pain in lower limbs, and burning sensation in soles of feet.

Autonomic neuropathy is characterized by gastrointestinal tract disturbances such as dysphagia, abdominal fullness, delayed gastric emptying and constipation. Genitourinary symptoms include difficulty in micturition and recurrent bladder infection.

(C) Macrovascular Disease (Accelerated Atherosclerosis)

Atherosclerosis is a common long-term complication in diabetes. It may lead to diabetic foot (gangrenous infection of the feet). Coronary artery disease and stroke are also complications of atherosclerosis in diabetics.

(D) Diabetic Coma

Diabetic coma is a state of unconsciousness that develops in severe and inadequately treated case of diabetes mellitus or after extreme hypoglycemia. Diabetic coma of hyperglycemia develops in association with one of the following conditions:
a. Genitourinary tract infection
b. Emotional upsets
c. Dehydration
d. Failure to take dose of insulin

Diabetic coma following extreme hypoglycemia is caused due to the following:
a. Insulin overdose
b. Decreased food intake
c. Increased exercise

Symptoms that precede the onset of coma are as follows:
a. Sweating

b. Headache
c. Convulsions
d. Diplopia
e. Palpitations
f. Anxiousness
g. Hunger

(E) Diabetic Nephropathy (Renal Failure)

Diabetic nephropathy is a major cause of mortality in diabetics and affects 50% of the patients with Type 1 diabetes. It is the most common cause of end-stage renal failure.

(F) Alterations in Wound Healing

(G) Cardiovascular (Coronary artery disease)

(H) Cerebrovascular (Stroke)

ORAL MANIFESTATIONS

Oral manifestations of diabetes mellitus are as follows:
1. The specific oral manifestation associated with diabetes is median rhomboid glossitis. It is characterized by well-circumscribed, non-ulcerated, smooth red area on the middle third of the tongue.
2. Increased incidence of gingivitis
3. Periodontal disease involving alveolar bone loss
4. Delayed wound healing
5. Dry socket after tooth extraction
6. Burning sensation of the oral mucosa
7. Increased incidence of oral candidiasis
8. Coated tongue and cracked lips
9. Acetone breath due to excretion of ketone bodies through lungs
10. Rarely, xanthomas may occur intraorally and on the face of patient with diabetes mellitus.
11. Painful burning sensation in the tongue
12. Taste dysfunction may also occur in diabetes mellitus.
13. White patch on lips-about 14 percent of patients with uncontrolled diabeties mellitus of long duration have white patch on the lips (Fig. 25.1).

TREATMENT (MANAGEMENT)

Main aim is to achieve normal or close to normal blood sugar and prevention of diabetic complications. Diet, exercise, weight control and medications are the mainstays of management.

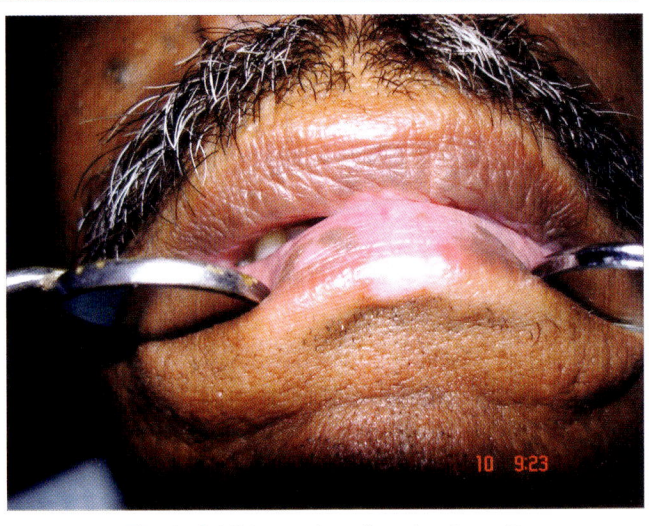

Fig. 25.1: White patch on lips of patient with uncontrolled diabeties of long duration

Type 1 Diabetes (IDDM)

Individuals with type 1 diabetes mellitus require treatment with insulin. Twice daily administration of a short acting and intermediate acting insulin is given in combination before breakfast and the evening meal.

Type 2 Diabetes (NIDDM)

Patients with NIDDM, who are obese require dietary control towards a balanced calorie intake and exercise leading to weight loss. If dietary management is ineffective, hypoglycemic drugs are prescribed. These drugs includes sulphonyl ureas, biguanides, thiazolidinediones and alpha-glucosidase inhibitors.

ORAL DISEASES IN DIABETES

Oral manifestations and oral diseases in diabetes are as follows:
1. Burning mouth syndrome.
2. Increased incidence of infection
3. Enlargement of parotid glands
4. Xerostomia—usually more from medication than the diabetes itself
5. Increased incidence of caries due to xerostomia and increased gingival crevicular fluid glucose levels.
6. If the sugar intake is reduced then the caries rate may be reduced.

Periodontal Health and Diabetes

Diabetes has following affects on periodontal health:
1. More periodontal diseases in diabetics

2. Increased gingival inflammation
3. Three times more periodontal attachment loss and alveolar bone loss
4. Increased prevalence and severity of periodontitis
5. Increased progression of bone loss and attachment loss
6. Delayed healing after periodontal surgery
7. Increased tissue destruction and diminished repair potential
8. Changes in function of host defense cells such as PMNs, monocytes, and macrophages. PMN adherence, chemotaxis and phagocytosis are impaired.

DENTAL MANAGEMENT OF DIABETIC PATIENT

The dental surgeon must have a clear understanding of each diabetic patient's blood sugar level before starting treatment. If it is too much it should be controlled before starting treatment:

1. Appointments should be of short duration and in the morning.
2. Patients should be encouraged to maintain their good oral hygiene and standard treatment regimens.
3. Patients with type 1 diabetes are more prone to develop glucose imbalance during treatment
4. Glucose drinks should be available in dental clinic in case patient complains of or show symptoms of hypoglycemia.
5. Local anesthetics without epinephrine should be used in dental surgical procedures.
6. After extractions, sockets should be sutured to aid in hemostasis.
7. If dental treatment is planned under general anesthesia, physician's advice should be taken.
8. Complicated oral surgery procedures except in dental emergencies should be avoided in patients with uncontrolled diabetes.
9. During immediate emergency, simple surgical drainage of acutely inflamed tissues and antibiotic administration is preferred. Further treatment can be carried out on blood glucose stabilization.
10. All types of dental treatment can be safely performed on controlled diabetic patient.

Diabetic Emergencies in the Dental Clinic

The most common diabetic emergency in dental clinic is hypoglycemia, which is a potentially life-threatening complication. Signs and symptoms are as follows:
a. Confusion
b. Excessive sweating
c. Tremors
d. Anxiety
e. Agitation
f. Dizziness
g. Tingling
h. Numbness
i. Tachycardia

Severe hypoglycemia may result in seizures or loss of consciousness.

Management of Emergency

a. Blood sugar level should be at once checked by a glucometer
b. If glucometer is not available then it should be presumed hypoglycemic condition
c. About 15 gm of glucose or sugar should be at once given.
d. If patient is not is a position to take orally than IV drip of 25 to 50 ml of 50% dextrose solution (D50) or 1 mg of glucagon can be given intravenously. In place of IV drip, 1 mg of glucagon can be given subcutaneously or IM injected anywhere in the body site. Usually signs and symptoms of hypoglycemia should disappear in 10 to 15 minutes. After recovery patient be kept under observation for ½ to 1 hour. Before releaving patient blood glucose level should be checked by glucometer.

Hypoglycemia

Predisposing factors are:
1. No or less food intake
2. Excessive intake of antidiabetic drugs or the doses have been taken too close to each other
3. Excessive exercise before meals
4. Accidental ingestion of wrong medication.

The response of these patients to any treatment is rapid.

Treatment

When the Patient is Conscious

1. Establish adequate airway, breathing and circulation by loosening his shirt/dress near the neck and putting on the fan/air conditioners, etc. and placing the patient in the head-low–feet-up position.
2. Administer oral carbohydrates.
   – 1 to 2 teaspoons of sugar taken directly or dissolved in a glass of water.
   – Sweetened orange juice, cola beverage or chocolate bars.
   – Placement of a small amount of honey/sweet syrup in the buccal fold.

Patient should be kept under observation for approximately 1 hour after this attack before allowing him to leave the dental clinic.

When the Patient is Unconscious

1. Establish (A) Airway, (B) Breathing, (C) Circulation
2. Administer parenteral carbohydrate.
   - Inj. Glucagon 1 mg IM
   - 50 ml of dextrose in 50% concentration.
3. 0.5 mg dose of a 1:1000 concentration of epinephrine may be administered subcutaneously or intramuscularly and repeated every 15 minutes as needed, if dextroses and glucagons are not available. Epinephrine increases blood glucose levels.
4. In the absence of parenteral route, a thick paste of concentrated glucose can be used with a degree of safety, i.e. strips of sweet chewing gum, jelly sweets or a strip of jaggery can be placed in the buccal fold of the patient. This makes the blood sugar level rise slowly during which basic life support is continued.

Prevention

Following precautions will help in the prevention of complications in the clinic:
1. Ask for the latest urine sugar and blood sugar reports.
2. Rely on the blood sugar postprandial and blood sugar fasting test reports rather than blood sugar random.
3. The readings must be: 60-100 mg/100ml for BSF TEST, 100-120 mg/100 ml for BSPP test. 180 mg/100 ml for urine sugar test.
4. In case of emergencies, i.e. accidents and uncontrolled diabetes, etc. the blood sugar values can be stretched to: 100-120 mg/100 ml for BSF test, 120-150 mg/100 ml for BSPP test.
5. Standby measures must be kept ready in the dental clinic at the time of the treatment.
6. Impart specific and clear instructions to the patient before calling him for his dental appointment, i.e. his antidiabetic drugs have to be taken at their regular time and he must come on a full stomach.
7. Following medical and dental evaluation of the diabetic patient, if any doubt persists as to the patient's medical status, patient's physician must be consulted.

BIBLIOGRAPHY

1. American Academy of Periodontology. Diabetes and periodontal diseases. Position paper. J Periodontal 1999;70:935-49.
2. American Diabetes Association. Standards of medical care for patients with diabetes mellitus. Diabetes Care 1998; 21 Suppl 1:s23-31.
3. Edelman SV. Type II diabetes mellitus. Adv Intern Med 1998; 43:449-500.
4. Mandrup-Poulsen T. Recent advances—diabetes. BMJ 1998;316:1221-5.
5. Mealey BL. Diabetes mellitus. In: Rose LF, Genco RJ, Mealey BL, Cohen DW, (Ed). Periodontal medicine. Toronto, Canada: BC Decker Inc. 2000.
6. Ragini. Diabetes and Dental Treatment. ITSCDSR News 2005;(7).
7. Scheen AJ, Lefebvre PJ. Oral antidiabetic agents. A guide to selection. Drugs 1998;55:225-36.
8. UK. Prospective Diabetes Study (UKPDS) Group. Effect of intensive blood-glucose control with metformin on complications in overweight patients with type 2 diabetes (UKPDS 34). Lancet 1998;352:854-65.

Hematological Disorders

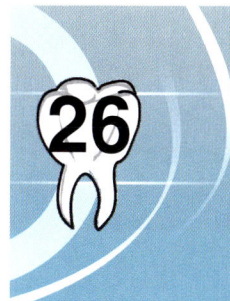

HEMATOPOIESIS

Hematopoiesis is the process of formation of cellular components of the blood from pluripotential stem cells. These cells are formed in embryonic life and persist through self-regeneration. The following hematological disorders are of interest in orodental practice.

DISORDERS OF THE WHITE BLOOD CELLS

White blood cells or leukocytes originate either from the bone marrow or lymphoid tissues. White blood cells (WBC) protect against foreign invaders like fungi, bacteria, viruses and parasites. There are five types of leukocytes. Granulocytes (neutrophils, eosinophils and basophils) and monocytes originate in the bone marrow, whereas lymphocytes are derived from lymph nodes. Peripheral blood contains approximately 4,000 to 11,000 leukocytes per cubic millimeter. Increase in absolute neutrophil count above 30,000/mm^3 is called as Leukemoid reaction.

This chapter is mainly concerned with diseases of granulocytes. Disorders of the granulocytes can be divided into following three groups:

Qualitative Disorders

These disorders result from poor functioning of the white blood cells.

Quantitative Disorders

Quantitative disorders result from abnormal number of white blood cells.

Myeloproliferative Disorders

Myeloproliferative disorders result from abnormal bone marrow cells present in peripheral blood and include myeloid metaplasia, myelofibrosis and leukemia. They are characterized by medullary and extramedullary proliferation of bone marrow constituents.

QUALITATIVE DISORDERS

Chronic Idiopathic Neutropenia

The disease is characterized by decreased production of neutrophils in the bone marrow. The disease is predominant in females.

Clinical Features

i. Most of the patients are asymptomatic.
ii. Few patients may exhibit recurrent bacterial infections including upper respiratory tract infections, bronchitis and otitis media.
iii. Oral ulcers, sinusitis and periodontal disease may also occur.

Treatment

i. Alternate day corticosteroid therapy.
ii. Antibiotics for bacterial infections.

Orodental Considerations

i. Recurring oral ulcers are also common in patients with chronic idiopathic neutropenia.
ii. The most common oral manifestation of chronic idiopathic neutropenia is severe, rapidly advancing periodontal disease.
iii. Disease is characterized by intense red gingiva with granulomatous margins, gingival recession, bone loss, mobility and loss of teeth.
iv. Recurring oral ulcers are also common in patients with chronic idiopathic neutropenia.
v. Advanced periodontal disease can be treated by repeated debridement and splinting of teeth.

Lazy Leucocyte Syndrome

Lazy leucocyte syndrome is caused due to inability of neutrophils to migrate from the bone marrow to peripheral blood. The patients are prone to infections due to severe neutropenia.

Clinical Features

i. Absolute neutrophil count is as low as 100 to 200/mm^3.
ii. Clinical features appear at 1 to 2 years of age.
iii. The common infections are stomatitis, gingivitis, bronchitis and otitis media.

Orodental Considerations

i. The early and common signs in lazy leucocyte syndrome are stomatitis and gingivitis.
ii. Disease is also associated with periodontal disease.

Chediak-Higashi Syndrome

It is a congenital disease characterized by presence of abnormal granules in renal tubular cells, nerve cells and fibroblasts due to defects in granulocytes and melanocytes. These abnormal granules result in decreased chemotactic and bactericidal activity of neutrophils.

Clinical Features

i. Hypopigmentation of skin and hair during infancy.
ii. Recurrent bacterial infections of skin and respiratory tract mainly by gram-positive bacteria such as *S. aureus* and beta-hemolytic streptococcus.
iii. Patients usually die before the age of 10 years due to recurrent infections.

Treatment

i. Infections are managed by antibiotics.
ii. Functions of neutrophils may be enhanced by ascorbate.
iii. Advanced stage of disease is treated by vincristine and prednisone therapy.

Orodental Considerations

i. The common oral findings in this syndrome are gingival and periodontal diseases.
ii. There is early loss of teeth due to caries and periodontal disease.
iii. Few patients may exhibit severe gingivitis, periodontal pockets and mobility of teeth.

QUANTITATIVE DISORDERS

Granulocytosis

Granulocytosis is characterized by elevation in number of white blood cells. It is usually associated with infections, neoplastic diseases, allergic reactions, inflammatory diseases and tissue necrosis. Stress and exercise may also increase the number of white blood cells. A constant elevation of leucocyte count with absolute neutrophil count above 30,000/mm^3 is called as Leukemoid reactions.

Cyclic Neutropenia

Cyclic neutropenia is caused by abnormality in regulation of bone marrow precursor cells leading to periodic failure of stem cells in bone marrow. The absolute neutrophil count falls below 500/mm^3. This period of neutropenia lasts for 3 to 7 days and usually follows a cycle of 21 days. The patient remains healthy between the neutropenic period as the peripheral blood is replenished with mature neutrophils.

Clinical Features

i. The disease is commonly seen in infancy or childhood.
ii. The common clinical signs are fever, pharyngitis, stomatitis and skin abscess.
iii. Some patients may exhibit lung and urinary tract infections and rectal and vaginal ulcers.

Treatment

i. Antibiotic therapy during neutropenic periods minimizes the infection.
ii. White blood cell count can be improved by recombinant colony stimulating factor.

Orodental Considerations

i. Oral mucosal ulcers and periodontal disease are the most common and major clinical manifestations of cyclic neutropenia.
ii. The oral ulcers appear as large deep scarring ulcers.
iii. Bacterial infection may result in marginal gingivitis to rapidly advancing periodontal bone loss.
iv. Routine dental procedure should be performed when absolute neutrophil count is above 2,000/mm^3.
v. Oral hygiene should be maintained and patient's oral prophylaxis should be done every two to three months.

Hematological Disorders

Agranulocytosis and Neutropenia

The term agranulocytosis refers to condition when no neutrophils are seen in peripheral blood smear. Neutropenia refers to decrease in number of neutrophils.

Neutropenia may be categorized as follows:
a. Mild neutropenia—1,000/mm^3 to 2,000/mm^3 neutrophils
b. Moderate neutropenia—500/mm^3 to 1,000/mm^3 neutrophils
c. Severe neutropenia—less than 500/mm^3 neutrophils.

Causes of Neutropenia

Decrease in neutrophil count is seen in following conditions:
  i. Deficiency of vitamin B$_{12}$ and folic acid.
 ii. Infection with viruses such as hepatitis A, HIV-1 and Epstein-Barr virus.
iii. Diseases like systemic lupus erythematosus and Felty's syndrome.
 iv. The most common cause of neutropenia is drug reaction. These drugs include cancer chemotherapeutic drugs, sulphonamides, phenothiazides, phenylbutazone, chloramphenicol, benzene and alcohol.

Clinical Features

  i. The most common complication in neutropenia is infection involving lungs, skin, urinary tract and mouth.
 ii. Acute bacterial infection by *Staphylococcus aureus*, *Klebsiella*, *Pseudomonas* and *Proteus* is most common
iii. The common sign of infection is fever.
 iv. Other manifestations include acute pharyngitis, mucosal ulcers and lymphadenopathy.

Treatment

  i. Underlying cause of neutropenia should be determined and managed.
 ii. If drugs are responsible for neutropenia, they should be stopped or alternative drugs should be prescribed.
iii. Infection should be controlled by antibiotic therapy.
 iv. Corticosteroids and cytotoxic agents increase the neutrophil count.

Orodental Considerations

  i. Severe rapidly advancing periodontal disease. In spite of neutropenia gingiva is red with granulomatous margins. Severe gingival recession, early periodontal disease and advanced bone loss, mobility, denuded roots, and teeth loss may be present in neutropenia.
 ii. The most common oral manifestation of neutropenia is ulcers of the oral mucosa, characterized as painful, large, irregular deep necrosed lesions without surrounding inflammation.
iii. There may also be pericoronitis, pulpal infections and advanced periodontal diseases.
 iv. Appropriate combinations of parenteral antibiotics should be prescribed for treatment of infections. Topical application of antibacterial mouthwash is beneficial for oral ulcers.

MYELOPROLIFERATIVE DISORDERS

Leukemia

Leukemia is a neoplastic proliferation of white blood cells found in hematopoietic tissues. The neoplastic process is characterized by differentiation and proliferation of malignantly transformed hematopoietic stem cells, resulting into suppression of normal cells. Leukemia can be categorized as either acute or chronic leukemia or by the types of cells involved.

Etiology

The etiology of leukemia is not known, but following factors increase the risk of disease:
  i. Genetic disorders such as Down, Klinefelter's and Fanconi's syndromes are associated with increased risk of leukemia.
 ii. Excessive radiations may increase the risk of leukemia.
iii. Exposure to certain chemicals such as benzene and drugs such as phenylbutazone, chloramphenicol and anticancer drugs is also associated with high incidence of leukemia.
 iv. Human T-cell leukemia viruses (HTLV-1 and HTLV-2) are suspected to be the cause of leukemia.

Acute Leukemia (AL)

Acute leukemia are malignancies of hematopoietic progenitor cells. These cells fail to mature and differentiate. Acute leukemia is characterized by presence of immature or blast cells in the circulating blood. Acute leukemias are divided into two groups: acute myelogenous leukemia (AML) and acute lymphocytic leukemia (ALL).

Clinical Features

a. ALL is usually found in children and AML occurs mostly in adults

b. Bone marrow suppression in acute leukemia leads to anemia, thrombocytopenia and decrease in normally functioning neutrophils
c. Anemia results in shortness of breath, pallor and fatigue
d. Thrombocytopenia results in petechiae, epistaxis, ecchymosis, melena, increased gingival and menstrual bleeding
e. Recurrent infection of skin, mouth, lungs, urinary tract and upper respiratory tract is frequent complication of disease
f. Leukemic cells get infiltrated into organs resulting in hepatomegaly, splenomegaly and lymphadenopathy
g. Large, irregular foul smelling oral ulcers surrounded by pale mucosa.

Treatment

a. Acute leukemia can be treated by antileukemic chemotherapeutic drugs. Chemotherapy is divided into three stages (a) Induction (b) Consolidation (c) Maintenance
b. ALL can be treated by combination of drugs such as prednisone, vincristine and daunorubicin
c. AML has worse prognosis due to toxicity of the combination of drugs used to treat AML. The common drug combination used is daunorubicin, 6-thioguanine and arabinosyl cytosine
d. Supportive treatment is provided to control bleeding, anemia and infections
e. Bone marrow transplantation can be used to treat acute leukemia. This treatment eradicates all malignant cells and replaces them with normal transplanted marrow.

Chronic Leukemia

Chronic leukemia is characterized by presence of large number of mature (well differentiated) cells in the peripheral blood, bone marrow and tissues. Chronic leukemia is divided into two major types.

Chronic granulocytic (CGL) or chronic myelocytic leukemia (CML) and chronic lymphocytic leukemia (CLL). They differ in natural history, clinical presentation, prognosis and treatment.

Chronic Granulocytic or Myelocytic Leukemia (CGL or CML)

In chronic granulocytic leukemia there is presence of large number of granulocytes in circulating blood, bone marrow and various tissues. It is closely associated with exposure to ionizing radiations and toxic chemicals.

Clinical Features

a. It occurs most frequently in individuals between 30 to 40 years of age
b. Early signs and symptoms are weakness, fatigue, dyspnea and abdominal pain
c. Thrombocytopenia causes petechiae, ecchymosis and hemorrhage
d. In late stages of disease, there may be involvement of liver, skin and lymph nodes.

Treatment

Treatment of CML or CGL is usually successful.
a. The treatment involves administration of busulfan and other alkylating agents
b. Size of enlarged spleen can be reduced by radiation therapy.

Chronic Lymphocytic Leukemia (CLL)

Chronic lymphocytic leukemia is characterized by uncontrolled proliferation and enlargement of lymphoid tissues.

Clinical Features

a. It occurs most frequently in males of 40 to 60 years of age
b. Anemia and thrombocytopenia result in pallor, dyspnea, weakness and purpura
c. Infiltration in tissues causes splenomegaly, hepatomegaly and lymphadenopathy
d. Head and neck involvement in CLL is characterized by cervical lymphadenopathy and tonsillar enlargement
e. Bacterial and viral infections are also common
f. Leukemic infiltration in last stages results in liver dysfunction, pulmonary obstruction, intestinal malabsorption and skin masses.

Treatment

a. CLL is mainly treated by alkylating agents such as chlorambucil or cyclophosphamide
b. Localized manifestations of the disease can be controlled by radiations.

Orodental Considerations in Leukemia

Oral complications are common throughout the clinical course of the disease. The mouth is a potential source of morbidity and mortality. Usually dental surgeon is first to suspect disease.

i. Leukemic infiltration and bone marrow failure in leukemia result in gingival infiltrates, oral bleeding, oral ulcers and oral infection.
ii. Thrombocytopenia and anemia result in petechiae, ecchymosis, pallor of mucosa and gingival bleeding.
iii. Oral hemorrhage may result due to decrease in number of platelets.
iv. Leukemic infiltrates may also involve palate, alveolar bone and dental pulp, which causes oral sign and symptoms due to disorders of fifth and seventh cranial nerves.
v. Oral infection is also one of the fatal complications in neutropenic leukemic patients. The most common oral infection in leukemic patient is candidiasis.
vi. Children with ALL below 5 yrs of age, who have received chemotherapy and radiation to the cranium may develop dental anomalies and craniofacial deformities. The most common anomalies are dental agenesis, microdontia, enamel dysplasia and arrested root development.
vii. Bone marrow transplant patients also exhibit oral lesions including keratotic lesions, desquamative gingivitis, atrophy and ulceration. These patients may also develop xerostomia.

ORAL ULCERS

Leukemic patients taking chemotherapy exhibit oral mucosal ulcers, which involve intraoral mucosa and lips.
a. The cause of oral ulceration is mainly recurrent Herpes simplex virus infection.
b. The ulcers are large, irregular, foul-smelling and surrounded by pale mucosa.
c. HSV oral ulcers can be treated by parenteral acyclovir administered intravenously or by mouth.
d. Oral ulcers due to bacterial infections can be treated by povidone-iodine solution, bacitracin-neomycin creams or chlorhexidine mouth washes.

MULTIPLE MYELOMA (MM)

Multiple myeloma is a malignant neoplasm of plasma cells that originates in bone marrow. It is characterized by the production of abnormal myeloma protein, kidney disease, bone lesions, hypercalcemia and hyperviscosity.

Clinical Features

a. The disease occurs most frequently in men older than 50 years of age.
b. The most common symptom is skeletal pain that is caused by bone lysis.
c. Most of the patients (more than 80%) have bone lesions that result in pathologic fractures
d. Abnormal myeloma protein coating platelets may result in clotting defects.
e. Hypercalcemia, amyloidosis and infiltration of malignant cells may result in renal failure.

Oral Manifestations

a. In about 5 to 30% of the cases of multiple myeloma jaw lesions occur, mainly in the mandible. The clinical signs and symptoms are pain, swelling, epulis formation and mobility of teeth.
b. Amyloidosis of tongue may also occur in few patients with multiple myeloma. The tongue appears enlarged with small garnet-colored enlargements.
c. Hemorrhage may result due to abnormal platelet function, abnormal coagulation and thrombocytopenia. So, before carrying out oral surgical procedures, recent platelet count, prothrombin time and bleeding time should be obtained.

Treatment

Multiple myeloma is treated by administration of alkylating agents such as cyclophosphamide or melphalan. Local symptomatic lesions can be treated by radiotherapy.

LYMPHOMA

Lymphoma are the neoplasm of lymphoid tissue involving cells of lymphoreticular or immune system such as B-lymphocytes, T-lymphocytes and monocytes. They are divided into Hodgkin's disease and non-Hodgkin's lymphoma.

Hodgkin's Disease (HD)

Hodgkin's disease is a malignant disease characterized by progressive involvement of lymphoid tissues. Etiology of disease is not known, but may be associated with infections. Viruses are possible etiological agents.

Clinical Features

i. The common clinical feature is painless enlargement of the lymph nodes.
ii. On palpation the lymphnodes are non-tender and rubbery.
iii. In older patients systemic symptoms such as malaise, fever and night sweats may occur.

iv. With the progression of disease, sign and symptoms arise due to obstruction caused by enlarged lymph-nodes such as dysphagia and ureteral obstruction.
v. A cyclic spiking fever called as Pel-Ebstein fever and generalized severe pruritus are characteristic features of Hodgkin's disease.

Treatment

Hodgkin's disease was considered to be a uniformly fatal disease. But modern diagnostic methods and treatment have given a newly diagnosed patient more than 70% chance of cure.

Hodgkin's disease can be treated by chemotherapy, radiotherapy or combination of both. Chemotherapeutic drugs include combination of nitrogen mustard, procarbazine, prednisone and vincristine.

The recommended doses of radiation is 3,500 to 4,500 cGy delivered to involved lymphnodes and contiguous areas.

The radiation can be delivered in three distinct fields (A) the mantle (B) para-aortic and (C) pelvic. The following are included in the mantle area (a) submandibular region (b) neck (c) axillae and (d) mediastimum.

Non-Hodgkin's Lymphoma

Non-Hodgkin's lymphoma (NHL) is a malignant disease arising from B or T-lymphocytes.

Clinical Features

i. It is most commonly found in patients older than 40 years of age.
ii. The common clinical feature is painless enlargement of lymphnodes.
iii. Extranodal lesions in gastrointestinal tract, skin, spleen and bone marrow are commonly found in Non-Hodgkin's lymphoma.
iv. Renal obstruction, bone marrow involvement, liver infiltration and neurologic impairment may also occur during the disease.

Treatment

Non-Hodgkin's lymphoma can be successfully treated by radiotherapy and chemotherapy. Localized NHL can be best treated by radiations between 3,000 to 4,000 cGy. The intermediate and high-grade NHL are treated by chemotherapeutic drugs including bleomycin, cyclophosphamide, prednisone and methotrexate.

Burkitt's Lymphoma (BL)

Burkitt's lymphoma is a rapidly growing tumor of jaw and abdominal lymphnodes. The disease is associated with a virus, mainly Epstein-Barr virus.

Clinical Features

i. The disease mostly affects young children.
ii. The tumor is rapidly growing and common site of involvement is jaws.
iii. Tumor may also involve kidneys or ovaries.
iv. Tumor expands rapidly and size can be doubled in 1 to 3 days.

Treatment

Burkitt's lymphoma can be managed by chemotherapy, especially cyclophosphamide. Surgical removal of large localized jaw lesion or abdominal tumor prior to chemotherapy is beneficial.

Orodental Considerations of Lymphoma

a. Extranodal lesions in Hodgkin's lymphoma may also occur in oral cavity involving tongue, palate or major salivary glands.
b. Dental abnormalities may occur due to radiotherapy administered to young children, with Hodgkin's disease. These abnormalities include hypoplasia, agenesis, blunted or thin roots.
c. Oral NHL are commonly found in immunocompromised patients, mostly on the palate. Tumor appears as slow growing, painless, soft bluish masses.
d. Paresthesia of face, major salivary gland enlargement and isolated loose teeth are also found in NHL.

DISORDERS OF RED BLOOD CELLS

POLYCYTHEMIA

Polycythemia refers to an abnormal increase in the erythrocyte count in the circulating blood along with increase in hemoglobin and hematocrit. Polycythemia is of two types—(a) Primary polycythemia or polycythemia vera and (b) secondary polycythemia or erythrocytosis.

Polycythemia Vera (PV)

Polycythemia vera is a myeloproliferative disorder. It is a chronic form of polycythemia characterized by increase in bone marrow elements and megakaryocyte and granulocytic cells. The RBC count increases to 6 to 12 million/mm^3 with hemoglobin concentration of 18 to 24 g/dl. There is increased blood viscosity, increase in number of platelets and platelet abnormality.

Clinical Features

i. Cyanosis of face and extremities due to deoxygenated blood in cutaneous vessels.
ii. Headache, tinnitus, dizziness and pruritus.
iii. Patients with polycythemia vera exhibit thrombosis and hemorrhage in the later stages of disease.
iv. Splenomegaly may also be noted.

Oral Manifestations

i. Purplish red discoloration of tongue, cheeks and lips.
ii. Petechiae and ecchymosis on oral mucosa may be present in patients with platelet abnormalities.
iii. Gums appear red and may bleed spontaneously.

Treatment

Treatment of polycythemia vera mainly involves repeated phlebotomy. Elderly patients and patients with severe disease may be treated by myelosuppressive agents and chemotherapeutic agents.

Orodental Considerations

i. Patients with polycythemia vera may face complications during dental treatment due to chances of bleeding and thrombosis. So, complete blood count should be obtained prior to treatment.
ii. Hemoglobin should be reduced below 16 g/dl and hematocrit below 52% to prevent complications.

Secondary Polycythemia

Secondary polycythemia refers to an increase in erythropoietin production which occurs in response to hypoxia. This condition is seen in patients with congenital heart disease, renal disease and chronic pulmonary disease. It is also associated with some tumors especially lung, renal and brain carcinoma. It may also occur in people living at high altitude. There is increased blood viscosity leading to thrombosis and coagulation defects. Treatment mainly includes phlebotomy.

ANEMIA

Anemia is defined as state in which there is decrease in normal amount of circulating hemoglobin in the blood. The decrease in the hemoglobin level may be due to (a) loss of blood as in iron deficiency anemia (b) decreased production of RBCs as in pernicious anemia or (c) destruction of RBCs as in hemolytic anemia.

Anemia may also be classified according to the size (microcytic, normocytic or macrocytic) of the erythrocytes or their hemoglobin concentration (hypochromic, normochromic). The common symptoms of all anemias include (a) pallor of the skin, nail beds and palpebral conjunctiva (b) dyspnea and (c) fatigability.

Anemia due to Blood Loss

Iron-deficiency Anemia

Iron-deficiency anemia (microcytic hypochromic anemia) is the most common of all anemias. It may result due to following factors:

a. Chronic blood loss as in menstrual or menopausal bleeding, bleeding hemorrhoids or bleeding ulcer in gastrointestinal tract
b. Impaired absorption of iron as in partial or complete gastrectomy or in malabsorption syndrome
c. Inadequate dietary intake of iron.

Clinical Features

a. Pallor of skin, palpebral conjunctiva and nail beds
b. Splitting and cracking of nails
c. Weakness and dyspnea on exertion.

Oral Manifestations

a. Pallor of oral mucosa
b. Tongue becomes smooth due to atrophy of filiform or fungiform papillae
c. Dysphagia may result due to oesophageal strictures or webs
d. Painful tongue may be the presenting symptom.

Dental Considerations

a. Elective oral surgical and periodontal procedures should not be carried out in anemic patients because of risk of abnormal bleeding and impaired wound healing
b. General anesthesia should not be administered if hemoglobin is less than 10 g/dl.

Treatment

Identification of etiology and its removal. Iron supplementation should be done.

Plummer-Vinson Syndrome

Plummer-Vinson syndrome is also called as Sideropenic dysphagia and is characterized by microcytic hypochromic anemia.

Clinical Features

a. The common clinical features are dry mouth, smooth and sore tongue, angular stomatitis and concavity of nails (koilonychia) or spoon shaped nails
b. Pallor, listlessness, dyspnea and ankle edema are also present
c. Most of the patients are edentulous, they may complain of sore mouth and inability to wear dentures
d. Dysphagia may occur due to muscular degeneration of oesophagus. Patient may complain of 'spasm in the throat'
e. Pharyngeal and intraoral carcinoma are the common complications in Plummer-Vinson syndrome
f. There is atrophy of the tongue papillae but less severe than in pernicious anemia.

There are atrophic changes in the oral mucosa, the pharynx, the upper esophagus and the vulva.

Anemia due to Decreased Erythrocyte Production

Pernicious Anemia

Pernicious anemia is caused by vitamin B_{12} deficiency. It is caused due to failure of absorption of vitamin B_{12} due to atrophy of gastric mucosa resulting in lack of secretion of intrinsic factor.

Clinical Features

a. Weakness and dyspnea on slight exertion
b. Neurologic symptoms such as numbness and tingling.
c. Anorexia and fever
d. Diarrhea and loss of weight.

Oral Manifestations

a. The classic oral symptoms of pernicious anemia are glossitis and glossodynia. Tongue appears "beefy red" and inflamed with erythematous area on tips and margins
b. Erythematous macular lesions may also involve buccal and labial mucosa
c. Dysphagia and taste abnormalities
d. Secondary fungal infection of mucosa by *Candida albicans*

Treatment

Treatment includes administration of parenteral cyanocobalamin.

Folic Acid Deficiency Anemia

Deficiency of folic acid causes severe anemia. Folic acid deficiency is seen in following conditions:
  i. Patients whose diet does not include leafy vegetables.
  ii. Alcoholics and drug abusers
  iii. Patients with increased requirement of folic acid, such as pregnant women and young children.
  iv. Cancer chemotherapeutic drugs also cause folic acid deficiency.

Oral manifestations include ulcerative stomatitis, pharyngitis and angular cheilitis. Folic acid deficiency anemia is treated by administration of oral folic acid tablets. Recommended dose of folic acid for most of the patients is 1 mg/day. In patients with intestinal malabsorption, the required dose is 5 mg/day.

Aplastic Anemia

Aplastic anemia is caused due to failure of bone marrow to produce red blood cells. The etiology is unknown, but in most of the cases it is associated with chemical substances like paint solvents, benzol and chloramphenicol or exposure to excessive X-ray radiations.

Orodental Considerations

a. Infection and bleeding are two major problems faced during the treatment of patients with aplastic anemia
b. Teeth, salivary gland, periodontium and soft tissues should be thoroughly examined when diagnosis of aplastic anemia is confirmed
c. Systemic antifibrinolytic agents can be used to reduce gingival bleeding
d. Chlorhexidine mouthwash 0.12 to 0.2% in aqueous solution should be used to reduce amount of plaque and microorganisms
e. Nerve block anesthesia and intramuscular injection should be avoided because of thrombocytopenia and bleeding tendency.

Hemolytic Anemia

Hemolytic anemia occurs due to excessive destruction of red blood corpuscles. Factors responsible for destruction of erythrocytes may be classified into intracorpuscular defects and extracorpuscular factors.

Intracorpuscular Defects

a. Hereditary spherocytosis
b. Glucose-6-phosphate dehydrogenase deficiency
c. Paroxysmal nocturnal hemoglobinuria
d. Sickle-cell anemia
e. Thalassemia.

Extra Corpuscular Factors

a. Infections and toxins
b. Transfusion reactions
c. Rh factor incompatibility
d. Systemic lupus erythematosus
e. Chronic liver disease.

Oral Manifestations

i. Pallor of the tongue, soft palate and sublingual tissues.
ii. Hemolytic anemia produces jaundice which exhibits as icterus of soft palate and tissues of floor of mouth.
iii. Hyperplasia of erythroid elements of bone marrow produces characteristic appearance of dental radiograph. The trabeculae becomes more prominent, resulting in increased bone radiolucency with prominent lamellar striations.

Sickle-Cell Anemia

Sickle-cell anemia is an autosomal recessive anemia characterized by sickle shaped erythrocytes which lead to stasis and hemolysis of the red cells. The sickling of erythrocytes is due to lower oxygen tension or increased blood pH.

Clinical Features

a. Patients show underdevelopment and often die before 40 yrs of age.
b. Jaundice, pallor or cardiac failure may result due to hemolysis, stasis of blood and vasoocclusion.
c. Chronic leg ulcers, cerebral vascular thromboses, splenic infarcts, abdominal and bone pain also occur
d. Increased susceptibility to bacterial infections. Infections and hypersensitivity reactions may lead to aplastic crisis in which patient becomes severely ill, RBC production stops and hemoglobin concentration drops.

Oral Manifestations

a. Pallor of the oral mucosa
b. Delayed eruption and hypoplasia of dentition

c. Patients with sickle cell anemia are more prone to develop osteomyelitis due to hypovascularity of the bone marrow.
d. Increased radiolucency is observed in dental radiograph due to decreased number of trabeculae, especially in the alveolar bone between the roots of the teeth.

Treatment

There is no specific treatment for sickle-cell anemia except symptomatic treatment such as antibiotics for infections and analgesics.

Orodental Considerations

a. Elective dental procedures should not be carried out unless extremely necessary because of chronic anemia and slow healing.
b. The oral hygiene and dentition should be maintained healthy and free from infection, as the oral infection may lead to aplastic crisis.
c. General anesthesia should be avoided in patients with sickle cell anemia. If it is a must then physician of the patient must be consulted.

Thalassemias

Thalassemia is a group of inherited disorders of hemoglobin metabolism in which there is impaired synthesis of one or more of the polypeptide chains of globin in hemoglobin molecule.

α (Alfa)-Thalassemia

In α (alfa)-thalassemia, synthesis of α-chain of Hb is affected. In most severe cases, the red blood cells of fetus contain hemoglobin that is composed of γ (gamma)-chain only. In such condition, hemoglobin lacks oxygen carrying capacity, which may lead to fetal death.

β (Beta)-Thalassemia

In β (Beta)-thalassemia, synthesis of β-chain of hemoglobin is affected. Imbalance in β-chain production may result in hemolysis and reduced erythropoiesis.

β (Beta)-Thalassemia Major (Cooley's Anemia)

It is the most severe form of thalassemia. Hemoglobin level may reach below 2 to 3 g/dl with hematocrit less than 20. There is extensive hemolysis.

There is retarded growth and development in children. The color of skin becomes ashen grey due to combination of pallor, jaundice and hemosiderosis. Patients may also exhibit hepatomegaly, splenomegaly and cardiomegaly.

Treatment

Thalassemia is mainly treated by blood transfusions. The hemoglobin concentration should be maintained between 10 and 14 g/dl. Hypertransfusion treatment results in iron overload due to which patient may develop abnormalities in cardiac, endocrine and hepatic function. This iron overload is treated by intravenous administration of iron-chelating agents such as deferoxamine.

Oral Manifestations

a. Bimaxillary protrusion and malocclusion are common in patients with thalassemia major
b. Spacing of teeth with marked open bite
c. Prominent malar bone and short and depressed nose
d. Cranial nerve palsy may also develop due to pressure on nerves due to extramedullary hematopoiesis
e. Discoloration of teeth in β-thalassemia major patients due to high concentration of iron.

BIBLIOGRAPHY

1. Besa EL, Kim PW, Havran FL. Treatment of primary defective iron-reutilization syndrome: revisited. Ann Hematol 2000;79; 465-8.
2. Papayannopoulou T, Abkowitz J, D' Andrea A. Biology of erythropoiesis, erythroid differentiation and maturation. In: Hoffman R, Benz EJ, Shatil SJ, et al, (Ed.). Hematology: basic principles and practice. (3rd edn). New York: Churchill Livingstone; 2000; p.202.
3. Shibutani T, Gen K, Shibata M, et al. Long-Term follow up of periodontitis in a patient with Chediak- Higashi syndrome. A case report. J Periodontal 2000;71;1024-8.
4. Stock W, Hoffman R. White blood cells I: non-malignant disorders. Lancet 2000;355:1351-7.

27

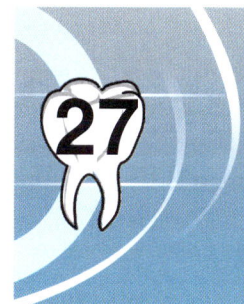

Disorders of Hemostasis and Oral Medicine

Dental surgeons are occasionally required to provide dental care to the persons with bleeding and clotting disorders due to inherited or acquired diseases. Among the inherited coagulopathies, von-Willebrand's disease (vWD) is most common. Hemophilia A, caused by coagulation factor (F) VIII deficiency is next most common followed by hemophilia B, caused by a factor IX deficiency. Acquired coagulation disorders may result from drug actions or side effects or underlying systemic disease.

NORMAL CLOTTING MECHANISM

After any injury, the blood vessels get opened, resulting in extravasation of blood. The normal clotting mechanism follows three steps:

Vascular Reaction

Vascular reaction is characterized by spasm of smooth muscles of arterioles and precapillary sphincters. Due to this, the blood flow ceases in the ensuing capillaries.

Formation of Platelet Plug

After blood vessel injury, the endothelial cells are lost. This exposes the subendothelial layer at which the platelets adhere. These platelets release adenosine diphosphate which draws further platelets and the platelets get stuck together, forming a mass of platelets known as Platelet Plug.

Coagulation of Blood

When blood clots, numerous thread like structures called fibrin are formed. Fibrin is developed from its precursor fibrinogen, which occurs naturally in the plasma. Fibrinogen is acted upon by thrombin. Thrombin is not a naturally occurring substance but its precursor prothrombin is present in normal blood.

The conversion of prothrombin to thrombin occurs when prothrombin is acted upon by (i) activated factor x (xa), (ii) activated factor v (va), (iii) phospholipids and (iv) Ca^{++} ions. All these are together called Prothrombin activator.

Coagulation of blood takes place in following three steps:

Stage I: In stage I, the procoagulants that help in coagulation of blood become active. The prothrombin activators are available at the end of this stage.

Stage II: The prothrombin activator converts prothrombin into thrombin.

Stage III: Thrombin converts the fibrinogen into fibrin and then the fibrin subsequently becomes firm in texture.

LABORATORY INVESTIGATIONS

Bleeding Time

Bleeding time provides information about platelet function and platelet deficiency. The normal bleeding time is between 3 to 7 minutes.

Clotting Time

The time taken by blood to clot is obtained by this investigation. Normal values are between 9 to 11 minutes.

Prothrombin Time

This test measures the normal levels of clotting factors I, II, V, VII, and X. The normal prothrombin time is 11 to 14 seconds.

Platelet Count

Platelet count is the clinical test used to evaluate primary hemostasis.

The normal platelet count is between 1,50,000 to 4,50,000 cells/ mm^3. Clinical hemorrhage is not observed with platelet count above 15,000 to 20,000/mm^3. Surgically related or traumatic hemorrhage occurs when platelet count is below 50,000 to 80,000/mm³.

Thrombin Clotting Time

It is used to measure the levels of fibrinogen and its conversion to fibrin. The normal level of circulating fibrinogen is 250 mg/dl. Normal range of thrombin clotting time is 9 to 13 seconds.

HEMOSTATIC DISORDERS

Coagulation Disorders

Hemophilia A

Hemophilia A is caused by deficiency of factor VIII, the antihemophilic factor. It is inherited as a sex-linked recessive trait that affects males. Females are clinically normal carriers. Severe bleeding occurs when factor VIII is less than 1% of normal. Factor (F) VIII levels between 1% to 7% of the normal lead to moderate bleeding. Mild symptoms such as prolonged bleeding after tooth extraction on severe trauma may occur when levels are between 7% and 50% of normal.

Hemophilia B

Hemophilia B is caused due to deficiency of factor IX (Christmas factor) plasma thromboplastin component. Catastrophic bleeding occurs in hemophilia B. Concentrates for treatment of hemophilia A (F VIII) and B (F IX) deficiencies are specific for each type of hemophilia. Therefore a correct diagnosis is a must for effective replacement therapy.

von-Willebrand's Disease (vWD)

von-Willebrand's disease is caused due to defect in factor VIII protein complex. Both males and females are affected. There is prolonged bleeding time but normal platelet count. The clinical features are mucosal bleeding, soft-tissue hemorrhage and bleeding from joints. von-Willebrand's disease (vWD) can be divided into following four types based on von-Willebrand Factor (vWF) subunits of varying molecular weight.
a. Type I vWD
b. Type II vWD
c. Type III vWD
d. Platelet type vWD

Factor V Deficiency

It is rare autosomal recessive disorder. The clinical symptoms of the disease may be moderate to severe. Soft tissue hemorrhage occurs occasionally. Bleeding in the joints may rarely occur.

Factor XI Deficiency

Factor XI deficiency is a mild disorder which is transmitted as an autosomal dominant trait. Bleeding may occur following trauma or major surgery.

Thrombocytopenic Disorders

Classification

Acquired Disorders

Thrombocytopenic:
- Idiopathic thrombocytopenia purpura (ITP)
- Thrombotic thrombocytopenia purpura (TTP)
- Diffuse intravascular coagulation (DIC)
- Systemic lupus erythematosus (SLE)
- Leukemia
- Hypersplenism
- Myelodysplasia.

Non-Thrombocytopenic:
- Uremia
- Liver disease
- Aspirin and other drugs
- Myeloma, myeloproliferative disorder, macroglobulinemia.

The most common acquired platelet disorders are idiopathic thrombocytopenia purpura (ITP) and thrombotic thrombocytopenia purpura (TTP).

Clinical features

i. Petechiae and purpura over limbs, chest and neck.
ii. Mucosal bleeding from oral cavity.
iii. Bleeding may also occur in gastrointestinal and genitourinary tract.
iv. Clinical features of TTP also include hemolytic anemia, neurologic abnormalities and renal dysfunction.
v. Microvascular infarcts occur in gingiva and other mucosal surfaces in most of the patients.

Treatment

Hemophilia A and B
  i. Recombinant factor VIII replacement therapy is safe and effective for the treatment of hemophilia A.
  ii. Mild to moderate hemophilia A can be treated by desmopressin acetate.
  iii. Virally inactivated factor IX concentrates and factor IX complex concentrates are used for treatment of Hemophilia B.

Congenital Disorders

Thrombocytopenic:
- Isoimmune neonatal thrombocytopenia
- May-Hegglin anomaly
- Wiskott-Aldrich syndrome.

Non-thrombocytopenic:
- von-Willebrand's disease
- Homocystinuria
- Thrombocytopathia (PF.3 Deficiency)
- Bernard-Soulier syndrome.

von-Willebrand's Disease

  i. Type I is treated by desmopressin acetate.
  ii. Type II and III require intermediate-purity factor VIII concentrates.
  iii. Bleeding in patients with platelet type von-Willebrand's disease is controlled by platelet concentrate infusions.

Postoperative bleeding in mild to moderate factor X deficiency can be managed by fresh frozen plasma.

IDENTIFICATION OF THE PATIENT WITH BLEEDING DISORDERS IN DENTAL CLINIC

Thorough medical history must be taken specially for the following:
a. Past bleeding experiences
b. Current medications
   i. Anticoagulants if any like aspirin, heparin.
   ii. Cytotoxic chemotherapy and
   iii. NSAIDs

Active medication of hepatitis, cirrhosis, kidney disease, hematologic malignancy and thrombocytopenia may cause excessive bleeding. Excessive alcohol intake may cause excessive bleeding. History of hemorrhagic diatheses, frequent epistaxis, excessive menstrual bleeding and hematuria is important.

ORAL MANIFESTATIONS OF BLEEDING DISORDERS

Vascular wall defects and platelet deficiency cause extravasation of blood into connective and epithelial tissues of the skin and mucosa. This create small pin point hemorrhages called 'petechiae'. The larger patches are called Ecchymosis. There is spontaneous gingival bleeding. The important are the following:

1. The major oral manifestation of hemophilia is oral bleeding. The locations of oral bleeding are labial frenum, tongue, buccal mucosa, gingiva and palate.
2. The bleeding is mostly caused due to traumatic injury.
3. Bleeding is also induced due to poor oral hygiene.
4. Oral hemorrhage in patients with factor VIII and factor IX deficiencies occurs in gingiva, dental pulp, tongue, lip, palate and mucosa.
5. Bleeding in the temporomandibular joint may also occur in few patients.
6. Patients with bleeding disorders may also exhibit higher caries rate and severe periodontal disease.

DENTAL MANAGEMENT OF HEMOPHILIC PATIENTS

Pain Control

a. Hypnosis and sedation by IV injection of diazepam reduce the need for LA solution but anesthetic solution with vasoconstrictor such as epinephrine should be used.
b. In severe hemophilia, during mandibular block injection there is risk of extravasation of blood into tissues of oropharyngeal areas that may produce pain, swelling, dysphagia and respiratory obstruction.
c. Block injections, if necessary, should be given after coagulation factor replacement therapy.
d. Intramuscular injections should be avoided because of the risk of hematoma formation.
e. Aspirin and other non-steroidal anti-inflammatory drugs for pain control are contraindicated, as they may inhibit platelet function.

Periodontal Treatment

a. Periodontal probing, supra gingival scaling and polishing can be done without any risk.
b. Subgingival scaling should be done with great care by fine scaler.
c. Inflamed and swollen tissues can be treated by gross debridement by ultrasonic or hand instruments, that leads to shrinkage of gingiva and thus aids in deep scaling.

d. Root planing should be performed in one quadrant per day, preferably per week to reduce bleeding.
e. Local pressure and antifibrinolytic oral rinses can be used to control bleeding.

Pedodontic Therapy

The child patient with bleeding disorder may complain of spontaneous continuous bleeding from exfoliating primary teeth. The following treatment modalities may be used in such patients:
a. Administration of plasma products for hemorrhage control.
b. Deciduous tooth should be extracted by gradual curettage or with rubber band which gradually pushs the tooth out.
c. Topical fluoride application and pit and fissure sealant should be used to avoid pulpal exposure and extraction of teeth.

Prosthodontic and Restorative Treatment

a. Rubber dam should be used to avoid laceration of soft tissue by high-speed rotating instruments and ecchymosis or hematoma formation by evacuators or saliva ejectors.
b. Tooth clamp should be carefully selected to avoid gingival trauma.
c. Denture should be carefully adjusted during post insertion to minimize trauma.

Endodontic Treatment

a. Endodontic therapy can be carried without any risk in patients with severe bleeding disorder.
b. Instrumentation and filling should not extend beyond the apex.
c. Hemostasis in the apical area can be provided by administration of epinephrine by the tip of the paper point through root canal.

Orthodontic Treatment

a. Orthodontic bands, wires and brackets should be carefully used to avoid mucosal laceration.
b. Fixed orthodontic appliances are preferred over removable orthodontic appliances as the latter may cause bleeding from chronic tissue irritation.
c. Use of extraoral force and short treatment durations decrease the risk of bleeding complications.

Oral Surgical Procedures

There are lot of chances of hemorrhage during and after oral surgical procedures. So following measures should be taken:
a. Replacement therapy for missing coagulation factors to levels of 50% to 100% prior to surgery, provides assurance of hemorrhage control.
b. Postoperative factor maintenance in extensive surgery may be accomplished by infusion of factor concentrates, desmopressin acetate, cryoprecipitate or fresh-frozen plasma.
c. Topical thrombin may be used at extraction site which converts fibrinogen into fibrin.
d. Absorbable gelatin sponge with intrinsic hemostatic properties can be used at surgical site.
e. Local hemostasis can be maintained by pressure, vasoconstrictors, surgical packs, sutures and absorbable hemostatic materials.
f. Antifibrinolytic drugs such as tranexamic acid and epsilon-aminocaproic acid should be used post operatively. These drugs inhibit fibrinolysis resulting in clot stabilization. To prevent postextraction bleeding in hemophiliacs oral rinse of 4.8% tranexamic acids is very effective with very few side effects.
g. Fibrin sealants (fibrin glue) are effective to control bleeding at wound or surgical sites. When used in combination with antifibrinolytics, its use has allowed reduction in factor concentrate replacement levels in hemophiliacs undergoing dental surgeries. In severe hemophiliacs the use of fibrin glue does not eliminate the need for factor concentration replacement. On simultaneous dispensing over the wound from separate syringes (a) the cryoprecipitate and (b) calcium chloride precipitate almost instantaneously to form a clear gelatinous adhesive gel.
h. Liquid diet for initial 24 to 48 hours, followed by soft diet for 1 to 2 weeks, should be instructed to protect the clot.

MANAGEMENT OF PLATELET DISORDERS

1. Thrombocytopenias are managed by transfusion of platelets at the level of 20,000/mm^3 to prevent spontaneous bleeding.
2. During oral surgical procedure, level of platelets should be maintained at 50,000/mm^3.

3. Hemorrhagic symptoms in idiopathic thrombocytopenia purpura can be managed by corticosteroids.
4. Thrombotic thrombocytopenia purpura is managed by plasma exchange therapy in combination with aspirin or dipyridamole or corticosteroids.
5. Microfibrillar collagen and antifibrinolytic drugs can be used in patients undergoing dental extractions.

Platelet Transfusion

When it is not possible to restore platelet counts to above the level of 50,000/mm^3 required for surgical hemostasis, platelet transfusions are required prior to extraction or other surgical procedures. Usually six units of platelets are infused at one time. By one unit of infusion usually 10,000 to 12,000/mm^3 are increased.

The antiplatelet activity of aspirin remains for the 8 to 10 days lifetime of the affected platelets. Hence the aspirin should be avoided for 1 to 2 weeks prior the major oral surgical procedure.

In Emergency (Unplanned) Surgery Controlling the Affect of Aspirin

Minor Oral Surgery: Adjunctive local hemostatic agents like adrenaline and tincture ferric perchlor are used to prevent postoperative oozing when aspirin therapy is in use.
Major Oral Surgery: In major emergency oral surgery 1-deamino-8-D- arginine vasopressin (DDAVP) is used to reduce the aspirin-induced prolongation of the BT and also to treat aspirin-related postoperative oozing of blood which usually require platelet infusion.

Controlling the Affect of Chemotherapy

Oral hemorrhage associated with chemotherapy in case of thrombocytopenia are managed by transfusion of HLA matched platelets and FFP along with topically applied clot promoting agents. DDAVP is also useful for the prevention and treatment of bleeding in patients having thrombocytopenia along with hematologic malignancy.

Hemophilias A and B and von-Willebrand's Disease

Procedures of Oral Surgery—Nowadays proper precautions make surgery safe. Although chances of bleeding are more in oral surgery procedures, but since 1980 due to precautionary measures the episodes of hemorrhages have reduced to only 8% even in hemophilic patients.

For outpatients to make certain the preoperative factor levels of atleast 40 to 50% of normal activity have been maintained, transfusion recommendations for replacement of missing coagulation factors to level of 50 to 100%. This will provide safety against hemorrhage control. For extensive surgery additional postoperative factor maintenance is used. Depending upon the individual patient's deficiency state infusion of factor concentrate, cryoprecipitate, FFP or DDAVP can be done.

If the postsurgical bleeding starts after 3 to 5 days it occurs due to fibrinolysis. It can be controled by local measures and by antifibrinolytics.

To maintain the circulating factor level minimum of 20% which is necessary for hemostasis during surgery and healing phases three months of replacement therapy are being used. These methods are:
a. Continuous intravenous factor infusion therapy.
b. Intermittent replacement therapy and
c. Single preoperative factor concentrate infusion along with an antifibrinolytic mouthwash.

In patient with mild to moderate hemophilia A and vWD, factor VIII levels can be sufficiently raised by DDAVP for dental extraction without transfusion.

Local Hemostatic Agents and Techniques

Local hemostatic agents and techniques include pressure, surgical packs, topical thrombin, use of absorbable hemostatic materials, vasoconstrictors, sutures and surgical stents. Surgical acrylic stents must be carefully prepared, finished and polished to avoid any type of irritation to the surgical site.

Diet Restriction

For first two days total liquid diet and then soft food for 2 weeks should be taken. This will protect the clot from chewing disturbances and provide proper time and environment for healing.

MANAGEMENT OF DISSEMINATED INTRAVASCULAR COAGULATION (DIC)

1. Initial therapy for disseminated intravascular coagulation (DIC) includes administration of intravenous heparin to prevent thrombin from acting on fibrinogen and thus preventing clot formation.
2. Underlying triggering disease or condition should be identified and treated for long-term survival.

3. Deficient coagulation factors should be replaced before emergency surgical procedure for improvement or prophylaxis of bleeding tendency of DIC.

MANAGEMENT OF DRUG-RELATED COAGULATION DISORDERS

Drug-related coagulation diseases are mostly caused due to anticoagulant medications such as dicumarol and heparin. The following treatment modalities should be undertaken to manage these coagulation disorders.

1. Dicumarol, a long-term anticoagulant has adverse effects on hemostasis, which can be completely reversed by parenteral injection of vitamin K.
2. Nonsurgical dental treatment can be successfully carried out without any change in dicumarol regimen, if prothrombin time is not above the therapeutic range and trauma is minimal.
3. During oral surgical procedure, dicumarol therapy should be discontinued at the time of surgery and reinstituted postoperatively.
4. Continuous intravenous heparin is discontinued 6 to 8 hours prior to surgery to allow surgical hemostasis. If bleeding occurs, action of heparin can be reversed by protamine sulphate.
5. Aspirin should be avoided 1 to 2 weeks prior to oral surgical procedure.
6. 1-deamino-8-D- arginine vasopressin (DDAVP) can be administered to reduce aspirin-induced prolongation of bleeding time.
7. Oral hemorrhage associated with chemotherapeutic drugs can be managed by transfusion of HLA matched platelets and fresh-frozen plasma.
8. Coagulopathy due to vitamin K deficiency can be treated by supplements with vitamin K injections.

MANAGEMENT OF DISEASE-RELATED COAGULATION DISORDERS

1. Bleeding in hepatic disease due to deficiency of vitamin-K dependent clotting factors may be reversed by vitamin K injections for 3 days.
2. Infusion of fresh frozen plasma may be required prior to dental extraction for immediate hemorrhage control.
3. Patients suffering from cirrhosis with moderate thrombocytopenia and platelet defects may be treated with DDAVP therapy.
4. In uremic patients bleeding can be controlled by dialysis.
5. Chronic abnormal bleeding in uremic patients can be managed by conjugated estrogen preparations and recombinant erythropoietin.

Patients on Anticoagulants

All nonsurgical dental treatment can be performed without any change in anticoagulant regimen, if the PT/INR is within therapeutic range. The extent of the bleeding expected is very important factor for the preparation of the patient on anticoagulants. Physician must be consulted for surgical procedures specially in high risk cardiac patients. Such patients must be hospitalized. Surgery should be performed when the prothrombin time/international normalized ratio (PT/INR) and a PTT are within the normal limit.

BIBLIOGRAPHY

1. Bodner L, Weinstein JM, Baumagartner AK. Efficacy of fibrin sealant in patients on various levels of oral anticoagulant undergoing oral surgery. Oral Surg Oral Med Oral Pathol Oral Radiol Endod 1998;86:421-4.
2. Christensen GJ. Nosebleeds may mean something much more serious: An introduction to HHT. J Am Dent Assoc 1998;129: 635-7.
3. Federici AB. Diagnosis of von Willebrand's disease. Haemophilia 1998;4:654-60.
4. George JN, Raskob GE, Shan SR. Drug-induced thrombocytopenia. A systematic review of published case reports. Ann Intern Med 1998;129:886-90.
5. Lusher J. Ingerslev J, Roberts H, et al. Clinical experience with recombinant factor VIIa. Blood Coagul Fibrinolysis 1998;9: 119-28.
6. Merry C, McMahon C, Ryan M, et al. Successful use of protease inhibitors in HIV-Infected haemophilia patients. Br J Haematol 1998;101:475-9.
7. Moake JL, Chow TW. Thrombotic thrombocytopenic purpura: Understanding a disease no longer rare. Am J Med Sci 1998;316: 105-19.
8. Patton LL. Hematologic abnormalities among HIV-infected patients. Association of significance for dentistry. Oral Surg Oral Med Oral Pathol Oral Radiol Endod 1999;88:561-7.
9. Throndson RR, Walstad WR. Use of the Argon Bean Coagulator for control of Postoperative Hemorrhage in an Anticoagulated patient, J Oral Maxillofac Surg 1999;57:1367-69.
10. Throndson RR, Walstad WR. Use of the Argon Beam Coagulator for control of Postoperative Hemorrhage in an anticoagulated patient, J Oral Maxillofac Surg 1999;57:1367-69.

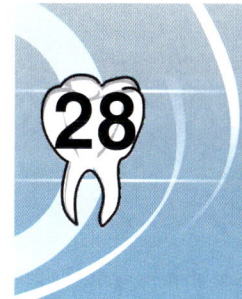

28. Infectious Diseases Related to Oral Medicine

The number of deaths due to non-sexually transmitted infectious diseases has decreased and the number of deaths due to sexually transmitted blood born infections has increased, specially in the developing and developed countries.

BACTERIAL INFECTIONS

TUBERCULOSIS (TB)

In the developed and developing countries the incidence of TB has decreased.

Signs and Symptoms

The following are seen in pulmonary tuberculosis:
1. Production of cough for more than 3 weeks.
2. Mild fever—specially in night
3. Night sweating
4. Chills—occasionally
5. Fatigue

Predisposing Factors

1. HIV infections
2. Closeness to infectious patients
3. Alcoholics
4. Poverty with congested and unhygienic living conditions and habits

Oral Manifestations and Considerations

Oral manifestations appear only in about 3% of the patients. Tuberculous lesions can be seen in oral tissues and lymph nodes. Oral lesions can be seen in the soft tissues, supporting bone, extraction socket, tongue and floor of the mouth. The risk of TB infection from patients to the dental care providers (DCP) and vice versa has very much reduced due to the precautions taken by the DCP.

SEXUALLY TRANSMITTED INFECTIONS

The terms sexually transmitted infections or sexually transmitted diseases (STD) are used to describe those infections which are exclusively transmitted through sexual contact. The infectious material gets transmitted due to deep contact and friction between skin and mucosa and transfer of oral and genital secretions during sexual intercourse.

Sexually transmitted infections are of concern to dental surgeon because of their oral manifestations and risk of their blood borne transmission from infected patient to dental care providers.

BLOOD BORNE INFECTIONS

The term blood borne infections is used for following contexts:
A. Sexually transmissible infections acquired by intravenous or percutaneous routes.
B. Infections resulting from transfusion of blood or blood products.
C. Infections transmitted due to accidental puncture of skin by a needle or other instruments contaminated with infected blood.
D. Infections secondary to invasive procedures involving tissues that are naturally colonized by bacterial flora.

The two major categories of sexually transmitted and blood borne infections that are of particular interest to the dental surgeon are described in this chapter: (a) The bacterial and chlamydial STDs and (b) viral STDs.

BACTERIAL AND CHLAMYDIAL INFECTIONS

GONORRHEA

Gonorrhea is caused by gram-negative bacteria *Neisseria gonorrheae*. Initial infection occurs on genitourinary, rectal and oropharyngeal mucosal surfaces.

Clinical Features

a. The main presenting symptom of gonorrhea is profuse purulent urethral discharge, which responds readily to appropriate antibiotic therapy.
b. Disease if not treated may lead to inflammation of periurethral glands, prostatitis and epididymitis in the males and periurethral inflammation, salpingitis or pelvic inflammatory disease in females.

Treatment

The treatment of gonorrhea includes administration of single dose of the broad spectrum cephalosporin antibiotic, ceftriaxone 125 to 250 mg intramuscularly plus doxycycline 100 mg orally twice a day for seven days or intramuscular administration of fluorinated quinolones (e.g., ciprofloxacin) plus doxycycline.

Oropharyngeal Manifestations of Gonorrhea

Pharyngeal Gonorrhea

Pharyngeal gonorrhea is characterized by sore throat and exudative pharyngitis. It is usually caused due to orogenital contact, but may also be due to autoinoculation and mouth-to-mouth contact.

Pharyngeal gonorrhea can be treated by single dose of ceftriaxone 125 mg intramuscularly or a single dose of ciprofloxacin 500 mg.

Gonococcal Stomatitis

Gonococcal stomatitis is a rare oral manifestation of gonorrhea. It is characterized by isolated mucosal ulcers, gingivitis and membranous gingivostomatitis.

CHLAMYDIAL INFECTIONS

Chlamydia trachomatis is one of the species of the genus chlamydia that is associated with sexually transmitted disease. It causes non-gonococcal urethritis and post-gonococcal urethritis. Most of the infections with *C. trachomatis* are asymptomatic. Complications of chlamydial infections include Reiter's disease and pelvic inflammatory diseases.

Reiter's disease is characterized by arthritis, conjunctivitis, balanitis and thickening of skin of soles of the hands and feet. There may also be oral ulcers and psoriasiform lesions.

Dental Treatment

Oropharyngeal secretions of patients with Reiter's disease are not infectious, whether oral lesions are present or not so, dental surgeon can carry out oral and dental procedures without risk.

SYPHILIS

Syphilis is a chronic infectious systemic disease caused by the spirochaete *Treponema pallidum*. Syphilis may be categorized into (a) acquired syphilis and (b) congenital syphilis. Majority of syphilitic infections are acquired by sexual contact in adult life, which are referred to as acquired syphilis. Congenital syphilis is caused by transmission of infection from mother to child in utero. Acquired syphilis can be again classified into (a) primary, (b) secondary and (c) tertiary syphilis.

Clinical Features of Acquired Syphilis

Primary Syphilis

i. The initial manifestation of the disease is slightly raised, ulcerated, firm plaque known as chancre which occurs mostly on genitalia.
ii. The regional lymph nodes become firm, enlarged and non-tender.

Secondary Syphilis

i. The secondary lesions appear within 3 to 6 weeks after the primary lesion.
ii. These lesions occur on mucous membrane and moist skin areas and are of three types: Mucous patch, split papule and condylomata.

Tertiary Syphilis

i. The characteristic lesion of tertiary syphilis is gumma, a chronic destructive granulomatous process occurring anywhere in the body.
ii. There is involvement of cardiovascular and nervous system leading to serious damage.

Clinical Features of Congenital Syphilis

i. Initial manifestations of congenital syphilis appear within the first 2 years of life characterized by rhinitis, chronic nasal discharge, maculopapular eruption and loss of weight.
ii. Mucocutaneous lesions including bullae, vesicles, superficial desquamation and mucous patches also appear.

iii. Late manifestations of congenital syphilis develop after 2 years of age and are characterized by interstitial keratitis and vascularization of cornea, arthropathy and gummatous destruction of palate and nasal septum.

Treatment

Treatment of syphilis includes administration of long acting penicillin, benzathine penicillin, aqueous crystalline penicillin, tetracycline, and erythromycin.

Oral and Facial Manifestations of Syphilis

Primary Syphilis

i. The oral lesion of primary syphilis is chancre, which occurs on oral mucosa, tongue, lips, soft palate and gingiva.
ii. Intraoral chancres are usually painful due to secondary infection and are covered with grayish white film.
iii. Chancre on the lips have brown-crusted appearance and may occur as multiple lesions.

Secondary Syphilis

The oral lesions of secondary syphilis are mucous patches, split papules and condylomata lata.

Mucous patches:
i. Syphilitic mucous patches are found on tongue, buccal mucosa, lips and the tonsillar and pharyngeal regions.
ii. They are highly infectious lesions of syphilis and appear as slightly raised, grayish white lesion surrounded by an erythematous base.
iii. They are often painless but may be moderately painful when they occur on movable tissues.

Split papules:
i. They are raised papular lesions at the commissures of the lips that split to separate upper lip portion of the papule from lower lip portion.
ii. They may also appear on the dorsum of the tongue.

Condylomata:
i. They are flat, silver gray, wart-like pustules having an ulcerating surface.
ii. They are usually painless.

Tertiary Syphilis

i. The characteristic oral lesion of tertiary syphilis is gumma, that occurs most frequently on the palate and tongue.
ii. Gumma may also involve salivary glands and facial and jaw bones.
iii. Severe neuralgic pain in head and neck region may occur due to involvement of nervous system.
iii. There may be loss of taste and spontaneous necrosis of the alveolar bone.
iv. Painless ulcerations of the palate and nasal septum may rarely occur.

Congenital Syphilis

Syphilitic rhagades and postrhagadic scars:
i. Syphilitic rhagades are cracks or fissures occurring at mucocutaneous junction. They are most prominent on the lower lip near the angle of the mouth.
ii. Postrhagadic scars are linear lesions that occur around the oral orifice. They result from diffuse syphilitic involvement of the skin in these areas from third to seventh weeks after birth.

Changes in the teeth:
i. There may be abnormalities in color, size and shape of the deciduous dentition with retarded root resorption.
ii. Dental hypoplasia in congenital syphilis affects the permanent incisors, cuspids and first molars as they are formed during the period of acute syphilitic infection.
iii. "Screw driver" and "peg-shaped" incisors are found in congenital syphilis, which are produced due to constriction of crown towards the incisal edge.
iv. Molars are characterized by positioning of the cusp towards the central portion of the crown, known as "mulberry molar".

Dentofacial abnormalities:
i. The most frequent dentofacial change in congenital syphilis is malocclusion and open bite.
ii. There may be frontal bossing, saddled nose and lack of development of premaxilla.

GRANULOMA INGUINALE

It is an infectious granuloma caused by a gram-negative bacterium, Donovania granulomatis. Donovan bodies are found in cytological examination of granuloma inguinale. It is chronic, slowly progressive, mild contagious disease found in the inguinal and anogenital regions.

Clinical Features

a. The primary lesions begin as small papule that ulcerates and gives rise to velvety, granulating, spreading ulcers of inguinal and anogenital regions.

b. Secondary lesions involve mouth, lips, throat, face, liver and thorax.

Oral Manifestations

a. Lesions may appear on lips characterized by extensive superficial ulceration with a well-defined elevated granulomatous margin.
b. Necrotic or granulomatous ulcers, or friable granular areas may also occur in oral cavity.

LYMPHOGRANULOMA VENEREUM

Lymphogranuloma venereum is caused by *Chlamydia trachomatis*, and is characterized by regional lymphadenitis.

Clinical Features

a. In males, there is firm tender enlargement of the inguinal lymph nodes, with redden overlying skin and multiple fistulas.
b. In females pararectal glands are involved. There is marked scarring and local edema secondary to suppurative lymphadenitis.

Oral Manifestations

a. Oral lesions mainly involve the tongue and appear as small, slightly painful, superficial ulcerations with non-indurated borders.
b. Other common symptoms are dysphagia, red soft palate, and small red granulomatous lesions accompanied by regional lymphadenopathy.

VIRAL INFECTIONS

HERPES SIMPLEX VIRUS INFECTIONS

Acute Ulcerative Herpetic Gingivostomatitis

Herpes simplex infection in children is characterized by ulcerative gingivostomatitis and sore mouth. It is a self-limiting infection with primary lesions and subsequent manifestations of recurrent infections restricted to oral cavity.

Oropharyngeal Herpes Simplex Virus Infection

Primary oropharyngeal herpes infection is caused due to either HSV-1 or HSV-2 which are acquired by orogenital contact with an infected individual.

Clinical Features

i. Acute gingivostomatitis
ii. Pharyngitis
iii. Perioral vesicular rash
iv. Fever, malaise and muscle pain

Treatment

Treatment includes oral administration of acyclovir 400 mg five times daily for 5 days.

EPSTEIN-BARR VIRUS INFECTIONS

Initial infection with Epstein-Barr virus (EBV) is usually acquired as a mild, nonspecific illness or asymptomatically in childhood. EBV may occur as a blood borne infection following blood transfusion or tissue transplantation. EBV infection is mostly associated with infectious mononucleosis.

Infectious Mononucleosis

It is a self-limiting, mild to severely debilitating condition characterized by fever, malaise, pharyngitis and lymphadenopathy.

Clinical Features

i. Sore throat accompanied by fever and fatiguability
ii. Enlarged palatine tonsils and anterior and posterior cervical lymph nodes.
iii. Nausea, vomiting or diarrhea
iv. Oral ulcerations and petechial hemorrhages

Treatment

Infectious mononucleosis is mainly treated by supportive therapy. EBV infection can be treated by acyclovir as well as ganciclovir and alpha interferon.

ORAL CYTOMEGALOVIRUS INFECTION

The majority of infections with cytomegalovirus (CMV) are symptomatic, but may be accompanied by severe illness with neurologic abnormalities, hepatosplenomegaly, jaundice, petechial hemorrhages and chorioretinitis.

Oral infections with CMV are observed in salivary glands, gingiva, non-keratinized oral mucosa and bone. CMV is also an etiological agent in oral ulcers, gingival hyperplasia, acute necrotizing ulcerative gingivitis (ANUG) and granulation tissue.

MOLLUSCUM CONTAGIOSUM (MCV) INFECTION

Molluscum contagiosum infection is characterized by multiple or isolated, small waxy papules occurring on the skin of lower abdomen, inner thighs and external genitalia. Most of the lesions of molluscum contagiosum resolve spontaneously in 1 to 2 months. Lesions are mostly asymptomatic.

Intraoral lesions are characterized by papillary eruptive lesions on the lips, cheeks and other regions in the oral cavity.

Treatment includes curettage, cryotherapy or topical application of caustics and irritants such as phenol, podophyllin, cantharidin and trichloroacetic acid.

ORAL CONDYLOMA ACUMINATUM

Condyloma acuminatum is characterized by small keratotic warts occurring alone or in clusters on the oral mucosa and is associated with human papilloma virus infections. Condyloma acuminatum of the oral cavity may involve cheeks, lips, gingiva, tongue, hard palate and floor of the mouth.

Treatment includes surgical excision, cryotherapy or carbon dioxide laser therapy and topical podophyllin.

Viral Infections

Currently there are six viral agents A, B, C, D, E and G which cause hepatits and new information is emerging to expand this list (Table 28.1).

Hepatitis C Virus (HCV)

HCV is a single—stranded positive-sense ribonucleic acid (RNA) virus.

Risk to Dental Health Care Workers (DHCW)

1. There is a risk for exposure to patient blood and possible subsequent infection from blood borne diseases.
2. Percutaneous accidental injuries from infected sharps (needles and knife blades) have been associated with resulting onset of both hepatitis B and C. HCV infected blood transfusion can readily cause infection. HCV infections carries the increased possibility of chronic liver disease. The virus infection can cause hepatic cirrhosis and hepatocellular carcinoma hence is a real challenge to infection control for DHCW.

Table 28.1: Important clinical features of hepatitis viruses

Features	Hepatitis A Virus (HAV)	Hepatitis B Virus (HBV)	Hepatitis C Virus (HCV)	Hepatitis D Virus (HDV)	Hepatitis E Virus (HEV)	Hepatitis G Virus (HGV)
Incubation period	15 to 40 days	50 to 180 days	1 to 5 months	21 to 90 days	2 to 9 weeks	NA
Transmission	Fecal-Oral; unhygienic sanitation usually seen in developing and underdeveloped countries	Parenteral; sexual contact; perinatal; other secretions (e.g. saliva, tears)	Usually parenteral; Rarely sexual contact, perinatal	Usually parenteral; Rarely sexual contact	Fecal-oral; waterborne (usually seen in developing and underdeveloped countries)	Parenteral; perinatal frequent co-infection with HCV
Carrier state	No	Yes (5 to 10%)	Yes (> 85%)	Yes	No	Yes
Onset	Mostly acute	Mostly gradual	Mostly gradual	Mostly acute	Mostly acute	Gradual
Prodrome: arthritis/rash	Not present	Sometimes	Sometimes	Unknown	Not present	NA
Serious manifestations	None observed	Hepatocellular carcinoma; cirrhosis	Hepatocellular carcinoma; cirrhosis	Hepatocellular carcinoma; cirrhosis	None observed	None observed
Mortality rate (in percentage)	0.1 to 0.2	1 to 2; higher in adults > 40 yr	1 to 2	2 to 20	1 to 2 in general population; 18 to 22 in pregnant women	NA
Homologous immunity	Anti HAV	Anti HBsAg	Not clear	Anti-HBsAg	Anti-HEV	Anti-HGV

NA= Not Applicable
HBs Ag = Hepatitis B surface antigen
All above viruses also transmitted by blood-to-blood contact

HCV Prevention and Treatment

An effective vaccine is not yet commercially available. Universal precautions must be observed during patient care. Blood donors must be screened for all virus infections. Combination of chemotherapeutic agents has shown good results. Multidrug approaches like interferon and specific HCV enzyme inhibitors have also shown good results.

HIV Infection

HIV is one of the most devastating infectious diseases. It is estimated that about 70 million persons are infected with this virus all over the world and the rate of infection is increasing unchecked. Two types of HIV, e.g. HIV-1 and HIV-2 have been isolated. Both types cause AIDS and deteriorates immunity. The median time from infection to full blown AIDS is about 10 years with HIV-1 and 20 years with HIV-2. Majority of infection is due to HIV-1, hence when nothing is specified it means HIV-1. An effective vaccine is not yet commercially available.

Orodental Considerations

No dental treatment is modified for outdoor dental patients with AIDS. They can tolerate all common dental treatments. In advanced stages with neutrophil counts below 500 to 750 cells/mm^3, and patients with chances of developing subacute bacterial endocarditis require antibiotic prophylaxis.

Xerostomia is the side effect of the medications used to treat HIV. Therefore when doing restoration and fixed and removable prosthodontics, due consideration should be given to the restorative material, long-term use and maintenance of the restoration.

Oral Lesions

All oral lesions observed in HIV-positive patients are also found in other diseases associated with immune suppression. There is a clear correlation between oral lesions and a decreased immune system. When there is impaired immune response with CD4 cell counts below 200 cells/mm^3 then any or many of the following may be present:
a. Oral hairy leukoplakia
b. Oral candidiasis
c. Kaposi's sarcoma
d. Necrotizing ulcerative periodontal disease with sore throat and exudative pharyngitis.
   Clinically oral candidiasis is of following four types:
   1. Pseudomembranous candidiasis or thrush
   2. Erythematous or atrophic candidiasis
   3. Hyperplastic or chronic candidiasis
   4. Angular cheilitis

Drugs Induced Ulceration

Some drugs used for HIV infected patients develop oral ulceration on nonkeratinized mucosa. These drugs include zidovudine, zalcitabine, foscarnet, interferons and ganciclovir.

Oral Lesions in Children

In comparison of adults, in HIV infected children oral lesions affect more severely so much so that oral intake of food and medicines become painful. Oral candidiasis very frequently appears in HIV infected children. The first loading dose of fluconazole suspension (6 mg per kg of body weight) is given. This is followed by 3 mg per kg of body weight per day. It is more effective than nystatin oral rinses. Its topical application is also effective.

BIBLIOGRAPHY

1. AIDS epidemic update. December 2000. UNAIDS/WHO 2000.
2. American Health Consultants. Fasten your seat belts. Hospitals face a bumpy ride as hepatitis C cases peak. Hosp Infect Cont 2000;27:129.
3. Ensoli B, Sgadari C, Barillari G, et al. Biology of Kaposi's sarcoma. Eur J Cancer 2001:1251.
4. Eswar N, Gnanasundaram N. Rhino cerebral mucormycosis—A case report, JIAOMR 2006; 18:01.
5. Gao F, Bailes E, Robertson DL, et al. Origin of HIV-1 in the chimpanzee *Pan troglodytes*. Nature 1999;396:437.
6. Iscovich J, Boffetta P, Franceschi S, et al. Classic Kaposi sarcoma-epidemiology and risk factors. Cancer 2000;88:500-17.
7. Kuriari K, Capt. Elongovan Anith B, Shammugam S. Nasolabial cyst—A review and report of 2 cases. JIAOMR 2006;18:01.
8. Liang JT, Rhermann J, Seeff LB, et al. NIH conference: Pathogenesis, natural history, treatment and prevention of hepatitis C. Ann Intern Med 2000;132:296.
9. Nicolatou O, Theodoridou M, Mostrou G, et al. Oral lesions in children with perinatally acquired human immunodeficiency virus infection. J Oral Pathol Med 1999;28:49.
10. Patton LL, Glick M. Clinician's guide to treatment of HIV-infected patients. 3rd ed. American Academy of Oral Medicine 2001.
11. Patton LL. Sensitivity, specificity, and positive predictive value of oral opportunistic infections in adults with HIV/AIDS as markers of immune suppression and viral burden. Oral Surg Oral Med Oral Pathol Oral Radiol Endod 2000;90:182.
12. Quinn TC, Wawer MJ, Sewankambo N, et al. Viral load and heterosexual transmission of human immunodeficiency virus type I. N Engl J Med 2000;342:921.
13. Rajishwari A, Zammera A, Naik. Oral Crohn's disease—A rare case report with review JIAOMR 2006; 18:01.
14. Raghu obul Reddy, Shanshikanth MC Ab. IM: Radio immuno imaging and therapy JIAOMR 2006;18:01.
15. Sulabha AN, Seemanth KN, SS Chopra. Ophthalmic complications secondary to oral sepsis—A review JIAOMR 2006;18:01.
16. Suwarna B Dargore, Degvekar SS, Bhowate RR, Indurkor AD. Bilateral Transmigration of impacted mandibular canines—A rare case report JIAOMR 2006; 18:01.

29

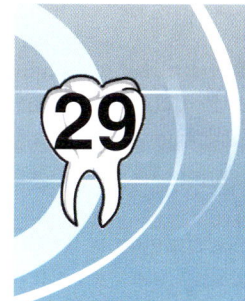

Endocrine Diseases and Orodental Health

Endocrine glands are ductless glands which produce internal secretions. There secretions are discharged into the blood or lymph for circulation to all parts of the body. Hormones are the active principles of the glands. Hormones affect the tissues which may be more or less remote from their place of origin. These glands include pituitary (Hypophysis), hypothalamus, adrenal, thyroid, parathyroid, islets of Langerhan's of the pancreas and gonads.

Endocrine dysfunction can be hyposecretion and hypersecretion. Secretion of endocrine glands are controlled by (a) the nervous system (b) chemical substances in the blood (c) by other hormones. Many pathological conditions are caused by or associated with malfunction of endocrine glands which effect orodental health.

HYPOTHALAMUS AND ANTERIOR PITUITARY

Pituitary adenomas secrete active hormones, in acromegaly and Cushing's disease. These hormones cause gradual changes in facial features and orofacial structures. The changes can be easily identified. Early recognition of pituitary dysfunction can prevent complication of dental treatment. This can provide a safe method for clinical and therapeutic treatment. Replacement therapy is indicated after partial destruction or resection of pituitary tissue.

The understanding of classic hypothalamic-pituitary thyroid axis is important to understand the dental clinical conditions. The deficiency or excess of cortisol caused by the long-term treatment of the patient with glucocorticoids or by its sudden withdrawal causes an iatrogenic disease.

ADRENAL DISEASES AND CONDITIONS

Adrenocorticotropic hormone (ACTH) secreted by pituitary tumors cause Cushing's disease. With similar symptoms like central obesity, cutaneous atrophy, muscle wasting, osteoporosis, diabetes mellitus, hypertension, immunosuppression and psychiatric symptoms are caused from iatrogenic glucocorticoids from adrenal tumors or from ectopic secretion of ACTH have Cushing's syndrome.

Orodental Considerations

Hemostasis

Patients taking glucocorticoid have decrease in subcutaneous collagen and the fibroblasts produce extracellular proteins. Wound healing and scar formation is delayed.

Prone to Infection

Patients taking heavy glucocorticoid treatment for longer period are immunocompromised and are more prone to infections. Choice of antibiotic depends on the basis of the underlying disease. Patients with Cushing's syndrome are prone to fungal infection and candida due to changes in mucosal and skin flora.

Tolerance to Dental Treatment

If the potential consequences of adrenal insufficiency are avoided then, patients taking low doses of glucocorticoid can tolerate dental treatment. If the patient is taking high doses of glucocorticoid for longer period then there may be following changes:
a. Delay in wound healing
b. Minor difficulty with hemostasis
c. Immunosuppression.

THYROID DISEASE

In the general population next to diabetes mellitus, thyroid is the most common endocrine problem. Under and over activity of thyroid may cause fatal cardiac problems. During examination of orofacial complex many signs and symptoms of thyroid disease can be observed. Dietary iodine regulates the functional activity of the thyroid gland. Thyroid gland depends on the intake of dietary iodine and produce the hormone called thyroxine. Thyroxine regulates the pace of metabolism in all cells. Iodine deficiency causes hypothyroidism and goiter in which there is increase in the size of thyroid gland. Goiter is also caused by autoimmune disease and excess production of TSH by pituitary adenoma.

Orodental Considerations

Enlarged tongue, facial myxedema and a hoarse voice are seen in hypothyroid state. In hyperthyroidism, goiter, exophthalmoses, lid lag and oculomotor defects are observed. Hyperthyroidism and hypothyroidism when well controlled do not present an excess risk for dental patients. Therefore complete history and physical examination of the patient having thyroid disease is a must before performing dental procedures. This will help in determining the states and stability of thyroid patients.

Hemostasis

Hyperthyroidism lead to raised blood pressure and heart rates. A longer duration of local pressure to stop bleeding is required for patient with high arteriolar pressure. Patient with hypothyroidism of long duration have decreased ability of small blood vessels to constrict when cut resulting into increased bleeding. Pressure pack for longer duration will control bleeding from small vessels.

Prone to Infection

Hypothyroid patients are not considered to be immunocompromised. Hypothyroidism lead to delayed wound healing which makes the tissues more prone to infection, because of prolonged exposure of the injured tissues open to pathogenic organisms.

Whenever history and physical examination reveal undiagnosed, untreated, unstable and uncontrolled endocrine disease physician of the patient must be consulted before performing dental procedures.

BIBLIOGRAPHY

1. Casanueva FF, Dieguez C. Neuroendocrine regulation and actions of leptin. Front Neuroendocrine 1998;20:317-63.
2. Freda PU, Wardlaw SL. Clinical review 110. Diagnosis and treatment of pituitary tumors. J Clin Endocrinol Metab 1999; 84:3859-66.
3. Greenspan SL, Greenspan FS. The effect of thyroid hormone on skeletal integrity. Ann intern Med 1999;130:750-8.
4. Koob GF. Corticotropin-releasing factor, norepinephrine, and stress.Biol Psychiatry 1999;46:1167-80.
5. Maurer RA, Kim KE, Schoderbek WE, et al. Regulation of glycoprotein hormone alphasubunit gene expression. Recent Prog Horm Res 1999;54:455-84.
6. Perry HM III. The endocrinology of aging. Clin Chem 1999; 45:1369-76.
7. Sapolsky RM. Glucocorticoids, stress and their adverse neurological effects. Relevance to aging. Exp Gerontol 1999;34:721-32.

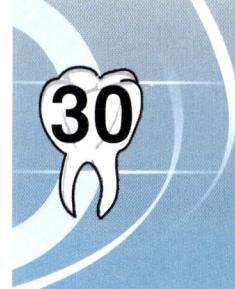

30. Orodental Medicine in Geriatrics

The percentage of geriatric population above 65 years of age is increasing specially in developing and developed countries due to family planning measures, development of medical sciences and availability of advanced medical services. Nowadays due to better medical facilities and health awareness among people, more number of people live longer and become aged. Therefore due to increase in number of aged population there is increase in diseases and chronic conditions that influence oral health of aged persons.

The common chronic diseases of old age are diabetes mellitus, hypertension, arthritis and heart diseases. These conditions have oral manifestations, especially in aged people. The treatment of these diseases with medications, chemotherapy and radiotherapy also affects the oral health.

COMMON SYSTEMIC CONDITIONS IN GERIATRICS AND THEIR ORODENTAL MANAGEMENT

In the developed and developing countries following is the incidence of common diseases in general population above the age of 65 years.

Name of diseases	Approximate percentage of people suffering
1. Arthritis	50
2. Hypertension	38
3. Cardiac diseases	32
4. Diabetes mellitus	12
5. Chronic sinusitis	13
6. Allergic rhinitis	08
7. Others	10

More than 80% of persons over the 65 years of age suffer from more than one diseases. Common disorders in aged persons are as follows:

Coagulation Disorders

Etiology: Anticoagulation treatment, chemotherapy, liver cirrhosis and renal disease.

Risk: Increased bleeding

Precautions: Limited surgery to be performed. Use of topical anticoagulant agents and change in anticoagulants treatment.

Immunosuppression

Etiology: Alcoholic cirrhosis of liver, diabetes, chemotherapy, organ transplant therapy, medications and renal disease.

Risk: Microbial infection

Precautions: Antimicrobial medicaments.

Radiation Hazard

Etiology: Head and neck radiation treatment for malignancy

Risks: Xerostomia, rampant caries, mucositis, osteoradionecrosis, dysphagia, dysgeusia, microbial infections, difficulty in mastication and poor denture retention

Precautions: Frequent topical fluoridation, salivary stimulants and proper oral hygiene.

Steroid Treatment

Etiology: Steroids are used in autoimmune diseases and in transplantation of organs.

Risks: Microbial infectious and increased risk for adrenal insufficiency.

Precautions: Antimicrobial medicaments and steroid supplementation.

Cardiac Problems

Etiology: Acquired and congenital heart defects and valvular transplants.

Risk: Subacute bacterial endocarditis

Precautions: Antibiotic cover.

Joint Replacement

Etiology: Arthritis and accidents

Risk: Joint infections

Precautions: Antibiotic cover

AGE-RELATED CHANGES IN ORAL HEALTH IN GERIATRICS

In Oral Mucosa

The appearance of oral mucosa in aged persons may get altered due to lifelong history of oral mucosal diseases (e.g., lichen planus), mucosal trauma (e.g., cheek biting), oral habits (e.g., smoking) and salivary disorders.

The mucosal surface appears dry, thin and smooth with loss of elasticity and stippling. These changes lead to trauma and infection of the oral mucosa when associated with denture use and salivary hypofunction. Process of wound healing and regeneration of tissues is also delayed in aged persons. Careful examination should be done for malignancy, ulcers and vesicles.

In Dentition

Age changes in dentition are due to normal physiologic processes and pathologic changes. These are as follows:
A. External tooth changes are discoloration and loss of enamel due to attrition, abrasion and erosion.
B. Thickness of cementum takes place and size of the pulp is also reduced with age.
C. Due to gingival recession, teeth develop cervical or root surface caries.
D. Previously restored teeth are more prone to recurrent decay due to fractured filling, defective restorations and poor oral hygiene.
E. Aged people develop plaque more rapidly than younger people resulting into caries. This occurs due to the following (a) diminished salivary gland function, (b) gingival recession, (c) disturbances in oral motor functions (d) difficulty in performing oral hygiene.

In Periodontium

A. Gingivitis, periodontitis and abscesses.
B. Gingival recession, loss of periodontal attachment and alveolar bone are the common periodontal changes related to age.
C. Systemic diseases such as osteoporosis and diabetes, and their medications prevalent among aged people are related with periodontal disorders.
D. Medications such as calcium channel blockers, antiseizure drug-phenytoin and immunosuppressant-cyclosporine are frequently prescribed in aged persons, which are associated with gingival over growth.
E. Deep periodontal pocket, smoking, stress, irregular dental visits and poor socioeconomic status are responsible for periodontal attachment loss in aged people.

Salivary Glands

Saliva plays a significant role in maintenance of oral health. Its deficiency can cause dental caries, speech dysfunction, oral mucosal infections, difficulty in chewing, swallowing and denture retention. In healthy aged people no significant changes are observed in salivary flow. Salivary glands should be carefully examined for obstructions, bacterial infections, hypofunctions and malignancy.

Mastication and Swallowing

The function of mastication and swallowing requires co-ordination of neuromuscular activities for transfer of food and fluids to gastrointestinal tract. The common oral motor disturbances in aged people are related to altered mastication. This altered mastication is due to partial or full edentulousness, painful and mobile teeth due to dental caries and periodontal diseases and decreased salivary flow.

The process of swallowing is also altered in aged people due to impaired neuromuscular processing and inadequate salivary production. Cerebrovascular and neurologic diseases, head and neck cancer and its treatment, other systemic diseases and disorders and their medications decrease salivary production and thus affect swallowing in aged people. Swallowing process should be examined for delayed swallowing and aspiration.

ORAL AND DENTAL DISORDERS IN ELDERLY PEOPLE

Oral Mucosal Diseases

Various oral mucosal diseases and lesions common in elderly people are as follows:
A. Most of the aged people have pigmented (lingual varicosities, melanotic macules) and benign soft-tissue conditions (fibromas, fordyce granules) and hard-tissue conditions (tori, exostosis)
B. Tongue diseases include geographic tongue, black-hairy tongue and atrophy of filiform and fungiform papillae.

Tongue may be fissured, coated or enlarged in edentulous patients.
C. There may be inflammation (denture stomatitis) and atrophy due to ill-fitting denture.
D. Low-grade irritation by ill-fitting denture leads to formation of epulis fissuratum.
E. Common oral vesicobullous diseases in adults include lichen planus, pemphigus vulgaris and primarily in older women cicatricial pemphigoid.
F. The most significant oral mucosal diseases in aged adults is oral cancer. Common sites of oral malignancy in aged persons are tongue, buccal mucosa, floor of mouth and posterior oropharynx.

Infectious Diseases

Aged individuals are more susceptible of developing oral infections.
A. The most common viral infection is of herpes simplex virus and varicella-zoster virus. Shingles, a varicella zoster infection characterized by incapacitating oral-facial lesions is common in older people. This infection is acquired from exposure to chickenpox during childhood, which reactivated in old age leading to vesicular eruptions on skin and mucous membrane. Post herpetic neuralgia occurs more frequently in aged patients.
B. The common oral fungal infection in aged individuals is caused by *Candida albicans*. Removable dentures, poor oral and denture hygiene, nutritional deficiencies, salivary gland hypofunction, endocrine disorders and medications are associated with fungal infection.

Dental Disorders

A. Root surface caries following gingival recession are common in elderly people. These lesions appear as well defined and discolored defects on cementum or cemento-enamel junction.
    Predisposing factors for root surface caries are salivary gland hypofunction, poor oral hygiene, gingival recession, poor diet, insufficient fluoride exposure and orofacial motor deficits.
B. Coronal caries is also more prevalent in elderly people. The lesion appears as discolored defect on occlusal and proximal tooth surface, and is of soft and rubbery texture. The risk factors are similar to those of root surface caries (except gingival recession).

Periodontal Diseases

A. The periodontal disease more likely to develop in older individuals is gingivitis which is caused due to oral and systemic factors. Predisposing factors are root caries, gingival recession, furcation involvement and tooth drifting and mobility.
B. Systemic conditions and medications common among adults have an adverse effect on periodontium e.g., gingival overgrowth is associated with use of phenytoin, cyclosporine and nifedipine. Diseases such as erosive lichen planus and cicatricial pemphigoid produce desquamative gingivitis; and diabetes may lead to periodontal breakdown.

Salivary Gland Dysfunction

Salivary gland dysfunction in older persons is a result of following conditions:
A. Obstruction and bacterial infection cause salivary dysfunction.
B. Sjogren's syndrome predominant in older females causes salivary dysfunction and is associated with dry mouth.
C. Systemic conditions such as Alzheimer's disease, diabetes and dehydration are common in elderly people which lead to salivary dysfunction.
D. Various drugs frequently taken by older persons such as antidepressants, antihypertensives, antipsychotics and antihistamines cause xerostomia and salivary dysfunction.
E. Extraoral manifestations of salivary dysfunction are candidiasis in the labial commissures and dry cracked lips.
F. Intraoral manifestations of diminished salivary production are dental caries, gingivitis, candidiasis, dysphagia, poorly fitting dentures and altered mastication and deglutition.

Smell and Taste Dysfunction

Smell and taste disorder in aged people may be due to chemosensory disorder or manifestation of an oral and systemic disease.
A. Oral conditions responsible for taste dysfunction are fungal infections, salivary hypofunction, gingivitis, halitosis, galvanism, dentoalveolar abscess and poorly fitting dentures.
B. Medical conditions such as Alzheimer's disease, multiple sclerosis, Parkinson's disease, diabetes, upper respiratory infections and ulcers in gastrointestinal tract result in smell and taste dysfunction.

Swallowing Disorders

A. Swallowing disorder such as dysphagia is common in elderly persons and is caused by various medical conditions such as
   a. immunologic disorders e.g., arthritis, diabetes
   b. neurologic disorders e.g., Parkinson's disease, stroke
   c. psychologic disorders e.g., dementia, depression.
B. Oral motor weakness of lips, tongue and buccal mucosa also results in poor swallowing reflex. Weakness of lips causes drooling from the lips that delays initiation of oral phase of swallowing. Tongue weakness impairs the formation of food bolus.

Edentulousness

A. Edentulism in elderly people is due to tooth loss due to dental caries and periodontal diseases and systemic conditions such as osteomyelitis and diabetes mellitus.
B. Due to tooth loss there is continuous alveolar bone resorption. Alveolar ridge atrophy in the mandible results in problems in denture fabrication and may also lead to mandibular fracture.
C. Edentulous patients with removable dentures have decreased masticatory forces and impaired chewing efficiency.

PREVENTION AND TREATMENT OF ORAL CONDITIONS IN AGED INDIVIDUALS

Oral Mucosal Diseases

A. The most significant and dangerous oral mucosal disease in older people is oral cancer and its prevention begins with elimination of risk factors such as, use of tobacco and alcohol.
B. Oral cancer is treated by surgery, chemotherapy and radiotherapy, which also have oral manifestations such as stomatitis, pain, paresthesia, dysphagia, oral motor dysfunction and salivary hypofunction. Dental management before, during and after treatment is essential to prevent complications.
C. Traumatic oral lesions prevalent in aged individuals are mostly due to sharp edges of attrited teeth and ill-fitting dentures. Their treatment involves rounding of sharp edges of attrited teeth and repair of ill-fitting denture flange or base or removal of an epulis fissuratum. Palliative topical medications and antibiotics to prevent secondary infection should be administered.
D. Vesicobullous and erosive lesions should be treated by topical steroids and systemic steroids. If the aged patient has medical problems such as diabetes, coronary heart disease or hypertension, the patient must be referred to physician.

Infectious Diseases

A. Viral infections such as herpes simplex and herpes zoster are usually self-limiting. Supportive therapy is required to eliminate pain and to maintain nutritional and fluid intake.
B. Treatment of postherpetic neuralgia in aged patients includes administration of analgesics, tricyclic antidepressants and steroids.
C. Candidiasis can be managed by maintaining good oral and dental hygiene, use of antibiotics and immunosuppressants and elimination of underlying local and systemic etiologic factors.
D. Dentures are frequent source of fungal infections. They should be soaked in 1% sodium hypochlorite for 10 to 15 minutes and should be used with antifungal creams.

Dental Disorders

A. Dental caries in aged patients can be prevented by maintenance of oral hygiene by regular rinsing, brushing and flossing after each meal.
B. Fluoride containing dentifrices and rinses should be used, as they help in prevention and remineralization of carious lesions.
C. Aged persons should regularly visit dental surgeon for examination and prophylaxis.
D. Intake of carbohydrate rich diet and sugar-containing beverages should be reduced.
E. Tooth destroyed due to coronal and root surface caries, abrasion, attrition and erosion can be restored by various enamel and dentin-bonding techniques.
F. Aged persons with impaired manual dexterity and other motor disabilities can maintain their oral hygiene by electric or battery operated toothbrush.

Fluoride gels (1.0 or 1.1 % sodium fluoride or 0.4% stannous fluoride) and rinses with 0.12 to 0.2% chlorhexidine mouthwash are recommended for these patients.

Salivary Gland Disorders

A. Infection of salivary gland requires culture and sensitivity tests and appropriate antibiotic therapy. Amoxicillin and clavulanic acid (clindamycin, if patient is allergic to penicillin group) can be prescribed until culture and sensitivity reports are received.
B. Systemic diseases such as Sjogren's syndrome should be identified and managed.

C. Drug-induced xerostomia can be managed by elimination or reduction of the causative drug or by substituting another drug with less side effects.
D. Salivary hypofunction can be treated by administration of pilocarpine (5 to 7.5 mg three times daily) and cevemeline HCl (30 mg TDS). Pilocarpine and cevemeline are contraindicated in patients with congestive heart disease, glaucoma and pulmonary diseases.

Periodontal Disease

A. Periodontal health can be maintained by proper rinsing, tooth brushing and flossing after each meal and regular dental check-up.
B. Periodontal diseases in very old patients can be managed by non-surgical approach by scaling and root planing and daily oral hygiene maintenance.
C. A course of systemic antimicrobial therapy may be administered in very old patients, but after consultation with patient's physician.

Chemosensory (Smell and Taste) Dysfunction

Smell and taste disorders are due to various oral problems, such as oral mucosal infections (e.g., candidiasis), ill-fitting dentures, dentoalveolar infections, poor tongue hygiene, oral mucosal diseases and periodontal and dental diseases.

These disorders should be managed and their treatment may improve smell and taste function. Flavor enhancers such as herbs and spices that stimulate trigeminal nerve can be used by patients with chemosensory deficits.

Masticatory and Swallowing Disorders

A. Masticatory disorders are related to the status of dentition. Dental and periodontal problems should be eliminated and prosthesis should be constructed if required. Salivary dysfunction alters denture use; so salivary hypofunction should be treated in denture-wearing aged persons to improve mastication.
B. Management of swallowing disorder such as dysphagia requires efforts of both dental surgeon and physician. If dysphagia is due to salivary hypofunction, salivary flow can be increased by administration of 5 mg of pilocarpine or 30 mg of cevemeline HCl 30 minutes before meal time.

Edentulousness

Edentulousness or total tooth loss in aged patients can be compensated by preparing prosthesis. Regular assessment of dentures, denture-bearing ridges and all mucosal surfaces is required to reduce the risk of developing denture stomatitis, angular cheilitis, traumatic ulcerations and alveolar atrophy. Endosseous dentoalveolar implants for partially or completely edentulous adults can also be used. Continuous edentulousness for prolonged period lead to osteoporosis, atrophic mandible, denture difficulties and pain over the mental foramen due to excessively resorbed mandibular ridge.

In oral and pharyngeal mucosa. viral diseases, fungal diseases and bacterial diseases may occur.

Pain Sensation

Atypical facial pain, burning mouth syndrome, post-herpetic neuralgia and trigeminal neuralgia may occur in old age.

BIBLIOGRAPHY

1. Chavez EM, Ship JA. Sensory and motor deficits in the elderly. impact on oral health. J Public Health Dent 2000; 60(4):297-303.
2. Ghezzi EM, Ship JA. Systemic diseases and their treatments in the elderly. Impact on oral health. J Public Health Dent 2000; 60(4): 289-96.
3. Ghezzi EM, Ship JA. Dementia and oral health. Oral Surg Oral Med Oral Path Oral Radiol Endod 2000; 89(1):2-5.
4. Greenlee RT, Murray T, Bolden S, Wingo PA. Cancer statistics, 2000. CA Cancer J Clin 2000;50:7-33.
5. Morley J. The role of cosmetic dentistry in restoring a youthful appearance. J Am Dent Assoc 1999;130(8):1166-72.
6. Narhi TO, Meurman JH, Ainamo A. Xerostomia and hyposalivation. causes, consequences and treatment in the elderly. Drugs Aging 1999;15(2):103-16.
7. Riley JL 3rd, Gilbert GH, Heft MW. Health care utilization by older adults in response to painful orofacial symptoms. Pain 1999; 81 (1-2):67-75.

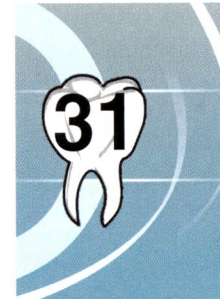

Orodental Considerations in Organ Transplantation

Life-threatening end-stage organ diseases can be treated by organ transplantation. Oral considerations in case of transplantation are important and very wide Table 31.1. The dental surgeon should have sound knowledge of medicine to avoid adverse outcome secondary to oral health care. Patients who have had an organ transplantation need routine oral and dental examinations. It is essential for the dental surgeon to know about the special needs of these patients.

Good orodental health is essential for all organ transplant patients. Their dental problems must be diagnosed and treated as early as possible. Regular topical fluoride application is essential for all patients with xerostomia. Oral ulcers can serve as a portal of entry for the pathogens to infect the immunocompromised host. Hence oral ulcers must be treated as early as possible.

Table 31.1: Main immunosuppressive drugs and their major side effects and orodental implications

Drug	Major side effects	Orodental implications
1. Antithymocyte globulin/anti-lymphocyte globulin (ATG/ALG)	Leukopenia, pulmonary edema renal dysfunction	Immunosuppressant
2. Azathioprine	Bone marrow suppression, hepatotoxicity	More chances of neoplasm
3. Corticosteroids	1. Induces diabetes, muscle weakness hyperlipidemia and osteoporosis, electrolyte imbalances, central nervous system effects including psychological changes, hyperlipidemia, and ocular changes like cataracts and glaucoma. 2. Aggravates high blood pressure, congestive heart failure and peptic ulcer disease and underlying infectious processes (e.g. tuberculosis). 3. Alters fat metabolism and distribution. 4. Suppresses the pituitary-adrenal axis, resulting in adrenal atrophy and the stress response.	Poor wound healing avoid NSAIDs and acetylsalicylic acid. Monitor CV system, more chances of neoplasm. Steroid supplement may be needed with stressful procedures
4. Cyclosporine	Nephro-toxicity, Hepatotoxicity, elevation of blood pressure, P-450 metabolized*, gingival hyperplasia, monitor CV system, may effect renal elimination of some drugs, more chances of neoplasm	Gingival hyperplasia
5. Daclizumab and basiliximab	Pulmonary edema, renal dysfunction	More chances of neoplasm
6. Muromonab- CD3	Cytokine release syndrome	Interact with indomethacin
7. Mycophenolate mofetil	Leukopenia	Absorption is altered by antibiotic, antacids, and bile acid binders, more chances of neoplasm
8. Sirolimus	Hyperlipidemia, Hypertriglyceremia P-450 metabolized * Monitor CV system, May effect renal elimination of some drugs	More chances of neoplasm
9. Tacrolimus	Neurotoxicity, hepatotoxicity P-450 metabolized monitor CV system, may effect renal elimination of some drugs, more chances of neoplasm, Nephrotoxicity Post transplants diabetes mellitus, elevation of blood pressure.	More chances of neoplasm

*1.Dental/oral pharmacotherapeutics which are metabolized by the liver's cytochrome P450 3A system alter this drug's serum levels.
*2.This group of medications includes, but is not limited to, erythromycin, clarithromycin, "azole" antifungals, benzodiazepines, carbamazepine, colchicines, prednisolone and metronidazole.
CV = cardiovascular; NSAIDs = nonsteroidal anti-inflammatory drugs.

ORAL LESIONS

Patients who have had organ transplantation are more susceptible to oral infection of bacterial, viral and fungal origin. These infections lead to the oral mucosal lesions or masses. The oral mucosal lesions can also be due to non-infectious process.

Viral Infections

Viral infections are common complication in immunosuppressed patients. *Herpes simplex* virus, *Epstein-barr* virus and *varicella-zoster* virus are involved in various oral diseases.

Oral hairy leukoplakia is also seen in transplant recipients. Viral infections can be treated by antiviral agents such as acyclovir, foscarnet and cidofovir.

Fungal Infections

Immunosuppressed patients are also susceptible to fungal infections. Fungal infections include candidiasis, cryptococcosis, mucormycosis, blastomycosis and aspergillosis. Candidiasis in these patients appears in pseudomembranous form, which responds to treatment with amphotericin B.

In the patients of hematopoietic cell transplantation, fungal infection manifest as necrotic plaques in the palatal areas. These fungal infections are treated by administration of intravenous antifungal agents such as amphotericin B.

Bacterial Infections

Bacterial infections in transplant patients do not manifest as in normal patients so, their treatment requires antibiotic therapy without delay. Culture and sensitivity test should be taken in severe infections. Dental caries, a bacterial infection, is associated with many end-stage diseases and is result of medications or therapy required to treat these diseases. Patients who have had hematopoietic cell transplantation or kidney transplantation have higher incidence of dental caries.

Non-Infectious Oral Lesions

The transplant recipients are also at a higher risk of developing lymphoma and carcinoma such as Kaposi's sarcoma and squamous cell carcinoma. Kaposi's sarcoma and lymphoma are found in mouth whereas epithelial malignancy involves the lips.

Graft-Versus-Host-Disease (GVHD)

GVHD is one of the complications in patients receiving hematopoietic cell transplantation. Oral GVHD clinically appears as an area of hyperkeratosis on an erythematous base on the oral mucosa. These lesions in severe case get eroded and lead to chronic mucosal ulcerations.

Oral GVHD can be treated by the following:
a. Topical azathioprine
b. Topical cyclosporine in a bioadhesive base
c. Ultraviolet A and B irradiation with oral psoralen.

Oral Mucositis

Patients on chemotherapy also complain of oral mucositis. Mucositis is also seen in patients of hematopoietic cell transplantation. It can be treated by topical application of mixture of an anesthetic, an antihistamine, and a coating agent.

Salivary Gland Dysfunction

Salivary gland dysfunction is also common in patients after hematopoietic cell transplantation due to chemotherapeutic drugs. Patients with chronic graft-versus-host-disease may have diminished salivary flow.

Gingival Enlargement

Drug-induced gingival enlargement is also seen in transplant recipients, who are on immunosuppressive agent, cyclosporine. Cyclosporine-induced gingival enlargement may be aggravated by co-administration of nifedipine used in treatment of hypertension which is a common post-transplantation problem. Severe gingival enlargement is usually treated by gingivectomy.

Developmental tooth defects such as altered root formation and dentofacial abnormalities are also observed in children who have received hematopoietic cell transplantation.

ORODENTAL MANAGEMENT

If the patient who is awaiting transplantation or who has had a transplant requires dental treatment, the treatment should be carried out in coordination with physician and surgeon who are performing or has performed transplantation. The physician and surgeon performing the transplantation should consult dental surgeon before transplantation to make sure that patient is free from any orodental infection that may complicate the transplantation. Dental management of such patients can be divided into the following.

Pre-transplantation Considerations

Patients who are preparing for transplantation are seriously ill and have end-organ damage. End-organ damage may pose various difficulties during dental procedures, so following precautions should be taken.

a. Patients who are preparing for kidney transplantation have end-stage renal disease and usually receive hemodialysis. These patients require antibiotic prophylaxis prior to dental treatment to prevent bacterial endocarditis (Table 31.2).
b. Patients preparing for lung transplantation are critically ill. They have difficulty in breathing and are on oxygen therapy. During carrying out any dental treatment, there should be no combustible sources near the patient if he or she is using oxygen therapy.
   Use of inhaled anesthetics is contraindicated. Narcotic medications are also contraindicated as they may cause respiratory distress.
c. Antibiotic prophylaxis prior to dental treatment is essential in patients preparing for hematopoietic cell transplantation (HCT) or heart or kidney transplantation. Patients for liver transplantation and HCT may require platelets and coagulation factors prior to dental treatment.
   Dental surgeon should be familiar with underlying disorder of his/her patient who is a transplantation candidate. He should consult the patient's physician and surgeon before carrying out any dental procedure. Dental surgeon should carry out detailed clinical examination of dentition, periodontium, oral mucosa, salivary glands and lymph nodes draining the head and neck region.

Table 31.2: Medicines to be avoided in patients with severe liver or kidney failure or both

Medicines which should be avoided in patients with liver failure	Medicines which should be avoided in patients with kidney failure	Medicines which should be avoided in patients with both liver and kidney failure
Acetaminophen	Acyclovir	Codeine
Clindamycin	Amoxicillin	Diazepam
Erythromycin	Cephalexin	Metronidazole
Ketoconazole	Clavulanic acid with amoxicillin	Naproxen
		Salicylates
Minocycline	Penicillin	Teracycline

Pretransplantation Dental Management

1. Dental consultation prior to transplant
2. Rule out and remove dental infection sources
3. Perform necessary treatment; this will require consultation with transplantation physician and surgeon to determine medical risk-to-benefit ratio
4. Obtain laboratory information/supplemental information as required
5. Become acquainted with specific management issues (e.g. blood products, prophylactic antibiotic) that may be required if treatment is rendered.

Post-transplantation Considerations

The post-transplantation period is divided into (a) immediate post-transplantation period, (b) the stable period and (c) chronic rejection period. Dental treatment in post transplant patients varies according to post transplant period.

Immediate Post-transplantation Period

This period begins immediately after the transplantation until the grafted organ starts functioning properly. In this period, there is increased level of immunosuppression used to avoid rejection, so elective dental procedures should not be performed. Emergency dental treatment should only be carried out after consultation with transplantation physician and surgeon.

Stable Post-transplantation Period

It is post-transplantation period when the grafted organ is stable. This period is appropriate for performing elective dental treatment since the organ is functioning properly. Patient taking cyclosporine as antirejection medication should be prescribed clindamycin instead of erythromycin. If the patient was on high-dose corticosteroid therapy, he may require corticosteroid supplements to avoid cardiovascular collapse during stressful dental procedure.

Chronic Rejection Period

The chronic rejection period starts when a grafted organ begins to fail. Only emergency dental treatment is indicated in this period with the consultation of the transplant surgeon and physician. All organ transplant patients must maintain excellent oral hygiene for this proper home care is very important. Oral hygiene instructions must be provided to all patients. The patients should be trained to do oral examination by himself at home. Small dental infection can be risky in these patients. Frequent professional dental check-up with topical fluoride application should be done.

BIBLIOGRAPHY

1. 1999 annual report of the US Scientific Registry of Transplants Recipients and the organ Procurement and Transplantation Network. transplant data 1989-1998. Rockville (MD) and Richmond (VA): HHS/HRSA/OSP/DOT and UNOS; accessed 2000; Feb 21.
2. Crespo M, Delmonic F, Saidman S, et al. Acute humoral rejection in kidney transplantation. Graft 2000; 3:12-7.
3. Comenzo RL. Hematopoietic cell transplantation for primary systemic amyloidosis. What have we learned. Luke Lymphoma 2000; 37:245-58.
4. Dykewicz CA, Jaffe HW, Kalpan JE, et al. Guideline for preventing opportunistic infections among hematopoietic stem cell transplants recipients. Recommendation of CDC, the infectious Disease Society of America and the American Society of Blood and Marrow Transplantation. MMWR Morb Mortal Weekly Rep 2000; 49:1-128.

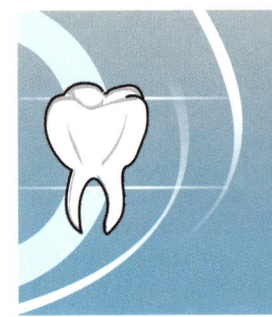

Multiple Choice Questions

ORODENTAL CONSIDERATIONS IN ORGAN TRANSPLANTATION

1. Which of the following transplant patient is more prone to have dental caries?
    a. Liver transplantation
    b. Kidney transplantation
    c. Hematopoietic cell transplantation
    d. Lung transplant

2. Which of the following drugs is/are associated with drug-induced gingival overgrowth?
    a. Cyclosporine
    b. Nifedipine
    c. Phenytoin
    d. All of the above

3. Multiresistant Herpes simplex virus infection can be successfully treated by:
    a. Acyclovir
    b. Foscarnet
    c. Cidofovir
    d. None of the above

4. Which of the following orodental manifestations may be present in children who have undergone Hematopoietic cell transplantation?
    a. Dental caries
    b. Altered root formation
    c. Dentofacial abnormalities
    d. All of the above

5. The best time to perform elective dental treatment in post-transplantation patient is:
    a. Immediate post-transplantation period
    b. Stable period
    c. Chronic rejection period
    d. Any of the above

6. Which of the following neoplasms is more likely to develop in transplant recipients?
    a. Malignant melanoma
    b. Kaposi's sarcoma
    c. Lymphangioma
    d. Nasopharyngeal carcinoma

7. "Wispy hyperkeratosis on an erythematous base" on the oral mucosa of the patient who has undergone hematopoietic cell transplantation is due to:
    a. Fungal infection
    b. Pre-transplant therapy
    c. Graft-versus-host disease
    d. Viral infection

8. Graft-versus-host disease in the oral mucous membrane can be treated by:
    a. Topical cyclosporine
    b. Topical azathioprine
    c. Cidofovir
    d. Both a and b

9. The most common viral pathogen cultured from oral infection in transplant recipient is:
    a. Herpes simplex virus
    b. Varicella-zoster virus
    c. Epstein-barr virus
    d. Cytomegalovirus

10. "Brittleinsulin-dependent diabetes" may be found in patients awaiting:
    a. Liver transplantation
    b. Kidney transplantation
    c. Pancreatic transplantation
    d. Intestinal transplantation

ULCERATIVE AND VESICULOBULLOUS LESIONS

1. Virus that causes oral ulcerations in immuno-suppressed patient is:
    a. Herpes simplex virus
    b. Varicella-zoster virus
    c. Cytomegalovirus
    d. Coxsackievirus

2. History of prodromal symptoms preceding the local lesions is found in:
   a. Erythema multiforme
   b. Herpes virus infection
   c. Allergic stomatitis
   d. Coxsackievirus infection

3. Acyclovir controls herpes simplex infections by:
   a. Inhibiting DNA replication in herpes simplex virus
   b. Dissolving protein capsid of virus
   c. Inhibiting DNA replication in HSV infected cells
   d. None of the above

4. Acute lymphonodular pharyngitis is caused by:
   a. Coxsackie A_5
   b. Coxsackie B_2
   c. Coxsackie A_9
   d. Coxsackie A_{10}

5. The required adult oral dose of acyclovir in the treatment of severe Herpes zoster is:
   a. 400 mg three times daily
   b. 800 mg five times daily
   c. 800 mg two times daily
   d. 400 mg five times daily

6. Large, irregular, deep and bleeding ulcers in the oral cavity are found in:
   a. Erythema multiforme
   b. ANUG
   c. Varicella-Zoster virus infection
   d. Herpangina

7. Necrotic, punched out ulcerations are the clinical feature of:
   a. Behcet's disease
   b. Pemphigus
   c. Recurrent aphthous stomatitis
   d. ANUG

8. Hyperreactivity to intracutaneous injection or a needlestick is found in the patients of:
   a. Pemphigus vulgaris
   b. Bullous pemphigoid
   c. Behcet's disease
   d. Allergic stomatitis

9. Nikolsky's sign is most frequently associated with:
   a. Epidermolysis bullosa
   b. Pemphigus
   c. Bullous pemphigoid
   d. Cicatricial pemphigoid

10. Use of corticosteroid is contraindicated in:
    a. Lichen planus
    b. Pemphigus
    c. Erythema multiforme
    d. Primary herpes

11. Formation of symblepharon and corneal damage is common in:
    a. Mucous membrane pemphigoid
    b. Bullous lichen planus
    c. Histoplasmolysis
    d. Blastomycosis

12. Indolent lesions of erosive lichen planus can be treated by:
    a. Topical corticosteroids
    b. Systemic corticosteroids
    c. Intralesional steroids
    d. All of the above

RED AND WHITE LESIONS OF THE ORAL MUCOSA

1. Which of the following is Non-keratotic white lesion?
   a. Stomatitis nicotina palati
   b. Linea alba
   c. Uremic stomatitis
   d. Focal epithelial hyperplasia

2. Which of the followings is not a histological feature of leukoedema?
   a. Thickened epithelium
   b. Keratinization
   c. Broad rete pegs
   d. Pyknotic nuclei

3. The number of Fordyce granule's present on oral mucosa:
   a. Increases with age
   b. Decreases with age
   c. Remains constant
   d. None of the above

4. Uremic stomatitis is caused in seriously ill patients with renal failure and blood urea nitrogen level-
   a. Less than 50 mg/dl
   b. More than 20 mg/dl
   c. Less than 20 mg/dl
   d. More than 50 mg/dl

5. Denture sore-mouth is:
   a. Not found under the mandibular denture
   b. Mostly found under the mandibular denture

c. Rarely found under the mandibular denture
d. Only found in maxillary denture

6. Dental hypoplasia and severe caries are common in:
   a. Candidiasis endocrinopathy syndrome
   b. Chronic hyperplastic candidiasis
   c. Acute atrophic candidiasis
   d. None of the above

7. Which of the following lesions does not have precancerous potential?
   a. Dyskeratosis congenita
   b. Actinic Keratosis
   c. Keratosis follicularis
   d. Erythroplakia

8. "Monro's abscesses" are found in:
   a. Focal epithelial hyperplasia
   b. Leukoedema
   c. Lichen planus
   d. Psoriasis

9. Orifices of palatal minor salivary glands appear as white, umblicated nodules with red centers in:
   a. Fordyce granules
   b. Denture sore-mouth
   c. Porokeratosis
   d. Stomatitis nicotina palati

10. "White epithelial pearls" or "Tobacco cells" or "cells-within-cells" occur most extensively in the cytologic examination of:
    a. Pachyonychia congenita
    b. Keratosis follicularis
    c. Hereditary benign intra epithelial dyskeratosis
    d. White sponge nevus

11. "Grains" and "corps ronds" can be examined in the cytologic smear of:
    a. Keratosis follicularis
    b. Dystrophic epidermolysis bullosa
    c. Acrodermatitis enteropathica
    d. Pseudoxanthoma Elasticum

12. Mixed red and white lesions are found in:
    a. Verrucous leukoplakia
    b. Nodular leukoplakia
    c. Homogenous leukoplakia
    d. Leukokeratosis

13. Major causative factor of leukoplakia is:
    a. Candidiasis
    b. Alcohol
    c. Tobacco
    d. Electrogalvanic current

14. Which of the following site in the mouth has highest rate for malignant transformation of oral leukoplakia?
    a. Buccal mucosa
    b. Lips and tongue
    c. Palate
    d. Floor of mouth

15. Which of the following diseases is/are correlated with tobacco use?
    a. Frictional keratosis
    b. Leukoedema
    c. Hairy tongue
    d. All of the above

16. White patches surrounded by a telangiectatic halo are found in:
    a. Erythema multiforme
    b. Systemic lupus erythematosus
    c. Discoid lupus erythematosus
    d. Pemphigus

17. "Wickham's striae" are found in:
    a. Reticular form of Lichen planus
    b. Papular form of Lichen planus
    c. Erosive lichen planus
    d. Bullous lichen planus

18. An association between oral lichen planus, diabetes mellitus and hypertension is found in which of the following syndromes?
    a. Ectodermal dysplasia syndrome
    b. Richter-Hanhart syndrome
    c. Grinspan's syndrome
    d. None of the above

19. Which of the following diseases does not exhibit Lichenoid tissue reaction?
    a. Erythema multiforme
    b. Secondary syphilis
    c. Lichen planus
    d. Leukoplakia

20. Which of the following syndromes is associated with vascular lesions?
    a. Sturge-Weber syndrome
    b. Gardner's syndrome
    c. Albright's syndrome
    d. Peutz-Jeghers syndrome

PIGMENTED LESIONS OF THE ORAL TISSUES

1. Which of the following is not a brown-melanotic lesion?
   a. Pigmented Lichen planus
   b. Ephulis
   c. Varices
   d. Blue Nevi

2. The most favoured oral site for Kaposi's sarcoma is:
   a. Gingiva
   b. Buccal mucosa
   c. Palate
   d. Lips

3. Which of the following is multifocal pigmentation of oral tissue?
   a. Hemochromatosis
   b. Hemangioma
   c. Melanoma
   d. Nevus

4. In the oral mucosa, blue nevi tend to exhibit:
   a. Blue color
   b. Red color
   c. Gray color
   d. Brown color

5. Which of the following drugs produces oral pigmentation?
   a. Acyclovir
   b. Fluconazole
   c. Minocycline
   d. Prednisone

6. "Café-au-lait" pigmentations are found in:
   a. Gardner's syndrome
   b. Neurofibromatosis
   c. Xanthomatosis
   d. Peutz-jeghers syndrome

7. The cause of patchy melanosis of the oral mucosa in Addison's disease is:
   a. Decreased secretion of ACTH
   b. Increased secretion of ACTH
   c. Decreased secretion of adrenal medullary hormone
   d. Increased secretion of adrenal medullary hormone

8. The most frequently affected site of HIV oral melanosis is:
   a. Buccal mucosa
   b. Gingiva
   c. Palate
   d. Tongue

9. Which of the following is the most common source of focal pigmentation in the oral mucosa?
   a. Ecchymosis
   b. Nevus
   c. Amalgam tattoo
   d. Graphite tattoo

10. The pigmentation due to heavy metal ingestion is usually found:
    a. At attached gingiva
    b. At interdental papillae
    c. Along the free gingival margin
    d. None of the above

11. Typical oral Kaposi's sarcoma lesions are:
    a. Focal
    b. Diffuse
    c. Multifocal
    d. None of the above

BENIGN ORAL TUMORS

1. Structural variants clinically appearing as slightly red nodular elevations are known as:
   a. Oral tori
   b. Oral tonsils
   c. Nodular fusciitis
   d. Fordyce granules

2. The inflammatory hyperplasia will not recur if:
   a. Lesion is excised
   b. Irritant is eliminated
   c. Irritant is eliminated with excision of lesion
   d. None of the above

3. Lesions developing on the hard palate due to dentures with relief areas or "suction chambers" are known as:
   a. Epulis fissuratum
   b. Palatal papillomatosis
   c. Denture-sore mouth
   d. Gumma of the palate

4. Pyogenic granuloma gradually converts into fibrous epulis when it becomes:
   a. More vascular and more collagenous
   b. More vascular and less collagenous
   c. Less vascular and less collagenous
   d. Less vascular and more collagenous

5. Which of the following is not a benign fibro-osseous lesion?
   a. Cherubism
   b. Aneurysmal bone cyst
   c. Osteitis deformans
   d. Ossifying fibroma

6. Cysts containing hair follicles, sweat glands and sebum are called as:
   a. Teratomas
   b. Epidermoid cyst
   c. Stafne's cyst
   d. Follicular cyst

7. Which of the following tumors is of mesodermal origin?
   a. Complex odontoma
   b. Ameloblastic fibroma
   c. Cementifying fibroma
   d. Ameloblastoma

8. Tumor occurring usually in children under 6 months of age is:
   a. Adenoameloblastoma
   b. Odontoameloblastoma
   c. Melanoameloblastoma
   d. None of the above

9. Virus-induced tumor characterized by soft, flat, sessile papules is found in:
   a. Heck's disease
   b. Darier's disease
   c. Keratoacanthoma
   d. Verruca vulgaris

10. "Floating teeth" are found in:
    a. Xanthomatosis
    b. Cherubism
    c. Tuberous sclerosis
    d. Acanthosis nigricans

11. The most frequent site of involvement in cervicofacial actinomycosis is:
    a. Masseter region
    b. Skull
    c. Submandibular region
    d. Parotid region

12. Mouth breathers mainly exhibit gingival enlargements in:
    a. Mandibular anterior region
    b. Maxillary anterior region
    c. Maxillary posterior region
    d. All of the above

13. Cyst that remains attached to the neck of the tooth enclosing the crown within the cyst is:
    a. Dentigerous cyst
    b. Primordial cyst
    c. Radicular cyst
    d. Eruption cyst

MALIGNANT ORAL TUMORS

1. The size of cervical lymph node of stage N2B is:
   a. More than 6 cm
   b. More than 8 cm
   c. Less than 6 cm
   d. None of the above

2. Virus most commonly present in oral squamous cell carcinoma is:
   a. HPV type 16
   b. HPV type 10
   c. HPV type 12
   d. HPV type 15

3. Treatment of choice for exophytic and well-oxygenated tumor is:
   a. Surgery
   b. Radiotherapy
   c. Chemotherapy
   d. All the above

4. Primary tumor of posterior third of the tongue is best treated by:
   a. Brachytherapy
   b. Intraoral cone therapy
   c. Interstitial therapy
   d. External beam therapy

5. Total dose of radiations given for treatment of malignant tumor is:
   a. 3500 to 5000 cGy
   b. 5000 to 5500 cGy
   c. 6000 to 6500 cGy
   d. 7000 to 8000 cGy

6. The most common symptom of nasopharyngeal carcinoma is:
   a. Neck mass
   b. Ear ache
   c. Pain
   d. Limited Jaw opening

7. Most rapidly increasing malignant disease in AIDS is:
   a. Kaposi's sarcoma
   b. Lymphoma
   c. Oropharyngeal carcinoma
   d. None of the above

8. Which of the following drugs can be used prophylactically to reduce complications of radiotherapy?
   a. Diphenhydramine HCl
   b. Sucralfate
   c. Benzydamine HCl
   d. Dyclonine HCl

9. Which of the following is not a complication of radiation therapy?
   a. Candidiasis
   b. Trismus
   c. Micrognathia
   d. Parotitis

10. Which of the following drugs is used in the treatment of radiation xerostomia?
    a. Bethanechol
    b. Pilocarpine
    c. Anetholetrithione
    d. All of the above

11. Bowen's disease occurs on skin as a result of:
    a. Mercury ingestion
    b. Arsenic ingestion
    c. Copper ingestion
    d. None of the above

DISEASES OF THE TONGUE

1. Which of the following syndromes have findings of cleft lip, cleft palate and congenital lip pit?
   a. Fraser's syndrome
   b. Meckel's syndrome
   c. van der Woude's syndrome
   d. Fetal face syndrome

2. Tongue with thick leathery coating in dehydrated and debilitated patients is referred to as:
   a. Hairy tongue
   b. Earthy tongue
   c. Geographic tongue
   d. Plicated tongue

3. Non ulcerating, irregular indurations on the tongue with leukoplakia are seen in:
   a. Interstitial glossitis
   b. Traumatic glossitis
   c. Median rhomboid glossitis
   d. Atrophic glossitis

4. Series of ulcers along the anterior third of the tongue on one side are seen in:
   a. Blastomycosis
   b. Primary herpes simplex gingivostomatitis
   c. Riga-Fede disease
   d. Herpes zoster infection

5. Purplish blue spots, nodules and ridges on anterior ventral surface of the tongue are referred to as:
   a. Neurofibromatosis
   b. Petechial hemorrhages
   c. Lingual varicosities
   d. Lingual hematomas

6. Lipoprotein lipase needed for digestion of fat in infants is secreted from:
   a. Glands of Blandin and Nuhn
   b. Lingual mucosal glands
   c. Glands of von Ebner
   d. None of the above

7. Rapid repetitive uncontrolled movement of the tongue is called as:
   a. Dystonia
   b. Tremors
   c. Myotonic dystrophy
   d. Tardive dyskinesia

8. Majority of tongue carcinomas occur on:
   a. Dorsum of the tongue
   b. Base of the tongue
   c. Anterior two-third of the tongue
   d. Ventral surface of the tongue

9. Carcinoma of the posterior tongue is mostly treated by:
   a. Surgery
   b. Radiation
   c. Combined radiation and surgery
   d. Chemotherapy

10. "Long and narrow" tongue as a result of hyperostosis and thickening of the mandible is seen in:
    a. Cystic hygroma
    b. Epidermolysis bullosa
    c. Cretinism
    d. Tuberous sclerosis

11. Riga's ulcers on the tongue of the infants occur on:
    a. Lateral border of the tongue
    b. Ventral surface of the tongue
    c. Lingual frenum
    d. Fimbriated folds

12. "Strawberry tongue" is a classic sign, found in infection with:
    a. Herpes simplex virus
    b. Capnocytophaga
    c. Salmonella lyphi
    d. Streptococcus pyogenes

13. Annular, circinate and serpiginous lesions of the tongue are found in:
    a. Hairy tongue
    b. Geographic tongue
    c. Scrotal tongue
    d. Depapillated tongue

SALIVARY GLAND DISEASES

1. An aberrant salivary gland is found:
    a. Posterior to the first molar in the mandible
    b. Posterior to the first molar in the maxilla
    c. Anterior to the first molar in the mandible
    d. None of the above

2. Sialoliths most frequently occur in:
    a. Parotid gland
    b. Sub-lingual gland
    c. Minor salivary gland
    d. Sub-mandibuar gland

3. Mucous-extravasation cysts are usually found on:
    a. Lower lip
    b. Tongue
    c. Floor of mouth
    d. Palate

4. In sialadenitis, viscosity and turbidity of the saliva:
    a. Decrease
    b. Increase
    c. Remain normal
    d. None of the above

5. Which of the following is not an inflammatory disease of salivary gland?
    a. Mumps
    b. Sarcoid sialadenitis
    c. Sialadenosis
    d. Bacterial sialadenitis

6. Acute non suppurative parotitis can be caused by:
    a. Paramyxovirus
    b. Para influenza type 1
    c. Para influenza type 3
    d. All the above

7. Purulent discharge with sulphur granules is milked from salivary gland duct when it is infected by:
    a. Staphylococcus aureus
    b. Escherichia coli
    c. Actinomycetes
    d. Proteus

8. Chemical constituents of saliva in sialosis are characterized by:
    a. Increased salivary K and decreased salivary Na
    b. Increased salivary Na and decreased salivary K
    c. Both salivary Na and K are decreased
    d. None of the above

9. A "salt and pepper" appearance of the salivary glands on MRI suggests:
    a. Sialadenosis
    b. Necrotizing sialometaplasia
    c. Heerfordt's syndrome
    d. Sjogren's syndrome

10. Disorder associated with decreased salivary flow in debilitated patient is:
    a. Sjogren's syndrome
    b. Sarcoidosis
    c. Acute parotitis
    d. Chronic parotitis

11. Dose of intraductal erythromycin for the treatment of chronic bacterial sialadenitis is:
    a. 25 mg/ml for 5 days
    b. 20 mg/ml for 5 days
    c. 15 mg/ml for 7 days
    d. 15 mg/ml for 5 days

TEMPOROMANDIBULAR JOINT DISORDERS

1. The lateral mandibular motion ranges from:
    a. 10-12 mm
    b. 5-7 mm
    c. 8-10 mm
    d. 6-8 mm

2. Eagle's syndrome is associated with:
    a. Pain in eye
    b. Pain in sinuses
    c. Pain due to elongated styloid process
    d. None of the above

3. The muscles most often involved in MPDS are:
    a. Digastric and medial pterygoid
    b. Geniohyoid and mylohyoid
    c. Temporalis and geniohyoid
    d. Lateral pterygoid and masseter

4. Ely's cyst is found in:
   a. Rheumatoid arthritis
   b. Degenerative joint disease
   c. Psoriatic arthritis
   d. Septic arthritis

5. Chronic pain or pain of increased intensity due to internal derangements in the TMJ can be treated by:
   a. Maxillary occlusal splint
   b. Mandibular protrusive splint
   c. Fixed orthodontic treatment
   d. All the above

6. Synovial chondromatosis is characterized by:
   a. Inflammation of synovial membrane
   b. Rupture of synovial membrane
   c. Cartilaginous nodules of the synovial membrane
   d. None of the above

7. Micrognathia and anterior open bite are found in:
   a. Septic arthritis
   b. Juvenile rheumatoid arthritis
   c. Rheumatoid arthritis
   d. Psoriatic arthritis

8. Pitting of the nails is a characteristic clinical feature of:
   a. Gout
   b. Septic arthritis
   c. Psoriatic arthritis
   d. Rheumatoid arthritis

9. Large and tender cervical lymphnodes are found in:
   a. Septic arthritis
   b. Psoriatic arthritis
   c. Gout
   d. None of the above

10. Flatness of face on one side is found in:
    a. Condylar hyperplasia
    b. Fracture of condyle
    c. Condylar hypoplasia
    d. Bifid condyle

11. Unilateral pain in preauricular region which becomes worse on awakening is a clinical feature of:
    a. Degenerative joint disease
    b. Myofascial pain dysfunction syndrome
    c. Chondrometaplasia
    d. Disc displacement

OROFACIAL PAIN AND ABNORMALITIES OF TASTE

1. Painful syndrome characterized by faulty identification and localization of stimulus is:
   a. Causalgia
   b. Anesthesia dolorosa
   c. Hyperpathia
   d. Hyperalgesia

2. The recommended dose of carbamazepine for treatment of trigeminal neuralgia is:
   a. Initial dose of 200 mg/day increased to 800 to 1200 mg/day
   b. Initial dose of 400 mg/day increased to 600 to 1200 mg/day
   c. Initial dose of 1200 mg/day decreased to 600 mg/day
   d. Initial dose of 800 mg/day decreased to 200 mg/day

3. Geniculate neuralgia results from herpetic inflammation of:
   a. Cranial nerve V
   b. Cranial nerve VII
   c. Cranial nerve X
   d. Cervical spinal nerve

4. Conjunctival reddening is observed in:
   a. Migraine headache
   b. Tension-type headache
   c. Cluster headache
   d. Mixed headache

5. Drug used prophylactically for preventing migraine headache is:
   a. Nifedipine
   b. Nadolol
   c. Indomethacin
   d. Prednisone

6. "Claudication" of the masticatory muscles is found in:
   a. Carotodynia
   b. Causalgia
   c. Cranial arteritis
   d. Geniculate neuralgia

7. Cluster headache is triggered by:
   a. Mastication
   b. Talking
   c. Smoking
   d. None of the above

8. Signs and symptoms present is stage 2 sympathetic dystrophy are:
   a. Diminished pain, muscle wasting and tissue damage
   b. Edema, increased skin temperature and decreased heat tolerance
   c. Cold intolerance, hyperesthetic pain and decreased skin temperature
   d. Burning and aching with sympathetic denervation.

9. Loss of the ability to classify or identify a given taste stimulus refers to:
   a. Cacogeusia
   b. Gustatory agnosia
   c. Phantogeusia
   d. Torquegeusia

10. Which of the following is not a "true taste disorder"?
    a. Transport disorders of taste
    b. Secondary dysgeusias
    c. Sensorineural disorders of taste
    d. None of the above

11. Familial dysautonomia is a rare disorder associated with:
    a. Hypersalivation
    b. Abnormal taste sensation
    c. Excessive sweating
    d. All of the above

12. Deficiency of which of the following minerals is associated with taste dysfunction:
    a. Chromium
    b. Selenium
    c. Zinc
    d. Manganese

13. Olfactory and gustatory sensations are lost in head injury due to damage to:
    a. Frontal lobe
    b. Occipital lobe
    c. Parietal lobe
    d. Temporal lobe

CARDIOVASCULAR DISEASES RELATED TO ORAL MEDICINE

1. Risk of coronary heart disease can be reduced by:
   a. Lowering LDL level and increasing HDL level
   b. Raising LDL level and lowering HDL level
   c. Decreasing both LDL and HDL levels
   d. Increasing both LDL and HDL levels

2. Chest pain occurring at rest mostly at night or during ordinary activity is:
   a. Classic angina
   b. Variant angina
   c. Unstable angina
   d. None of the above

3. Severe crushing pain in the left side of the jaw that is brought on by exertion and is relieved by rest and lasts for few seconds to few minutes is seen in:
   a. Multiple sclerosis
   b. Trigeminal neuralgia
   c. Angina pectoris
   d. MPDS

4. The skin eruptions found in rheumatic fever are known as:
   a. Erythema multiforme
   b. Erythema marginatum
   c. Erythema circinata migrans
   d. None of the above

5. Characteristic clinical feature found in Endocarditis is:
   a. Subcutaneous nodules on the extensor surface of the wrist
   b. Ecchymosis of the eyelids and sclera
   c. Petechial hemorrhage in the conjunctivae
   d. Bluish skin pigmentation

6. Cardiac condition in which Endocarditis prophylaxis in not recommended before dental treatment is:
   a. Rheumatic fever with valvular involvement
   b. Prosthetic cardiac valves
   c. Congenital heart diseases
   d. Cardiac pacemakers

7. Drug of choice for patient with rheumatic heart disease undergoing surgical procedure in the oral cavity is:
   a. Penicillin
   b. Ampicillin
   c. Amoxicillin
   d. None of the above

8. Diastolic pressure in stage-2 hypertension ranges between:
   a. 110 to 119 mm Hg
   b. 100 to 109 mm Hg
   c. 90 to 99 mm Hg
   d. 120 to 130 mm Hg

9. Antihypertensive drug that may cause gingival enlargement is:
    a. Furosemide
    b. Prazosin
    c. Diltiazem
    d. Methyldopa

10. Cyanosis of the oral mucosa with severe marginal gingivitis is clinical feature in:
    a. Coarctation of the aorta
    b. Tetralogy of fallot
    c. Persistent ductus arteriosus
    d. Atrial septal defects

11. The early signs of congestive heart failure are:
    a. Cyanosis of the oral mucosa with tongue edema
    b. Pain in the jaw and teeth
    c. Shortness of breath and headache
    d. Cyanosis of the oral mucosa with ankle edema

12. Which of the following antihypertensive drugs may cause ulcerations in the oral mucous membrane?
    a. Nifedipine
    b. Methyldopa
    c. Diltiazem
    d. Furosemide

DISEASES OF THE RESPIRATORY SYSTEM RELATED TO ORAL MEDICINE

1. Micro-organism responsible for sinusitis particularly in children is:
    a. Streptococcus pneumoniae
    b. Staphylococcus aureus
    c. Streptococcus pyogenes
    d. Haemophilus influenza

2. Persistent hoarseness of voice with acute pain and dysphagia is found in:
    a. Acute laryngitis
    b. Pharyngitis
    c. Tuberculous laryngitis
    d. None of the above

3. The commonest cause of chronic bronchitis is:
    a. Air pollution
    b. Smoking
    c. Chronic recurrent infections
    d. Occupational inhalants

4. In immunosuppressed patients, pneumonia is mostly caused by:
    a. Pneumocystis carinii
    b. Klebsiella pneumoniae
    c. Streptococcus pneumoniae
    d. Legionella pneumophila

5. Drug of choice for treatment of Pneumocystis Carinii pneumonia is:
    a. Tetracycline
    b. Erythromycin
    c. Penicillin
    d. Pentamidine

6. Which of the following infectious diseases is also referred to as "acid-fast infection"?
    a. Pneumonitis
    b. Histoplasmosis
    c. Tuberculosis
    d. Tonsillitis

7. Scrofula refers to:
    a. Tuberculous involvement of spine
    b. Tuberculous involvement of cervical lymph-nodes
    c. Tuberculous involvement of adrenal cortex
    d. Tuberculous involvement of parotid gland

8. Oral lesions in tuberculosis are characterized by:
    a. Small ulcers at the corners of the mouth
    b. Lesions at the lateral margin of the tongue
    c. Deep central ulcers of the tongue
    d. All of the above

9. Dental treatment in actively infected patient with tuberculosis can be carried out:
    a. After 2 to 3 weeks of antitubercular therapy
    b. After 4 to 5 weeks of antitubercular therapy
    c. After 1 to 2 months of antitubercular therapy
    d. After 3 months of antitubercular therapy

10. The most presenting oral manifestation of Wegener's granulomatosis is:
    a. Ulceration of the tongue
    b. Destruction of the hard palate
    c. Hemorrhagic gingival enlargement
    d. Oropharyngeal lesions

11. Destruction and perforation of hard and soft palates are found in:
    a. Wegener's granulomatosis
    b. Midline granuloma
    c. Pyogenic granuloma
    d. Giant-cell granuloma

12. Tetracycline staining of the teeth is commonly seen in patients of:
    a. Pneumonitis
    b. Actinomycosis

c. Recurrent aphthous ulcers
d. Cystic fibrosis

DISEASES OF GASTROINTESTINAL TRACT RELATED TO ORAL MEDICINE

1. Swallowing tablets or capsules without adequate amount of water may lead to:
   a. Gastric ulcer
   b. Esophageal ulcer
   c. Duodenal ulcer
   d. Peptic ulcer

2. Which of the following is the most frequent cause of peptic ulceration?
   a. Infection with Helicobacter.pylori
   b. Hypoglycemia
   c. NSAIDs
   d. Smoking

3. Which of the following drugs used in the treatment of peptic ulcer may lead to xerostomia?
   a. Sucralfate
   b. Omeprazole
   c. Ranitidine
   d. Atropine

4. Which of the following drugs may induce hepatitis?
   a. Nizatidine
   b. Pyrazinamide
   c. Isoniazid hydrochloride
   d. None of the above

5. Yellow discoloration of oral mucosa in hepatitis is most readily seen on:
   a. Palate
   b. Buccal mucosa
   c. Alveolar mucosa
   d. Muco-buccal fold

6. Chronic hepatitis B can be treated by administration of:
   a. Interferon beta-1b
   b. Interferon alpha-2b
   c. Interferon gamma
   d. Trophoblast interferon

7. Oral manifestation in Crohn's disease is characterized by:
   a. Pigmentation of the oral mucosa
   b. Gingival enlargement
   c. Aphthous like ulcerations
   d. Cracked lips

8. Hepatic dysfunction or severe jaundice may lead to:
   a. Severe bleeding following periodontal operation
   b. Spontaneous bleeding in the oral cavity
   c. Both a and b
   d. None of the above

9. Which of the following methods is not effective in inactivating Hepatitis B virus?
   a. Immersion in 100°C boiling water for 10 minutes
   b. Immersion in 1% solution of sodium hypochlorite for 10 minutes
   c. Immersion in solution of isopropyl alcohol for 15 minutes
   d. Dry heat at 106°C for 1 hour

10. Least amount of infected blood on dental instruments that may transmit Hepatitis virus to dental surgeon and other patients is:
    a. 0.04 ml
    b. 0.004 ml
    c. 0.0004 ml
    d. 0.4 ml

RENAL DISEASES AND ORAL MEDICINE

1. Which of the following is the second most common cause of renal failure?
   a. Polycystic renal disease
   b. Glomerulonephritis
   c. Pyelonephritis
   d. Nephrosclerosis

2. Anemia in patients with renal diseases is caused due to:
   a. Destruction of RBCs
   b. Failure of erythropoietin production
   c. Loss of blood during hemodialysis
   d. All of the above

3. Changes associated with renal osteodystrophy are most frequently seen in:
   a. Maxillary premolar region
   b. Maxillary molar region
   c. Mandibular molar region
   d. Mandibular premolar region

4. The giant cell lesions found in hyperparathyroidism and related to renal diseases are called as:
   a. Wilm's tumor
   b. Blood tumor
   c. Brown tumor
   d. Gray tumor

5. Which of the followings is not an oral manifestation in dialysis patients?
   a. Tooth erosion
   b. Bleeding from gingiva
   c. Enamel hypoplasia
   d. Hematoma formation

6. Uremic stomatitis occurs in oral cavity when:
   a. BUN level is greater than 50 mg/dl
   b. BUN level is greater than 75 mg/dl
   c. BUN level is greater than 100 mg/dl
   d. BUN level is greater than 150 mg/dl

7. Dental treatment of patient with renal disease should be performed:
   a. Before dialysis
   b. Within 24 hours of dialysis
   c. After 24 hours of dialysis
   d. During dialysis

8. The recommended dose of prednisolone used for anti-rejection therapy in kidney transplantation is:
   a. 5 to 10 mg/d
   b. 10 to 40 mg/d
   c. 40 to 60 mg/d
   d. None of the above

9. Administration of cyclosporine in kidney transplant patients may lead to:
   a. Hepatic dysfunction
   b. Kidney arteriolopathy
   c. Gingival hyperplasia
   d. All of the above

10. Which of the following drugs can produce stomatitis and xerostomia?
    a. Cyclosporine
    b. Azathioprine
    c. Prednisone
    d. Phenacetin

11. The first and most frequently involved area of cyclosporine-induced gingival hyperplasia is:
    a. Lingual gingiva in the posterior teeth
    b. Lingual gingiva in the anterior teeth
    c. Labial gingiva in the anterior teeth
    d. Buccal gingiva in the posterior teeth

RELATION OF IMMUNOLOGIC DISEASES WITH ORAL MEDICINE

1. X-linked gamma globulinemia is caused by defect in-
   a. T-cell function
   b. B-cell function
   c. Both B and T-cell functions
   d. None of the above

2. B-lymphocyte deficiencies are associated with:
   a. Viral infections
   b. Fungal infections
   c. Bacterial infections
   d. All of the above

3. Congenital defects of the mouth and jaws are seen in:
   a. X-linked agammaglobulinemia
   b. Severe combined immunodeficiency
   c. Secondary immunodeficiency
   d. Thymic hypoplasia

4. AIDS patients become susceptible to infections when T_4 lymphocytes count is below:
   a. 200 mm^3
   b. 75 mm^3
   c. 100 mm^3
   d. 150 mm^3

5. Persistent generalized lymphadenopathy occurs in AIDS patients during:
   a. Acute infections
   b. Opportunistic infections
   c. Asymptomatic phase
   d. None of the above

6. An initial opportunistic infection in AIDS patients is of:
   a. Candida albicans
   b. Pneumocystis carinii pneumonia
   c. Mycobacterium tuberculosis
   d. Cryptococcus

7. The second most common tumor in AIDS patients is:
   a. Non-Hodgkin's lymphoma
   b. Hodgkin's lymphoma
   c. Kaposi's sarcoma
   d. Cervical carcinoma

8. The drug used in management of AIDS is:
   a. Azidothymidine
   b. Pentamidine
   c. Didanasine
   d. All of the above

9. The most common oral manifestation in patients with systemic lupus erythematosus is:
   a. Oral ulceration
   b. Petechiae
   c. Edema
   d. Xerostomia

10. Hard and rigid tongue and lips with narrow mouth opening are oral findings in:
    a. Dermatomyositis
    b. Lupus erythematosus
    c. Scleroderma
    d. Rheumatoid arthritis

11. Which of the following muscles get weakened in dermatomyositis?
    a. Masticatory muscles
    b. Pharyngeal muscles
    c. Palatal muscles
    d. All of the above

12. The recommended dose of epinephrine for treatment of generalized anaphylaxis is:
    a. 0.2 ml intravenously
    b. 0.5 ml subcutaenously
    c. 0.3 ml subcutaneously
    d. 0.5 ml intravenously

13. Uniform thickening of periodontal membrane around posterior teeth is found in:
    a. Progressive systemic sclerosis
    b. Linear localized scleroderma
    c. Dermatomyositis
    d. Lupus erythematosus

NEUROMUSCULAR DISEASES AFFECTING THE ORO-FACIAL REGION

1. The most frequent site of brain involvement in cerebral abscess is:
   a. Frontal lobe
   b. Parietal lobe
   c. Temporal lobe
   d. Occipital lobe

2. Impairment of vision, muscular incoordination and bladder dysfunction are found in:
   a. Amyotrophic lateral sclerosis
   b. Parkinson's disease
   c. Guillain-Barre syndrome
   d. Multiple sclerosis

3. Rapid vision loss following an increase in body temperature associated with heavy exercise is known as:
   a. Marcus Gunn's pupillary sign
   b. Uthoff's sign
   c. Ewing sign
   d. None of the above

4. Impaired swallowing or paresthesia of the mouth and face is found in:
   a. Peutz-Jegher syndrome
   b. Guillain-Barre syndrome
   c. Sjogren's syndrome
   d. Stevens-Johnson syndrome

5. Atrophy of sternomastoid muscles is found in:
   a. Myasthenia gravis
   b. Huntington's chorea
   c. Myotonic dystrophy
   d. Duchenne's dystrophy

6. Epileptic seizures found in children are called as:
   a. Grand mal
   b. Petit mal
   c. Status epilepticus
   d. Tonic-clonic

7. Which of the following phases of epilepsy is associated with cyanosis?
   a. Tonic phase
   b. Postictal stage
   c. Clonic phase
   d. Status epilepticus

8. Bacteria isolated from cerebral abscess in immunocompromised patient is:
   a. Staphylococci
   b. Streptococcus milleri
   c. Peptostreptococcus
   d. Nocardia

9. Which of the following is the main clinical feature of Parkinson's disease?
   a. Hyperkinesia
   b. Bradykinesia
   c. Muscular atrophy
   d. None of the above

10. Mild form of Parkinson's can be managed by:
    a. Levodopa
    b. Carbidopa
    c. Trihexyphenidyl
    d. Bromocriptine

11. Increased incidence of enamel defects in children is found in:
    a. Bell's palsy
    b. Cerebral palsy
    c. Birth palsy
    d. All of the above

12. In Bell's palsy, food is retained in upper and lower buccal and labial folds due to weakness of following muscle:
    a. Buccinator muscle
    b. Risorius muscle
    c. Temporalis muscle
    d. Masseter muscle

13. Which of the following is the initial clinical sign in myasthenia gravis?
    a. Diplopia and colour blindness
    b. Periorbital edema
    c. Cataract
    d. Diplopia and ptosis

14. Gingival hyperplasia induced by phenytoin first starts in:
    a. Attached gingiva
    b. Unattached gingiva
    c. Interdental papillae
    d. Any of the above

DIABETES AND ITS ORAL MANIFESTATIONS

1. Which of the following viruses is not related to onset of Insulin dependent diabetes mellitus?
    a. Coxsackie B4 virus
    b. Cytomegalovirus
    c. Epstein Barr virus
    d. Rubella

2. Rapid weight loss with salt and water depletion is found in:
    a. Type 1 diabetes
    b. Type 2 diabetes
    c. Gestational diabetes
    d. Drug-induced diabetes

3. Which of the following is the clinical feature of type 2 diabetes?
    a. Loss of skin turgor
    b. Chronic fatigue and malaise
    c. Rapid weight loss
    d. None of the above

4. Burning sensation in soles of feet in diabetic patient is caused due to:
    a. Atherosclerosis
    b. Ketoacidosis
    c. Peripheral neuropathy
    d. Autonomic neuropathy

5. Which of the following is the pathognomonic oral manifestation of diabetes?
    a. Oral candidiasis
    b. Burning tongue
    c. Gingival disease
    d. Median rhomboid glossitis

6. Dry socket after tooth extraction in diabetic patients is caused due to:
    a. Infection
    b. Delayed wound healing
    c. Atherosclerosis
    d. None of the above

7. Which of the following is the rare oral manifestation of diabetes mellitus?
    a. Burning tongue
    b. Median rhomboid glossitis
    c. Xanthomas
    d. Oral candidiasis

8. In diabetic patients, complicated oral procedures in dental emergencies:
    a. Should be avoided
    b. Can be performed on stabilization of blood glucose level
    c. Both a and b
    d. None of the above

HEMATOLOGICAL DISORDERS

1. Increase in absolute neutrophil count above 30,000/mm^3 is called as:
    a. Granulocytosis
    b. Leukemia
    c. Leukemoid reaction
    d. Myeloid metaplasia

2. Oral ulcers characterized by necrosis and without surrounding inflammation are found in:
    a. Leukemia
    b. Neutropenia
    c. Cyclic neutropenia
    d. Lymphoma

3. The large, irregular, foul smelling oral ulcers surrounded by pale mucosa are found in:
    a. Neutropenia
    b. Agranulocytosis
    c. Leukemia
    d. None of the above

4. Pel-Ebstein fever is found in the following disease:
   a. Non-hodgkin's lymphoma
   b. Multiple myeloma
   c. Burkitt's lymphoma
   d. Hodgkin disease

5. Slow-growing, painless, bluish, soft masses on palate are found in:
   a. Multiple myeloma
   b. Non-hodgkin's lymphoma
   c. Neutropenia
   d. All of the above

6. Multiple myeloma is characterized by:
   a. Amyloidosis of tongue
   b. Glossitis
   c. Ulcers on the tongue
   d. Glossodynia

7. Purplish red discoloration of oral mucosa is observed in:
   a. Primary polycythemia
   b. Secondary polycythemia
   c. Plummer-vinson syndrome
   d. Chediak-Higashi syndrome

8. General anesthesia should not be administered in iron-deficiency anemic patient, unless the concentration of hemoglobin is atleast:
   a. 8 g/dl
   b. 10 g/dl
   c. 12 g/dl
   d. 14 g/dl

9. "Hair on end" appearance in skull radiograph is observed in:
   a. Sickle-cell anemia
   b. Thalassemia
   c. Both a and b
   d. None of the above

10. Delayed eruption and hypoplasia of dentition is found in:
    a. Paroxysmal nocturnal hemoglobinuria
    b. β-thalassemia major
    c. β-thalassemia minor
    d. Sickle cell anemia

11. The color of skin in patients with β-thalassemia major is ashen-gray due to:
    a. Jaundice
    b. Pallor
    c. Hemosiderosis
    d. Combination of all the above

12. The most frequent oral manifestation in Cooley's (Thalassemia major) anemia is:
    a. Spacing of teeth
    b. Saddled nose
    c. Bimaxillary protrusion
    d. Open bite

13. "Beefy red" tongue with erythematous areas is found in:
    a. Aplastic anemia
    b. Pernicious anemia
    c. Folic-acid deficiency anemia
    d. Sickle-cell anemia

14. Spontaneous hemorrhage from gingiva is characteristic feature of:
    a. Pernicious anemia
    b. Thalassemia
    c. Aplastic anemia
    d. Secondary polycythemia

15. Patient complains of "spasm in the throat" in:
    a. Lazy-leukocyte syndrome
    b. Plummer-vinson syndrome
    c. Chediak-Higashi syndrome
    d. None of the above

16. Which of the following is the characteristic clinical feature of polycythemia vera?
    a. Cyanosis of face
    b. Varicosities in tongue
    c. Pruritus
    d. All of the above

17. Hyperpigmentation of skin and hair is found in:
    a. Sjogren's syndrome
    b. Cowden's syndrome
    c. Chediak-Higashi syndrome
    d. Plummer-vinson syndrome

18. The most common oral infection in leukemic patients is of:
    a. Histoplasma
    b. Phycomycetes
    c. Candidiasis
    d. Aspergillus

19. The most common cause of oral ulcerations in leukemic patients on chemotherapy is:
    a. Coxsackie virus infection
    b. Varicella zoster virus infection
    c. Cytomegalovirus
    d. Herpes simplex virus infections

20. The etiology of Burkitt's lymphoma is most closely linked with:
    a. Varicella-zoster virus
    b. Epstein-Barr virus
    c. Cytomegalovirus
    d. Coxsackievirus

DISORDERS OF HEMOSTASIS AND ORAL MEDICINE

1. Clinical test used to evaluate primary hemostasis is:
   a. Prothrombin time
   b. Thrombin clotting time
   c. Fibrin degradation products
   d. Platelet count

2. The normal level of circulating fibrinogen in:
   a. 150 mg/dl
   b. 200 mg/dl
   c. 250 mg/dl
   d. 300 mg/dl

3. Hemophilia A is caused by deficiency of:
   a. Stuart factor
   b. Antihemophilic factor
   c. Christmas factor
   d. Hageman factor

4. Prolonged bleeding after tooth extraction in patients with hemophilia A is seen when level of factor VIII is:
   a. Less than 1% of normal
   b. 1% to 7% of normal
   c. 7% to 50% of normal
   d. 50% to 70% of normal

5. Microvascular infarcts in gingiva and other mucosal surfaces are found in:
   a. Thrombotic thrombocytopenic purpura
   b. Thrombocytopathia
   c. Hemophilia
   d. None of the above

6. Mild moderate hemophilia A can be managed by administration of:
   a. Fresh frozen plasma
   b. Cryoprecipitate
   c. Desmopressin acetate
   d. Factor IX concentrates

7. Which of the following oral structures exhibits most frequently bleeding in hemophilia?
   a. Tongue
   b. Labial frenum
   c. Buccal mucosa
   d. Gingiva

8. Which of the following oral manifestations occur in hemophilic patient?
   a. Bleeding from buccal mucosa
   b. Severe periodontal disease
   c. TMJ arthropathy
   d. All of the above

9. The management of thrombocytopenia includes:
   a. Transfusion of platelets
   b. Plasma exchange therapy
   c. Corticosteroids
   d. All of the above

10. Excessive bleeding caused due to anticoagulant medication such as heparin, during surgical procedure can be managed by administration of:
    a. Recombinant erythropoietin
    b. Infection of vitamin K
    c. Protamine sulphate
    d. Conjugated estrogen preparation

11. Chronic abnormal bleeding in uremic patients can be treated by:
    a. Conjugated estrogen preparation
    b. Recombinant erythropoietin
    c. Both (a) and (b)
    d. None of the above

12. Oral hemorrhages related to thrombocytopenia, associated with chemotherapeutic drugs, can be managed by:
    a. Desmopressin acetate
    b. Transfusions of HLA matched platelets
    c. Infusion of FFP (Fresh Frozen Plasma)
    d. Recombinant erythropoietin

13. Disseminated intravascular coagulation can be treated by administration of:
    a. Intravenous heparin
    b. Subcutaneous heparin
    c. Dicumarol
    d. None of the above

14. Which of the following drugs inhibits fibrinolysis by blocking the conversion of plasminogen to plasmin?
    a. Tranexamic acid
    b. Protamine sulphate
    c. Dipyrimadole
    d. None of the above

INFECTIOUS DISEASES RELATED TO ORAL MEDICINE

1. Treatment of pharyngeal gonorrhea includes administration of:
   a. Single dose of ceftriaxone 125 mg IM
   b. Ceftriaxone 125 mg IM twice a day
   c. Ceftriaxone 250 mg IM twice a day
   d. Single dose of ceftriaxone 250 mg IM

2. Reiter's disease is caused by:
   a. Treponema pertenue
   b. C. trachomatis
   c. N. catarrhalis
   d. Donovania granulomatosis

3. Slightly raised grayish white oral lesions surrounded by an erythematous base found in syphilis are known as:
   a. Chancre
   b. Gumma
   c. Mucous patches
   d. Split papules

4. Split papules are the oral lesions of secondary syphilis and are found on:
   a. Buccal mucosa
   b. Tongue
   c. Commissures of the lips
   d. All of the above

5. Oral manifestations of tertiary syphilis are:
   a. Gumma of palate and tongue
   b. Severe neuralgic pain in head and neck
   c. Paresthesia in the lips and tongue
   d. All the above

6. "Syphilitic rhagades" near the angle of the mouth are found in:
   a. Primary syphilis
   b. Secondary syphilis
   c. Tertiary syphilis
   d. Congenital syphilis

7. Oral manifestations of congenital syphilis are characterized by:
   a. "Peg-shaped" incisors
   b. "Mulberry molar"
   c. Death of the dental pulp
   d. Both (a) and (b)

8. Donovan bodies are found in cytological examination of:
   a. Gonorrhea
   b. Syphilis
   c. Granuloma inguinale
   d. Lymphogranuloma venereum

9. The recommended dose of acyclovir for the treatment of oropharyngeal HSV infection is:
   a. 100 mg five times daily
   b. 200 mg five times daily
   c. 400 mg five times daily
   d. 400 mg twice daily

10. Oral ulcerations with pharyngitis, tonsillitis and cervical lymphadenopathy are found in:
    a. Cytomegalovirus infection
    b. Infectious mononucleosis
    c. Reiter's disease
    d. Burkitt's lymphoma

11. Oral condyloma acuminatum can be treated by:
    a. Surgical excision
    b. Cryotherapy
    c. CO$_2$ laser therapy
    d. All of the above

12. Isolated mucosal ulcers with membranous gingivostomatitis are the clinical features of:
    a. Herpetic stomatitis
    b. Gonococcal stomatitis
    c. Allergic stomatitis
    d. None of the above

13. Ulcerative gingivostomatitis with sore mouth are the clinical features of:
    a. Aphthous stomatitis
    b. Gonococcal stomatitis
    c. Herpetic stomatitis
    d. Allergic stomatitis

14. Extensive superficial ulceration on the lip with a well defined elevated granulomatous margin is found in:
    a. Molluscum contagiosum infection
    b. Lymphogranuloma venereum
    c. Granuloma inguinale
    d. None of the above

15. Dysphagia and red soft palate with regional lymphadenopathy are the oral manifestations of:
    a. Lymphogranuloma venereum
    b. Infectious mononucleosis
    c. Oral CMV infections
    d. Oropharyngeal HSV infection

16. Pharyngitis, perioral vesicular rash with acute gingivostomatitis are the clinical features of:
    a. Oral CMV infection
    b. EBV infections
    c. Oropharyngeal HSV infection
    d. MCV infection

Multiple Choice Questions

ORODENTAL MEDICINE IN GERIATRICS

1. Age-related changes in the oral-mucosa of an older individual is/are:
   a. Delayed wound healing
   b. Dry mucosa
   c. Loss of elasticity
   d. All of the above

2. Which of the following changes is/are not true about dentition of elderly people?
   a. Diminished tooth sensitivity
   b. Thickness of cementum increases
   c. Pulp dimensions decrease
   d. None of the above

3. Pigmented lesions common in elderly people is/are:
   a. Nevocellular nevus
   b. Melanotic macule
   c. Angiosarcoma
   d. All of the above

4. Oral vesiculobullous disease that primarily affects older women is:
   a. Lichen planus
   b. Cicatricial pemphigoid
   c. Pemphigus vulgaris
   d. Erythema multiforme

5. The most common viral infection in older persons is of:
   a. Cytomegalovirus
   b. Coxsackie virus
   c. Varicella-zoster virus
   d. None of the above

6. Root surface caries in elderly individuals may be caused due to:
   a. Gingival recession
   b. Salivary gland hypofunction
   c. Orofacial motor deficits
   d. All of the above

7. Which of the following diseases may produce desquamative gingivitis?
   a. Histoplasmosis
   b. Pemphigus vegetans
   c. Cicatricial pemphigoid
   d. Erythema multiforme

8. Which of the following is not an intraoral sequelae of insufficient salivary production in older individuals?
   a. Gingivitis
   b. Poorly fitting dentures
   c. Candidiasis in the labial commissures
   d. Dental caries

9. Postherpetic neuralgia in older patients can be treated by administration of:
   a. Analgesics
   b. Tricyclic antidepressants
   c. Immunosuppressants
   d. Both a. and b.

10. Which of the following drugs can be prescribed in salivary gland infection until its culture and sensitivity report is received?
    a. Ciprofloxacin
    b. Tetracycline
    c. Amoxicillin
    d. Metronidazole

11. Recommended dose of pilocarpine for the treatment of salivary hypofunction in older patients is:
    a. 2.5 to 5 mg two times daily
    b. 5 to 7.5 mg three times daily
    c. 5 to 7.5 mg two times daily
    d. 10 mg three times daily

12. Pilocarpine and cevimeline are contraindicated for patients with:
    a. Renal diseases
    b. Liver diseases
    c. Pulmonary diseases
    d. All the above

13. Which of the following systemic conditions is/are associated with microbial infections in elderly patients?
    a. Immunosuppression
    b. Steroid therapy
    c. Radiation sequelae
    d. All of the above

14. Which of the following drugs commonly prescribed in older patients may lead to lichenoid mucosal lesions?
    a. Azathioprine
    b. Cyclosporine
    c. Thiazide diuretics
    d. Prednisone

ANSWERS

Orodental considerations in organ transplantation
1. c 2. d 3. c 4. d 5. b
6. b 7. c 8. d 9. a 10. c

Ulcerative and vesiculobullous lesions
1. c 2. b 3. c 4. d 5. b
6. a 7. d 8. c 9. b. 10. d
11. a 12. c

Red and white lesions of the oral mucosa
1. c 2. b 3. a 4. d 5. c
6. a 7. c 8. d 9. d 10. c
11. a 12. b 13. c 14. d 15. d
16. c 17. a 18. c 19. d 20. a

Pigmented lesions of the oral tissues
1. c 2. c 3. a 4. d 5. c
6. b 7. b 8. a 9. c 10. c
11. c

Benign oral tumors
1. b 2. c 3. b 4. d 5. c
6. b 7. c 8. c 9. a 10. b
11. c 12. b 13. a

Malignant oral tumors
1. c 2. a 3. b 4. d 5. c
6. a 7. b 8. c 9. d 10. d
11. b

Diseases of the tongue
1. c 2. b 3. a 4. d 5. c
6. c 7. d 8. c 9. b 10. d
11. c 12. d 13. b

Salivary gland diseases
1. a 2. d 3. a 4. b 5. c
6. d 7. c 8. a 9. d 10. c
11. d

Temporomandibular joint disorders
1. c 2. c 3. d 4. b 5. b
6. c 7. b 8. c 9. a 10. c
11. b.

Orofacial pain and abnormalities of taste
1. c 2. a 3. b 4. c 5. b
6. c 7. c 8. c 9. b 10. b
11. d 12. c 13. d

Cardiovascular diseases related to oral medicine
1. a 2. b 3. c 4. b 5. c
6. d 7. c 8. b 9. c 10. b
11. d 12. b

Diseases of the respiratory system related to oral medicine
1. d 2. c 3. b 4. a 5. d
6. c 7. b 8. d 9. d 10. c
11. b 12. d

Diseases of gastrointestinal tract related to oral medicine
1. b 2. a 3. d 4. c 5. a
6. b 7. c 8. c 9. c 10. b

Renal diseases and oral medicine
1. c 2. d 3. c 4. c 5. c
6. d 7. b 8. b 9. d 10. b
11. c

Relation of immunologic diseases with oral medicine
1. b 2. c 3. d 4. a 5. c
6. b 7. a 8. d 9. d 10. c
11. d 12. b 13. b

Neuromuscular diseases affecting the oro-facial region
1. a 2. d 3. b 4. b 5. c
6. b 7. a 8. d 9. b 10. c
11. b 12. a 13. d 14. c

Diabetes and its oral manifestations
1. c 2. a 3. b 4. c 5. d
6. c 7. c 8. c

Hematological disorders
1. c 2. b 3. c 4. d 5. b
6. a 7. a 8. b 9. c 10. d
11. d 12. c 13. b 14. c 15. b
16. d 17. c 18. c 19. d 20. b

Disorders of hemostasis and oral medicine
1. d 2. c 3. b 4. c 5. a
6. c 7. b 8. d 9. d 10. c
11. c 12. b 13. a 14. a

Infectious diseases related to oral medicine
1. a 2. b 3. c 4. c 5. d
6. d 7. d 8. c 9. b 10. b
11. d 12. b 13. c 14. c 15. a
16. c

Orodental medicine in geriatrics
1. d 2. d 3. b 4. b 5. c
6. d 7. c 8. c 9. d 10. c
11. b 12. c 13. d 14. c

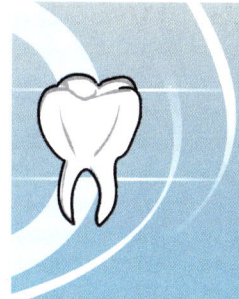

Appendices

Table 1: Blood values

Hematocrit	
• Men	38-54%
• Women	36-74%
Hemoglobin	
• Men	14-18 gm%
• Women	12-16 gm%
• Children	12-14 gm%
• Newborn	14.5-24.5 gm%

Table 2: Blood counts

Erythrocytes		
Men		$4.5\text{-}6.0 \times 10^6$
Women		$4.3\text{-}5.5 \times 10^6$
Reticulocytes		0.1%
Leucocytes, total	5,000 to 10,000	100%
• Myelocytes	0	0%
• Juvenile Neutrophiles	0 to 100	0-1%
• Band Neutrophiles	0 to 500	0-5%
• Segmented Neutrophiles	2500 to 6000	40-60%
• Lymphocytes	1000 to 4000	20-40%
• Eosinophiles	50 to 300	1-3%
• Basophiles	0 to 100	0-1%
• Monocytes	200 to 800	4-8%
Platelets	2,00,000 to 500,000	

Table 3: Blood miscellaneous

• Bleeding Time	1-3 min (Duke)
	2-4 min (Ivy)
• Circulation Time, arm to lung (Ether)	4-8 sec
• Circulation Time, arm to tongue, (sodium dehydrocholate)	9-16 sec
• Clot retraction time	2-4 hrs
• Coagulation time (venous)	6-10 min (Lee & White)
	10- 30 min (Howell)
• Fragility, erythrocyte (Haemolysis)	0.44-0.35% of NaCl
Prothrombin Time	70-110% of control value

contd...

contd...

• Sedimentation rate:	
• Men	0-9 mm per hr (Wintrobe)
• Women	0-20 mm per hr (Wintrobe)

Incidence of blood groups in normal population:
Group O–40%
         A–45%
         B–12%
         AB–4%
         Rh positive–85%
         Negative–15%

Table 4: Normal blood levels

Blood pressure	
Male: > 45 years	<140/90 mm/Hg
< 45 years	<130/85-90 mm/Hg
Female:	<140/90 mm/Hg
Hemoglobin	
Male: 13-18 gm/dl	
Female: 12-16 gm/dl	
Normal values	
Total cholesterol:	< 190 mg/dl with CHD
	< 160 mg/dl with CHD
HDL-C:	> 45 mg/dl for men
	> 55 mg/dl for women
LDL-C:	< 130 mg/dl with CHD
	< 100 mg/dl with CHD
VLDL-C	< 28 mg/dl
Triglycerides	< 130 mg/dl
Blood Sugar	
Fasting	< 120 mg/dl
Post prandial	< 160 mg/dl
Uric acid	< 8 mg/dl
Creatinine	< 1.5 mg/dl
Urea	20-40 mg/dl
Bilirubin (total)	0.2-0.8 mg/dl
SGOT	< 40 IU/litre
SGPT	< 40 IU/litre
Serum Alkaline	
Phosphatase	279 IU
Serum Albumin	4.5-6.0 gm/dl

Table 5: Urine-normal values

Volume/24 hrs	:600 to 2400 ml	Sugar	:Absent
		Creatinine	:0.8 to 1.8 gm/liter
Color	:amber yellow or straw color	Phosphates	:1.7 gm/liter
Turbidity	:clear	Potassium	:1.7 gm/liter
pH	:4.8 to 8	Sodium	:3.5 gm/liter
Specific gravity	:1.001 to 1.035	Urea	:25 to 30 gm/liter
Albumin/Protein	:Absent	Uric acid	:0.5 gm/liter

Table 6: Calorie consumption by activity per hour

Body weight in kgs

On the job	50	58	65	75	85	95
Driving (active)	180	204	228	252	276	300
Keyboarding	114	126	138	150	162	174
Managerial (desk)	180	204	228	252	276	300
Managerial (active)	198	222	246	270	294	324
Phoning (active)	174	198	222	246	270	294
Teaching	180	204	228	252	276	300
Writing (sitting)	90	102	120	132	150	168

Exercising

Badminton						
singles		276	312	348	384	420	456
doubles		234	270	306	342	378	414
Dancing						
aerobic (medium)	348	396	444	492	540	588
contemporary (rock)	198	228	258	252	318	248
Golf						
driving	198	228	258	288	318	348
putting	120	138	156	174	192	210
foursome	204	234	264	294	324	354
9 holes in 2 hrs twosome	276	318	360	402	444	486
Hill climbing	468	534	600	666	732	798
Run in placer						
50-60 steps per min (left foot only)	402	456	510	564	618	672
70-80 steps per min (left foot only)	438	498	558	618	678	738
Running						
9 Km per hr	516	594	660	732	804	876
11 Km per hr	552	624	696	768	840	912
12 Km per hr	540	672	816	960	1104	1188
Swimming (crawl)						
slow	234	270	306	342	388	414
medium	426	480	534	594	642	696
fast	540	618	696	774	832	930

contd...

contd...

Tennis						
singles	336	378	420	462	510	552
doubles	234	270	306	342	378	414
Walking						
3.2 Km per hr	144	168	192	216	240	264
4.8 Km per hr	234	270	306	342	378	414
6.4 Km per hr	270	312	354	396	438	480
8.0 Km per hr	438	498	558	618	678	738
Yoga	180	204	228	252	276	300

Others

Cooking	142	165	192	216	240	267
Card playing	78	90	102	114	132	144
Eating	78	84	90	96	102	108
Showering and dressing	156	180	204	228	252	276
Sitting quietly	66	72	84	96	108	120
Sitting talking	78	90	102	114	132	144
Sleeping	54	60	66	72	78	84
Waiting inline	78	90	102	114	132	144
Watching TV	66	78	90	96	102	108

Table 7: Recommended calorie intake (Kcal/Kg of ideal body weight) for different categories of physical activity

	Sedentary	Moderate	Strenuous
Normal Weight	30	35	40
Over Weight	20	30	35
Under Weight	35	40	45

Table 8: Height and weight standard (Based on insurance data)

Height ft. & inch	Height in cms	Weight (men) kg	Weight (women) kg
5′	152	56-58	50-54
5′1″	154	56-59	51-55
5′2″	157	56-60	53-56
5′3″	159	57-61	54-58
5′4″	162	59-63	56-59
5′5″	165	60-65	55-61
5′6″	167	62-66	58-63
5′7″	170	64-68	60-65
5′8″	172	65-70	62-66
5′9″	175	67-72	64-68
5′10″	177	69-74	65-70
5′11″	180	71-76	67-71
6′	182	73-78	68-72
6′1″	185	75-83	—
6′2″	187	77-83	—
6′3″	190	80-85	—

Table 9: Approximate daily allowances of various foods for an executive

Food group	Approximate size of serving	Number of servings per day at various Caloric Levels (Kcal)*			
		1200	1500	1800	2000
Skim or low fat dairy	I cup skim or low fat milk or yoghurt/40 gm. low fat cheese	2	2	2	3
Lean meat/Fish/poultry without skin or	80-100 gm. cooked lean meat, fish/poultry without skin	1	1	1	2
Pulses and legumes	Katori dal/beans cooked	2	3	3	4
Vegetables		3	3	3	4
Fruits	½ cup cut-up	3	4	4	4
Breads/cereals/starches	1chapati, 1slice whole bread or ½ cup cooked rice pasta 3 table spoon ready to eat cereal	6	8	10	11
Fats/Oils	1 tea spoon oil	5	5	6	6
Sugar	In moderation only				
Alcohol	In moderation only				

Table 10: Food values, calories and cholesterol per 100 gm

Food Cereals	Protein gm	Fat gm	Calcium mgm	Iron mgm	Vit 'C' mgm	Vit 'A' IU	Calories	Cholesterol mgm
Rice								
Raw milled	6.8	0.5	10	3.1	0	0	280	0
Par boiled	6.4	0.4	9	4.0	0	0	260	0
Flakes	6.6	1.2	20	20.0	0	0	280	0
Puffed	7.5	0.1	20	7.6	0	0	260	0
Wheat								
Whole flour	12.1	1.7	48	11.5	0	29	310	0
Flour refined	11.0	0.9	23	2.5	0	25	320	0
Suji	10.4	0.8	16	1.6	0	-	320	0
Bread white	7.8	0.7	11	1.1	0	0	280	0
Millets								
Bajra	11.6	5.0	42	5.0	0	132	350	2
Jowar	10.4	1.9	25	5.8	0	47	340	0
Maize	11.1	3.6	10	2.0	0	90	320	0
Dals								
Bengal gram	20.8	5.6	56	9.1	1	129	370	0
Black gram	24.0	1.4	154	9.1	0	38	340	0

contd...

contd...

Food Cereals	Protein gm	Fat gm	Calcium mgm	Iron mgm	Vit 'C' mgm	Vit 'A' IU	Calories	Cholesterol mgm
Green gram	22.5	1.0	75	6.5	0	49	300	0
Red gram	22.3	1.7	73	5.8	0	132	330	0
Whole Dal								
Bengal gram	17.1	5.3	58	10.2	3	189	360	0
Green gram	22.0	1.0	100	7.3	0	52	300	0
Lentil (Masure)	25.0	0.7	69	4.8	0	294	340	0
Peas dry	19.7	1.1	75	5.1	0	39	310	0
Rajmah	22.9	1.3	260	5.8	0	-	340	0
Soyabean	43.2	19.5	240	11.5	0	226	430	0
Nuts and Seed								
Groundnut	25.3	40.1	90	2.8	0	37	560	5
Til	18.3	43.0	1450	10.5	0	60	560	3
Cashew nut	21.2	47	50	5.0	-	-	596	5
Almond	20.8	59	230	4.5	-	-	655	5
Dry coconut	6.8	62	40	2.7	7	-	662	8
Milk and Products								
Milk cow	3.2	4.1	120	0.2	2	174	70	20
Milk buffalo	4.3	8.8	210	0.2	1	160	120	70
Milk goat	3.3	4.5	170	0.3	1	182	70	15
Curd	3.1	4.0	149	0.2	1	102	60	24
Butter milk	0.8	1.1	30	0.8	-	10	30	05
Cheese	24.1	25.1	790	2.1	-	200	348	08
Khoa	14.6	31.2	650	5.8	-	300	430	160
Whole milk powder	25.8	26.7	950	0.6	140	250	496	200
Skimmed milk powder	38.0	0.1	1370	1.2	5	10	350	16
Paneer buffalo	28	30	700	3	4	200	380	140
Paneer cow	22	25	600	2	3	150	300	100
Paneer skimmed	20	3	500	2	2	20	80	80
Egg and Meat								
Egg hen (boiled)	13.3	13.3	60	2.1	0	600	120	280

contd...

contd...

Food	Protein gm	Fat gm	Calcium mgm	Iron mgm	Vit 'C' mgm	Vit 'A' IU	Calories	Cholesterol mgm
Cereals								
Mutton	18.5	13.3	150	2.5	-	0	190	160
Goat meat	21.4	3.6	12	-	-	-	118	94
Chicken	26.0	0.6	25	-	-	-	109	85
Beef	22.6	2.6	10	0.8	0	0	114	90
Pork	18.7	4.4	30	2.2	0	0	114	80
Liver sheep	19.3	7.5	10	6.3	0	0	150	250
Fish								
Pomfrets (steamed)	17.0	1.3	200	0.9	-	-	100	30
Hilsa	21.8	19.4	180	2.1	24	-	273	50
Prawn fresh	19.1	1.0	323	5.3	-	-	89	30
Fish fresh high fat	11.2	5.8	240	2.3	-	-	138	80
Fish dry	5.5	2.7	315	3.5	-	-	255	40
Crab	8.9	1.1	1370	21.2	-	-	59	10
Vegetables								
Amranth	4.0	0.5	397	25.5	99	5520	45	0
Bathua	3.7	0.4	150	4.2	35	1700	30	0
Cabbage	1.8	0.1	39	0.8	124	1200	27	0
Coriander	3.3	0.6	184	18.5	135	6918	44	0
Methi	4.4	0.9	395	16.5	52	2300	49	0
Lettuce	2.1	0.3	50	2.4	10	990	21	0
Raddish leaves	3.8	0.4	265	3.6	81	5300	28	0
Palak (spinach)	2.0	0.7	73	10.9	28	5580	26	0
Beet root	1.7	0.1	18	1.0	10	0	43	0
Carrot	0.9	0.2	80	2.2	3	1890	48	0
Raddish	0.7	0.1	35	0.4	15	0	17	0
Onion	1.2	0.1	47	0.7	2	0	50	0
Potato	1.6	0.1	10	0.7	17	50	100	0
Tomato	0.9	0.2	48	0.4	27	420	20	0
Capsicum	1.2	0.3	10	1.0	137	125	24	0
Karela	1.6	0.2	20	1.8	88	0	25	0
Sitaphal (Kaddoo)	1.6	0.4	17	1.5	37	130	54	0
Beans French	1.7	0.1	50	1.7	24	200	26	0
Beans cluster	3.2	0.4	130	4.5	49	80	60	0
Peas	7.2	0.3	20	1.5	9		93	0
Fruits								
Amla	0.5	0.1	50	1.2	600	9	58	0
Guava	0.9	0.3	10	1.4	212	0	51	0
Grape	0.7	0.1	20	0.2	31	0	32	0
Lemon	1.0	0.9	70	2.3	39	0	57	0
Mosambi	0.8	0.3	40	0.7	50	0	43	0
Orange	0.7	0.2	26	0.3	30	20	65	0
Juice of orange	0.2	0.1	5	0.7	64	15	48	0
Lichi	1.1	0.2	10	0.7	31	0	61	0
Melon	0.3	0.2	32	1.4	26	5	17	0
Papaya	0.6	0.1	17	0.5	57	665	32	0
Pineapple	0.4	0.1	20	1.2	39	+	46	0
Strawberry	0.7	0.2	30	1.8	52	15	44	0
Apple	0.2	0.5	10	1.0	1	0	59	0
Bael fruit	1.8	0.3	85	0.6	3	55	137	0
Banana	1.2	0.3	17	0.9	7	78	116	0
Cherris	1.1	0.5	24	1.3	7	-	64	0
Figs	1.3	0.2	80	1.0	5	162	37	0
Jack fruit	1.9	0.1	20	0.5	7	175	88	0
Mango	0.6	0.4	14	1.3	16	1740	74	0
Chiku	0.7	0.1	28	2.0	6	95	98	0
Fats and Oils								
Butter	-		-	-	-	960	730	120
Ghee (cow)	-	81.0	-	-	-	600	900	100
Ghee (buffalo)	-	100	-	-	-	640	900	140
Vanaspati	-	100	-	-	-	550	900	100
Refined oil	-	100	-	-	-	550	900	80
Miscellaneous								
Dates	2.5	0.4	120	7.3	3	25	317	1
Coriander seeds	14.1	16.1	630	18.0	0	940	288	2
Methi	26.2	5.8	160	14.1	0	95	335	0
Chillies green	2.9	0.6	30	1.2	111	175	29	0
Betel leaves	3.1	0.8	230	7.0	5	5760	44	0
Biscuits salted	4.5	6.6					534	2
Biscuits sweets	5.4	6.4					450	2
Honey	0.3	0	5	0.9	4	-	320	0
Jaggerry	0.4	0.1	80	11.4	-	165	383	0
Mushroom	4.6	0.8	6	1.5	12	0	43	0
Papad	18.8	0.3	80	17.2	-	-	288	0
Sugar-cane juice	0.1	0.2	10	1.1	-	-	39	0

contd...

Table 11: Approximate values of common food

Food	Quantity	Wt grams	Calories	Protein	Fats grams	Cholesterol
Chapaties	2	57	193	5	5.5	0
Rice	1 plate	100	110	6	0.2	0
Pulse	1 cup	150	284	16	9	0
Omelette	1	39	77	5.8	5.7	300
Bread	2 slice	46	120	4.0	1.0	0
Biscuits	2	16	64	1.6	2.0	2
Milk	1 cup	703	300	9.0	6.0	20
Banana	1	100	99	1.2	0.2	0

contd...

contd...

Food	Quantity	Wt grams	Calories	Protein	Fats grams	cholesterol
Apple	1	66	42	0.2	0.3	0
Butter	Table spoon	20	158	0.1	18	2.2
Ghee	Table spoon	20	180	15	20	25
Sugar	1 teaspoon	5	20			0
Groundnut	30 gm	-	165	8	14	1.5

Index

A

Abfraction 33
Abnormalities of taste 150
Abrasion of the teeth 32
Acanthosis nigricans 94
Accelerated atherosclerosis 189
Accessory ducts 124
Accessory teeth 21
Acinic cell carcinoma 132
Acquired immunodeficiency syndrome 176
Actinomycosis of tongue 115
Acute apical periodontitis 40
Acute idiopathic polyneuropathy 183
Acute lymphonodular pharyngitis 47
Acute necrotising ulcerative gingivitis 48
Acute rhinitis 159
Adenoid cystic carcinoma 132
Adenomatoid odontogenic tumor 90
Adrenal diseases 215
Agenesis 124
Aglycogeusia 151
Agnathia 25
Agranulocytosis 195
Albright's syndrome or café-au-lait pigmentation 79, 94
Allergic sialadenitis 129
Allergy 180
Alterations in wound healing 190
Alveolar abscess 41
Amalgam tattoo 82
Ameloblastic fibroma 91
Ameloblastic fibro-odontoma 91
Ameloblastoma 90
Amelogenesis imperfecta 22
Amyloidosis 94, 116
Amyotrophic lateral sclerosis 184
Anemia 199
Aneurysmal bone cyst 89
Angioedema 180
Angioneurotic edema 116, 180
Angiosarcoma 81
Angular cheilitis 61
Ankyloglossia (tongue tie) 26
Ankylosis of jaw 141
Anodontia 21
Antifungal drugs 93
Aphthous stomatitis 53
Aplasia 124
Aplastic anemia 200
Asthma 161
Ataxia telangiectasia 175
Atresia 124
Attrition of the teeth 32
Atypical odontalgia 149
Atypical orofacial pain 149
Autoimmune diseases 177

B

Bacterial and chlamydial infections 209
Bacterial infections 209, 233
Bad taste and odor 171
Basal cell
    adenoma 131
    carcinoma 108
Behcet's syndrome 54
Bell's palsy 193
Benign lymphoid hyperplasia 86
Benign odontogenic tumors 89
Bilirubin pigmentation 83
Bismuth pigmentation 82
Blastomycosis 56
Bleeding time 203
Blisters 44, 48
Blocked taste bud pores 151
Blood borne infections 209
Blue/purple vascular lesions 80
Bowen's disease 103
Bronchitis 160
Brown heme-associated lesions 79
Brown melanotic lesions 76
Brush biopsy 101
Burkitt's lymphoma 198
Burning mouth syndrome 150
Burns of oral mucosa 62

C

Calcifying odontogenic cyst 90
Calculus 9
Candidiasis 57, 60, 61, 177
Carbohydrates
    functions 10
    role in dental caries 10
Carcinoma 102, 103
Carcinoma expleomorphic adenoma 132
Cardiac arrhythmia 156
Carotenemia 82
Carotodynia 148
Cavernous sinus thrombosis 158, 187
Cementifying fibroma 91
Cementoblastoma 91
Cementoma 91
Central odontogenic fibroma 91
Central pain 149
Cerebral abscess 184
Cerebral palsy 182
Cerebrovascular disease 185
Cervicofacial actinomycosis 93
Chediak-Higashi syndrome 194
Cheek biting 63
Cheilitis glandularis 27
Chemiluminescence 102
Chemotherapy 106, 107
Cherubism 89
Chicken pox 45
Chlamydial infections 210
Chronic idiopathic neutropenia 193
Chronic obstructive pulmonary diseases 160
Chronic renal failure
    manifestations 170
    management 171
Cleft lip 27
Cleft or bifid tongue 26
Cleft palate 27
Clotting mechanism 203
Clotting time 203
Cluster headache 148
Coagulation disorders 204
Coagulation of blood 203
Coarctation of aorta 157
Coated or hairy tongue 113
Collagenase 72
Combined immunodeficiency 174
Concrescence 22
Condylar hyperplasia 141
Condyloma acuminatum 93, 213
Congenital heart disease 156
Congenital lip pits 27
Congestive heart failure 155
Contact allergic stomatitis 47
Cooley's anemia 201
Coronary artery disease 190
Coronary heart (artery) disease
    angina pectoris 154
    myocardial infarction 155
Corticosteroid 72
Cowden's syndrome 94
Coxsackievirus infections 46
Cranial arteritis 148
Crohn's disease 169
Cross bite 25
Cyclic neutropenia 194
Cystic fibrosis 164
Cysticercosis 115
Cysts of the jaws 91
Cytologic examination 100
Cytomegalovirus infection 128

D

Darier's disease 124
Deep overbite 25
Degenerative joint disease 140
Delayed eruption 24
Dens evaginatus 22
Dens-in-dente 22
Dental caries 30
   oral mucosa 28
   etiology 30
   types and classification
      pit and fissure 30
      smooth surface 30
      root 30
      rampant 30
      nursing bottle rampant 31
      recurrent 31
      arrested 31
      chronic 31
      radiation 31
Dental plaque 9
Dentigerous cyst 92
Dentinal dysplasia 23
Dentinogenesis imperfecta 23
Denture sore mouth 61
Deposits on teeth 9
Dermatomyositis 178
Dermoid cysts 89
Dermoid/epidermoid/sebaceous cyst 88
Developmental disorders 21
   teeth
      size 21
      number 21
      shape 22
      structure 22
      eruption 24
   jaws 25
   tongue 26
   lips and palate 27
Diabetes mellitus 188
   etiological classification 188
   etiology
      type 1 diabetes 188
      type 2 diabetes 189
   clinical features 189
   complications 189
   oral manifestations 190
   treatment 190
   oral diseases in diabetes 190
   dental management 191
   diabetic emergencies 191
Diabetic coma 189
Diabetic neuropathy 189, 190
Diabetic retinopathy 189
Dialysis 171
Diastema 25
Dilaceration 22
Disaccharides 10

Disc displacement 141
Discoid lupus erythematosus 74
Discoloration of teeth
   causes 31
   treatment 32
Diseases of liver 167
Dislocation of the mandible 141
Disorders of red blood cells polycythemia 198
Disseminated intravascular coagulation 207
Diverticuli 124
Doctor-patient relationship 4
Double lip 27
Drug-induced melanosis 76
Drugs induced ulceration 214
Duchenne's pseudohypertrophic dystrophy 184
Ductal papilloma 131
Duodenal ulcers 166
Dysgeusias 150
Dyskeratosis congenita 74
Dysphagia 166
Dystonia 116

E

Ecchymosis 79
Ectopic eruption 24
Ectopic lymphoid nodules 84
Ectopic lymphoid tissue 74
Ectopic salivary gland 124
Edentulousness 220, 221
Emphysema 160
Enamel hypoplasia 23
Encephalotrigeminal angiomatosis 80
Endocrinopathic pigmentation 78
Endocrinopathy syndrome 62
Enlarged salivary gland 119
   physical examination
      parotid gland 119
      submandibular and sublingual glands 119
      minor salivary glands 119
   differential diagnosis 120
   examination 120
      collection of saliva sample 121
   imaging
      plain film radiography 121
      sialography 121
      ultrasonography 121
      radionuclide salivary imaging 122
      computed tomography 122
      magnetic resonance imaging 122
      biopsy of salivary glands 123
   staging 123
   specific diseases and disorders 124
   radiation induced pathology 125
   obstructive disorders 126

   inflammatory diseases
      bacterial infections 127
      viral infections 128
   inflammatory and reactive lesion 129
   allergic reaction or disease 129
   granulomatous conditions 129
   immunological disorders 130
   salivary gland tumors 131
Epidermolysis bullosa dystrophica 28
Epilepsy 186
Epstein-barr virus infections 212
Epulis fissuratum 85
Erosion 33
Erythema multiforme 47
Erythroplakia 64
Erythroplasia of Queyrat 64
Esophageal diseases 166
Esophageal ulcers 166
Excisional biopsy 101
Exfoliative cytology 101

F

Facial hemihypertrophy 26
Facioscapulohumeral dystrophy 184
Factor V deficiency 204
Familial dysautonomia 151
Fats in orodental health 11
Fibroma 84
Fibromatosis gingivae 28
Fibrous dysplasia of bone 89
Fibrous inflammatory hyperplasia 84
Fissured or scrotal tongue 26
Fissured tongue 117
Focal epithelial hyperplasia 28, 63
Folic acid deficiency anemia 200
Follicular cyst 92
Fordyce's granules (spots) 28, 59
Frictional keratosis 59
Fungal infections 223
Fungal ulcers 56
Fusion 22

G

Gardner's syndrome 93
Gastric ulcers 167
Gemination 22
Generalized anaphylactic reactions 180
Geniculate neuralgia 146
Geographic tongue 113
Giant cell granuloma 86
Gingiva 7
Gingival abscess 43
Gingival enlargement 35, 223
   inflammatory 35
   fibrotic 35
   associated with systemic conditions
      pregnancy 35
      puberty 36
      nutritional deficiency 36

Index

Gingivitis and gingival abscess 33
   etiological factors
      local 33
      systemic 34
   clinical features 34
   treatment 34
Glomerulonephritis 170
Glossodynia 150
Glossopharyngeal neuralgia 147
Gonococcal stomatitis 210
Gonorrhea 209
Graft-versus-host-disease 70, 223
Granular cell tumor 87
Granulocytosis 194
Granuloma inguinale 211
Graphite tattoo 82
Grey/black pigmentations 81
Guillain-Barré syndrome 183
Gustatory-olfactory confusion 150, 151

H

Habitual lip 63
Hairy leukoplakia 177
Hairy tongue 82
Hamartomas 86
Hand-foot-and-mouth disease 47
Healing of oral wound 17
Heavy metal ingestion 81
Hemangioma 80, 87
Hematopoiesis 193
Hemochromatosis 79
Hemodialysis 171
Hemolytic anemia 200
Hemophilia A 204
Hepatitis 167
Hereditary benign intraepithelial dyskeratosis 60
Hereditary hemorrhagic telangiectasia 81
Herpangina 46
Herpes simplex virus infections 212
Herpesvirus infection 44
Herpetiform ulcers 54
HIV infection 128
HIV-oral melanosis 78
Hodgkin's disease 175, 197
Huntington's chorea 183
Hyaluronidase 72
Hydrogen-ion concentration 8
Hyperplasia 16
Hyperplastic foliate papillae 117
Hypertension
   clinical features 153
   management 153
      oro-dental considerations 154
      rapid control 154
Hypertrophy
   physiologic 15

   compensatory 16
   pathologic 16
Hypothalamus and anterior pituitary 215

I

Idiopathic taste abnormality 150, 152
Immune defence mechanisms 16
Immunity 174
Immunodeficiencies
   primary 174
   secondary 175
Immunohistochemical techniques 102
Infection 16
Infectious mononucleosis 212
Infective endocarditis 157
Inflammation 14
   signs 14
   types
      acute 14
      chronic 14
      subacute 15
      chronic granulomatous 15
      acute 15
      chronic 15
   characteristics 15
Inflammatory disorders 140
   (reactive) hyperplasias 84
   diseases of the intestine 169
Intraoral skin grafts 63
Iron-deficiency anemia 199

J

Jaundice (Icterus) 167
Jaw jerk reflex 135
Juvenile periodontitis 36

K

Kaposi's sarcoma 80, 108
Keratinization 59
Keratoacanthoma 93
Keratosis follicularis 64
Kidney transplantation 172
Koplik's spot 63

L

Lamina propria 7
Langerhans' cell granulomatosis 94
Laryngitis 160
Lasers 102
Latex allergy 180
Lazy leucocyte syndrome 193
Leprosy (Hansen's disease) 93
Leukemia 176, 195
   acute 195
   chronic 196

   chronic granulocytic or myelocytic 196
   chronic lymphocytic 196
Leukocytic emigration 15
Leukoedema 58
Leukoplakia 66-68
Lichen planus 68
Lichenoid reactions 70
Light emitting diodes 102
Limb girdle dystrophy 185
Linea alba 58
Lingual thyroid nodule 27
Lingual varicosity 115
Lip, tongue and cheek biting 59
Localized anaphylactic reactions 180
Ludwig's angina 115
Lupus erythematosus 74
Lymphangioma 87
Lymphoma 197

M

Macrodontia 21
Macroglossia 26
Macrognathia 26
Macrovascular disease 189
Malignant melanoma 77, 108
Malignant neoplasm of salivary glands 108
Manifestations of anxiety 5
Materia alba 9
Median rhomboid glossitis 26, 114
Melanoameloblastoma 88
Microbial flora 8
Microdontia 21
Microglossia 26
Micrognathia 25
Midline fissure 117
Midline granuloma 163
Migraine 147
Migraine headache 148
Minerals and trace elements
   calcium 12
   phosphorus 13
   magnesium 13
   iodine 13
   iron 13
   fluoride 13
Mitral valve disease 155
Mixed connective tissue disease 179
Mixed headache 148
Molluscum contagiosum 93, 213
Moniliasis 60
Monosaccharides 10
Movement disorders 182
Mucocele 126
Mucoepidermoid carcinoma 132
Mucormycosis (phycomycosis) 56
Mucositis 109
Mucous extravasation cyst 126

Mucous retention cyst 126
Multiple mucosal neuroma syndrome 94
Multiple myeloma 176, 197
Multiple sclerosis 152, 183
Mumps (epidemic parotitis) 128
Muscular dystrophy 184
Myasthenia gravis 116, 185
Myeloproliferative disorders 195
Myoepithelioma 132
Myofacial pain dysfunction syndrome 137
Myotonic dystrophy 185

N

Nasopalatine cyst 92
Nasopharyngeal carcinoma 108
Necrosis of the pulp 39
Necrotizing sialometaplasia 129
Neoplasms 177
Nephrotic syndrome 176
Neuralgia 145
Neurilemmoma 88
Neurofibroma 88
Neurofibromatosis 78
Neuromuscular disorders 116
Neutropenia 195
Nevocellular and blue nevi 77
Nevoid basal cell carcinoma syndrome 94
Non-Hodgkin's lymphoma 176, 198
Non-infectious oral lesions 223

O

Occipital neuralgia 147
Odontogenic keratocyst 92
Odontogenic myxoma 91
Odontomas 91
Oncocytoma 131
Opportunistic infections 177
Oral cancer 95
   etiology and risk factors 95
   clinical features 95
   pathogenesis 100
   investigations 100
   differential diagnosis 100
   diagnosis 100
   prognosis 103
   nutritional prevention 104
   treatment 104
      surgery 105
      laser surgery 105
      radiation therapy 105
      chemotherapy 106
      anticancer drugs 106
      combined surgical and radiation therapy 108
      pretreatment dental and oral evaluation 109
      complications of cancer treatment 109
Oral cytomegalovirus infection 212

Oral lesions 214, 223
Oral management 72
Oral medicine 1
   hospital practice 2
   severe medical problems 2
Oral melanotic macule 76
Oral mucositis 223
Oral mucous membrane 6
Oral neoplasms 177
Oral squamous papilloma 84, 92
Oral submucous fibrosis 71
Oral ulcers 197
Orodental management 223
   pre-transplantation 224
   post-transplantation 224
Orofacial pain
   classification 143
   evaluation of pain 144
   assessment of patient
      history 144
      physical examination 145
      intraoral examination 145
      range of motion 145
      tests of sensory discrimination 145
      diagnostic studies 145
   specific orofacial pain conditions 145
Oropharyngeal dysphagia 116
Ossifying fibroma 89
Osteitis deformans 94
Osteoradionecrosis 109

P

Paget's disease of bone 94
Pain control 205
Pain-related terminology 143
Palatal papillomatosis 86
Parageusias 150, 151
Paralysis agitans 182
Parkinson's disease 182
Pemphigus 48
   vulgaris 49
   vegetans 50
   cicatricial pemphigoid 50
   parapemphigus 51
   erosive and bullous lichen planus 51
Peptic ulcers 166
Periapical abscess 40
Periapical cemental dysplasia 91
Periapical cementoma 23
Periapical granuloma 42
Periodontal abscess 42
Periodontal ligament 7
Periodontitis 36
Periodontium 7
Peritoneal dialysis 171
Permanent pacemakers 158
Pernicious anemia 200
Petechiae 79
Petechial hemorrhages 115

Petit mal seizure 186
Peutz-Jegher's syndrome 28, 78, 94
Phagocytosis 15
Pharyngitis 159
Physiological pigmentation 77
Pigmented lichen planus 79
Pindborg tumor 90
Placental extract 72
Platelet count 203
Platelet plug 203
Platelet transfusion 207
Pleomorphic adenoma 131
Plumbism 81
Plummer-Vinson syndrome 200
Pneumonia 162
Polycythemia vera 198
Polysaccharides 10
Post-traumatic neuropathic pain 149
Predeciduous teeth 22
Premature eruption 24
Procedure of oral diagnosis 18
   history taking and recording
      constituents of patient history 18
      examination of the patient 19
      general 19
      extraoral 19
      intraoral 19
   specialized examination 19
      laboratory investigations 20
   establishing the diagnosis 20
   treatment planning 20
Proteins 11
Prothrombin time 203
Pseudoepitheliomatous hyperplasia 86
Pseudohypoparathyroidism 151
Psoriasiform lesions 64
Psoriatic arthritis 140
Psychosomatic oral diseases 4
Pulp 7
   structure 8
Pulp calcification 39
Pulp diseases 38
Pulp polyp 39, 85
Pulp stones (denticles) 40
Pulpitis 38, 39
Pyelonephritis 170
Pyogenic granuloma 85

R

Radiation caries 109
Radicular cyst 42, 92
Recurrent oral ulcers 52
   herpes simplex virus infection 52
   aphthous stomatitis 53
Red lesions 57
Regional odontodysplasia 23
Renal diseases 170
Respiratory infections
   upper respiratory tract 159
   lower respiratory tract 160

Index

Reverse smoking 73
Rheumatic fever 156
Rheumatic heart disease 156
Rheumatoid arthritis 140, 179
Root resorption 42

S

Saliva 6
Salivary gland dysfunction 223
Salivary gland stones 126
Salivary hypofunction 151
Sarcoid sialadenitis 129
Sarcoidosis 163
Scleroderma 179
Scrotal tongue 117
Secondary polycythemia 199
Selective immunoglobulin deficiencies 174
Sensorineural taste disorders 150, 151
Septic arthritis 141
Severe acute respiratory syndrome 164
Sexually transmitted infections 209
Shock 16
    primary 17
    secondary 17
    etiology and types 17
    biochemical mechanism 17
Sialadenitis 127
Sialadenosis 130
Sialolithiasis 126
Sialorrhea 124
Sickle-cell anemia 201
Sinusitis 159
Sjögren's syndrome 130
Smoker's glossitis 117
Smoker's melanosis 77
Squamous cell carcinoma 96, 116
Squamous odontogenic tumor 90
Status epilepticus 186
Stomatitis nicotina palati 64
Stroke 185, 190
Sturge-Weber syndrome 80
Supernumerary teeth 21
Synovial chondromatosis 141
Syphilis 210
Syphilitic interstitial glossitis 115
Syphilitic mucous patch 63
Systemic conditions in geriatrics 217
    common disorders
        coagulation disorders 217
        immunosuppression 217
        radiation hazard 217
        steroid treatment 217
        cardiac problems 217
        joint replacement 218
    age-related changes
        in oral mucosa 218
        in dentition 218
        in periodontium 218
        salivary glands 218
        mastication and swallowing 218
    oral and dental disorders
        oral mucosal diseases 218
        infectious diseases 219
        dental disorders 219
        periodontal diseases 219
        salivary gland dysfunction 219
        smell and taste dysfunction 219
        swallowing disorders 220
        edentulousness 220
    prevention and treatment
        oral mucosal diseases 220
        infectious diseases 220
        dental disorders 220
        salivary gland disorders 220
        periodontal disease 221
        chemosensory (smell and taste) dysfunction 221
        masticatory and swallowing disorders 221
        edentulousness 221
        pain sensation 221
Systemic lupus erythematosus 178

T

Tardive dyskinesia 116
Taurodontism 22
Temporomandibular disorders
    functional anatomy of TMJ 134
    patient history 134
    examination of articulatory system 135
    etiology 135
    differential diagnosis 136
    diagnostic aids 136
    history taking for evaluating a patient 138
    intracapsular disorders 140
Tension-type headache 148
Teratomas 89
Tetralogy of Fallot 157
Thalassemias 201
Thrombin clotting time 204
Thrombocytopenic disorders 204
Thrush 60
Thymic hypoplasia 174
Thyroid disease 215
Toluidine blue 100
Toluidine blue staining 101
Tongue
    structure 112
    functions 112
    examination 113
    diseases
        mucosa 113
        body 115
Tonsillitis 159
Tori 84
Torus palatinus 28
Traction headache 148
Transport disorders 151
Traumatic disorders 140
Traumatic injuries on tongue 114
Traumatic keratosis 63
Traumatic ulcers 55
Trichinosis 115
Trigeminal neuralgia 145
Tuberculosis 129, 162, 209
Tuberculous sclerosis 94
Tumor biology 104
Tumors of ectodermal origin 90

U

Ulcerative colitis 169
Ulcers 44, 48
Uremic stomatitis 63
Urticaria 180

V

Valvular heart disease 155
Varicella-zoster virus infection 45
Varices 81
Vascular disease 116
Vascular pain 147
Verrucous carcinoma 96
Viral hepatitis 168
Viral infections 223
Virus induced benign tumors 92
Vitamins 11
    fat-soluble
        A 11
        D 11
        E 11
        K 12
    water soluble
        B complex 12
        C (ascorbic acid) 12
Von Recklinghausen's neurofibromatosis 94
von-Willebrand's disease 204, 205

W

Wegener's granulomatosis 163
White blood cells 193
White lesions 57
White sponge nevus 28
Witkop's disease 60

X

Xanthomas 94
Xerostomia 109, 120, 124, 151, 171
X-linked agammaglobulinemia 175